"This new edition of *The Meat Crisis* makes an even stronger case for radically rethinking our food and farming systems and transforming our diets."

– **Joanna Lumley**, OBE, actor and campaigner

"This new enlarged and enriched edition makes both enthralling and chilling reading. You will be in no doubt as to why factory farming is so unsustainable, not just for the animals, but for the health and survival of humanity and the planet."

– **Philip Lymbery**, Chief Executive, Compassion in World Farming, and author of *Farmageddon*

"If you care about climate change, suffering, sustainability, and rights, you need to care about the meat crisis. With hard data and compelling logic, the authors in this collection show just how little the meat industry cares for the consequences of their business model, one on which the planet is gradually becoming hooked. Happily, there are solutions here too – ones that are worth heeding. For a world without Big Meat, the ideas in this book are invaluable."

– **Raj Patel**, Research Professor, Lyndon B Johnson School of Public Affairs, University of Texas at Austin, US

THE MEAT CRISIS

Meat and dairy production and consumption are in crisis. Globally, 70 billion farm animals are used for food production every year. It is well accepted that livestock production is a major contributor to greenhouse gas emissions. The Food and Agriculture Organization of the United Nations (FAO) predicts a rough doubling of meat and milk consumption in the first half of the 21st century, with particularly rapid growth occurring in the developing economies of Asia. What will this mean for the health and well-being of those animals, of the people who consume ever larger quantities of animal products, and for the health of the planet itself?

The new edition of this powerful and challenging book explores the impacts of the global growth in the production and consumption of meat and dairy, including cultural and health factors, and the implications of the likely intensification of farming for both small-scale producers and for animals. Several chapters explore the related environmental issues, from resource use of water, cereals and soya, to the impact of livestock production on global warming and issues concerning biodiversity, land use and the impacts of different farming systems on the environment. A final group of chapters addresses ethical and policy implications for the future of food and livestock production and consumption.

Since the first edition, published in 2010, all chapters have been updated, three original chapters rewritten and six new chapters added, with additional coverage of dietary effects of milk and meat, antibiotics in animal production and the economic, political and ethical dimensions of meat consumption. The overall message is clearly that we must eat less meat to help secure a more sustainable and equitable world.

Joyce D'Silva worked for Compassion in World Farming from 1985 to 2016, including fourteen years as Chief Executive. She now does consultancy work. She lectures internationally and has published widely on farm animal welfare, including co-editing *Animals, Ethics and Trade* (Earthscan, 2006).

John Webster is Professor Emeritus at the University of Bristol, UK. He was a founding member of the Farm Animal Welfare Council and is a former President of both the Nutrition Society and the British Society for Animal Science. His books include *Animal Husbandry Regained* (Routledge, 2012), *Understanding the Dairy Cow*, *Animal Welfare: A Cool Eye Towards Eden* and *Animal Welfare: Limping Towards Eden.*

Other Books in the Earthscan Food and Agriculture Series

For further details please visit the series page on the Routledge website: www.routledge.com/books/series/ECEFA/

Sustainable Intensification in Smallholder Agriculture
An integrated systems research approach
Edited by Ingrid Öborn, Kwesi Atta-Krah, Michael Phillips, Richard Thomas, Bernard Vanlauwe and Willemien Brooijmans

Environmental Justice and Farm Labor
Rebecca E. Berkey

Plantation Crops, Plunder and Power
Evolution and exploitation
James F. Hancock

Food Security, Agricultural Policies and Economic Growth
Long-term dynamics in the past, present and future
Niek Koning

Agriculture and Rural Development in a Globalizing World
Challenges and Opportunities
Edited by Prabhu Pingali and Gershon Feder

Food, Agriculture and Social Change
The vitality of everyday food in Latin America
Edited by Stephen Sherwood, Alberto Arce and Myriam Paredes

Contract Farming and the Development of Smallholder Agricultural Businesses
Improving markets and value chains in Tanzania
Edited by Joseph A. Kuzilwa, Niels Fold, Arne Henningsen and Marianne Nylandsted Larsen

Agribusiness and the Neoliberal Food System in Brazil
Frontiers and fissures of agro-neoliberalism
Antonio Ioris

THE MEAT CRISIS

Developing more Sustainable and Ethical Production and Consumption

Second edition

Edited by Joyce D'Silva and John Webster

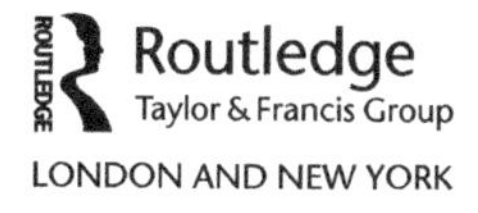

LONDON AND NEW YORK

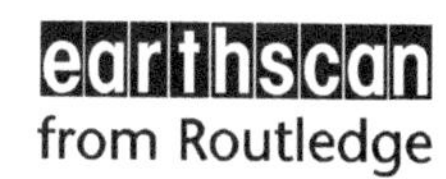

First published 2017
by Routledge
2 Park Square, Milton Park, Abingdon, Oxon OX14 4RN

and by Routledge
711 Third Avenue, New York, NY 10017

Routledge is an imprint of the Taylor & Francis Group, an informa business

British Library Cataloguing-in-Publication Data
A catalogue record for this book is available from the British Library

Library of Congress Cataloging-in-Publication Data
Names: D'Silva, Joyce, editor. | Webster, John, 1938– editor.
Title: The meat crisis / [edited by] Joyce D'Silva and John Webster.
Description: Abingdon, Oxon ; New York, NY : Routledge, 2017. |
Series: Earthscan food and agriculture | Earlier edition: 2010. |
Includes bibliographical references and index.
Identifiers: LCCN 2017007952| ISBN 9781138673281 (hardback) |
ISBN 9781138673298 (pbk.) | ISBN 9781315562032 (ebook)
Subjects: LCSH: Animal industry—Environmental aspects. |
Meat industry and trade—Environmental aspects. |
Sustainable agriculture. | Animal culture. | Livestock.
Classification: LCC HD9410.5 .M43 2017 | DDC 338.1/76—dc23
LC record available at https://lccn.loc.gov/2017007952

ISBN: 978-1-138-67328-1 (hbk)
ISBN: 978-1-138-67329-8 (pbk)
ISBN: 978-1-315-56203-2 (ebk)

Typeset in Bembo
by Apex CoVantage, LLC

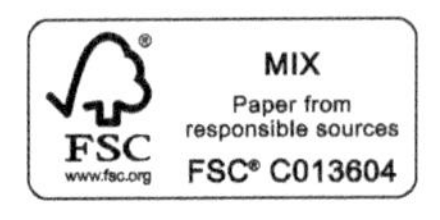

Printed and bound by CPI Group (UK) Ltd, Croydon, CR0 4YY

CONTENTS

TABLES

FIGURES

CONTRIBUTORS

Editors

Joyce D'Silva worked for Compassion in World Farming, the leading charity advancing the welfare of farm animals worldwide, for over thirty years, including fourteen years as Chief Executive. She is now Compassion's Ambassador Emeritus. Joyce has given oral evidence to the UK government's Advisory Committee on Climate Change and to the European Commission's European Group of Ethical Advisers on Science and New Technologies on the welfare aspects of cloning farm animals for food. She has written widely on the welfare of farm animals, including co-editing *Animals, Ethics and Trade* (Earthscan, 2006), publishing chapters in *The Future of Animal Farming* (Blackwell, 2008), *Global Food Insecurity: Rethinking Agricultural and Rural Development Paradigm and Policy*, (Springer, 2011), the UNCTAD Trade and Environment Review 2013, and *Faith in Food: Changing the World One Meal at a Time* (Bene Factum Publishing, 2014). In 2004 Joyce was the joint recipient of the RSPCA Lord Erskine Award in recognition of a "very important contribution in the field of animal welfare". In 2015 Joyce was conferred with an honorary Doctorate (D.Litt) by the University of Winchester, in recognition of her work for the welfare of animals. She is a Patron of the Animal Interfaith Alliance and a Trustee of the UK branch of Help in Suffering, a charity carrying out veterinary work in Jaipur, India.

John Webster graduated as a vet from Cambridge in 1963 and is now Professor Emeritus at the University of Bristol. His early career was spent in Scotland and Canada studying the nutrition and physiology of farm animals, especially in harsh environments. On appointment to the Chair of Animal Husbandry at Bristol (UK) in 1977, he established the unit for the study of animal welfare and behaviour, which is now over sixty strong. He was a founder member of the UK Farm Animal

Welfare Council and first propounded the "Five Freedoms" that have gained international recognition as standards for defining the elements of good welfare in domestic animals. He is a former president of the UK Nutrition Society and British Society of Animal Science. His most notable publications include two books on Animal Welfare: *A Cool Eye Towards Eden* and *Limping Towards Eden*. His most recent book, *Animal Husbandry Regained: The Place of Farm Animals in Sustainable Agriculture*, extends the principle of unsentimental compassion beyond that for farm animals to embrace all concerns for life on the land.

Chapter authors

Dr Emma Baxter is a researcher in the Animal Behaviour and Welfare Team at SRUC. She graduated in Zoology from the University of Manchester before completing the MSc in Applied Animal Behaviour and Welfare at Edinburgh University. Her PhD investigated the behavioural and physiological indicators of piglet survival in different farrowing systems. Pig welfare and behaviour continue to be her main research focus. Engagement with key stakeholders in industry has been a major part of her work to encourage uptake of high welfare systems and practices.

Dr Alberto Bernués Jal is a researcher at the Centre for Agrifood Research and Technology (CITA) in Spain. He has worked at the University of Edinburgh and the Norwegian University of Life Sciences. He has published scientific work in analysis of livestock and mixed farming systems, sustainability assessment, consumer quality perception and food chains, and valuation of ecosystem services. He is Section Editor (Farming Systems and Environment) of ANIMAL-International Journal of Animal Bioscience.

David Bryngelsson holds a post-doc position at the Dept. of Energy and Environment, Chalmers University of Technology, Sweden. Along with his co-authors in this volume he has recently published a major paper that assesses options for food and agriculture to meet EU climate targets (*Food Policy* 2016, 59: 152–164).

Dr Andy Butterworth, MRCVS, is Senior Lecturer, Clinical Veterinary Science, University of Bristol, teaching and doing research in the areas of animal disease and production, animal welfare and legislation, behavioural biology and animal welfare assessment. He is a member of the European Food Standards Agency Scientific Panel on Animal Health and Welfare, and chairs the EEER (Ethics, Economics, Education and Regulation) of the Farm Animal Welfare committee in the UK. He lectures widely and publishes in books and the academic and trade press, with over 160 publications to date.

Ian Duncan is Professor Emeritus and Emeritus Chair in Animal Welfare at the University of Guelph in Ontario, Canada. He has been investigating the welfare of poultry for fifty years and has published many papers on this topic.

Dr Tara Garnett is a researcher at the University of Oxford. Her work centres on the interactions among food, climate, health and broader sustainability issues. She has particular interests in livestock as an area where many of these converge. Tara founded the Food Climate Research Network in 2005. The FCRN is a network of thousands of individuals, drawn from over seventy countries, who share a common interest in food system sustainability. The FCRN provides integrative knowledge on food systems, and a space for diverse stakeholders to engage in the contested food arena.

Dr Michael Greger is a physician and internationally recognised speaker on nutrition, food safety, and public health issues. He is Director of Public Health and Animal Agriculture at the Humane Society of the United States. His latest book, *How Not to Die*, became an instant *New York Times* bestseller. More than a thousand of his nutrition videos are freely available at *NutritionFacts.org*, with new videos and articles uploaded every day.

Fredrik Hedenus is an Associate Professor at the Dept. of Energy and Environment, Chalmers University of Technology, Sweden. Along with his co-authors in this volume he has recently published a major paper that assesses options for food and agriculture to meet EU climate targets (*Food Policy* 2016, 59: 152–164).

Dr Arjen Y. Hoekstra is Professor in water management at the University of Twente, the Netherlands. Hoekstra was the first to quantify the water volumes virtually embedded in trade, showing the relevance of a global perspective on water use and scarcity. As creator of the water footprint concept, Arjen introduced supply-chain thinking in water management. His books include *The Water Footprint of Modern Consumer Society* (Routledge, 2013), *The Water Footprint Assessment Manual* (Earthscan, 2011) and *Globalization of Water* (Wiley-Blackwell, 2008).

Dr Steve Kestin has a degree in Agriculture and a PhD in Animal Welfare. His research career started at the AFRC Institute of Food Research and progressed to the University of Bristol at Langford. His research interests centre on animal welfare and food quality. He is best known for his work on the prevalence and welfare implications of lameness in broiler chickens and the welfare of fish at killing. He is now based in Cornwall where he farms bivalve molluscs.

Tim Lang is Professor of Food Policy at City, University of London's Centre for Food Policy. Hill farming in Lancashire, UK, in the 1970s formed his interest in the relationship between food, health, environment, culture and political economy. He is co-author of *Food Wars* (2015), *Unmanageable Consumer* (2015), *Ecological Public Health* (2012), *Food Policy* (2009), and most recently, *Sustainable Diets* (Routledge, 2017).

Dr Alistair Lawrence has a joint Chair in Animal Behaviour and Welfare with SRUC and the University of Edinburgh. His research interests include understanding and promoting both positive welfare in animals and young peoples' attitudes and behaviour to animals. He has always been involved with farming, having been brought up on a family farm. He graduated in Zoology (University of St Andrews) before studying for his PhD at Edinburgh under Professor David Wood-Gush, who introduced him to the study of farm animal behaviour and welfare.

Carol McKenna has worked with animal protection organisations in senior campaigning roles for over thirty years. Currently Carol is Special Advisor to the Chief Executive of Compassion in World Farming providing leadership for key projects. Previous positions include Director of Campaigns at Compassion and Director of Programmes at World Animal Protection, formerly WSPA. Additionally, Carol is a director of the Eating Better, a broad alliance and a Member of the Wild Animal Welfare Committee (WAWC).

Cóilín Nunan is a scientific adviser to the Soil Association and to the Alliance to Save Our Antibiotics. He campaigns against the overuse of antibiotics in farming and has co-authored numerous reports on antibiotic resistance and antibiotic residues that highlight the human-health impact of excessive antibiotic use in intensive livestock farming. This work aims to encourage a move to more responsible use of antibiotics in farming, through better regulation and improvements in production systems, which would also improve animal welfare.

Martin Palmer is Secretary General of the Alliance of Religions and Conservation (ARC). He is the author of many books and radio programmes on the interface between faith and the environment. ARC has helped launch tens of thousands of practical faith-based environmental programmes from China to the UK and from Mongolia to Mexico. He is a regular broadcaster with the BBC on faith and history issues as well as being a translator of Chinese classics for Penguin Classics.

Jonathon Porritt is Co-Founder of Forum for the Future, the UK's leading sustainable development charity. He was formerly Director of Friends of the Earth, Co-Chair of the Green Party and Chairman of the UK Sustainable Development Commission and is the Chancellor of Keele University. Recent books are *Capitalism as if the World Matters* (2007) and *The World We Made* (2013) – which seeks to inspire people about the prospects of a sustainable world in 2050. Jonathon received a CBE in January 2000 for services to environmental protection.

Dr Kate Rawles is a freelance writer, outdoor philosopher and environmentalist. A former university lecturer, she's passionate about using adventurous journeys to raise awareness and inspire action on our most urgent environmental challenges. *The Carbon Cycle: Crossing the Great Divide* (Two Ravens Press, 2012) is based on her Texas to Alaska bike ride exploring climate change. In December 2016 she started *The Life Cycle*, cycling from Costa Rica to Cape Horn with a focus on biodiversity. (www.outdoorphilosophy.co.uk)

Mike Rayner is Professor of Population Health at the Nuffield Department of Population Health of the University of Oxford and Director of the British Heart Foundation Centre on Population Approaches for Non-Communicable Disease Prevention. The Centre, which he founded in 1993, is a World Health Organisation Collaborating Centre and carries out research in two main areas: the burden of cardiovascular disease and the promotion of healthier and more sustainable diets.

Dr Peter Scarborough is University Research Lecturer at the Nuffield Department of Population Health, Oxford University. Pete leads a research programme on the relationship between public health and environmental sustainability. He specialises in developing models of the health and environmental impact of changes in diets and food systems. He is a principal investigator in the Oxford Martin School Future of Food programme and has authored over eighty research articles in journals including the *Lancet* and the *British Medical Journal.*

Peter Stevenson is Chief Policy Advisor to Compassion in World Farming. He studied economics and law at Trinity College Cambridge. He has written legal analyses of EU legislation on farm animals and of the impact of the WTO rules on animal welfare. Peter is lead author of the recent FAO study reviewing animal welfare legislation in the beef, pork and poultry industries. He has written reports on the economics of livestock production and on the detrimental impact of industrial farming on natural resources.

Colin Tudge is a biologist by education and a writer by trade, with a lifelong interest in food and farming. He is a co-founder of the Oxford Real Farming Conference and founder of the College for Real Farming and Food Culture (www.collegeforrealfarming.org), which develops the ideas of Enlightened Agriculture and Agrarian Renaissance. Recent books include *The Secret Life of Trees*, *Consider the Birds*, *Why Genes Are Not Selfish and People Are Nice* and *Six Steps Back to the Land.*

Dr Claire Weeks is a Senior Research Fellow at the University of Bristol whose recent publications include two co-authored papers examining farmer attitudes and consumer attitudes to injurious pecking in laying hens; and a PLoS ONE paper, "Implications for welfare, productivity and sustainability of the variation in reported levels of mortality for laying hen flocks kept in different housing systems: a meta-analysis of ten studies".

Stefan Wirsenius is Associate Professor at the Dept. of Energy and Environment, Chalmers University of Technology, Sweden. Along with his co-authors in this volume he has recently published a major paper that assesses options for food and agriculture to meet EU climate targets (*Food Policy* 2016, 59: 152–164).

Richard Young is Policy Director of the Sustainable Food Trust. He has farmed organically since 1974 and played a leading role in the development of organic standards and certification in the UK. He is a past editor of *New Farmer & Grower* (now *Organic Farming*) and has written widely on the overuse of antibiotics, livestock farming, soil degradation and sustainable food production. He runs a 400-acre farm in the Cotswolds with his sister Rosamund, producing grass-fed beef and lamb and bread-making wheat.

FOREWORD

I am delighted to write the Foreword to this new edition of *The Meat Crisis*, as I regard the book as providing a timely perspective on global food systems. Rising population, changing diet, and consumption patterns on the one hand, and the adverse impact of climate change on food systems on the other, are producing a global food crisis that constitutes a major global threat. To solve this upcoming crisis, the world seems faced with two widely different policy options relating to the future of food security: the first option favours agro-industry, resulting in a push for large-scale monoculture production and a supply and demand-oriented economic model that is put forward as a solution. Yet, we know that more food production does not necessarily result in fewer people suffering from hunger and malnutrition. The world already produces enough food, sufficient not only for the current population of 7.5 billion, but actually enough to meet the needs of the 9.7 billion or more people expected to inhabit the planet by 2050. Hunger in an age of plenty isn't a problem of production, efficiency, or even distribution. It is a matter of priorities, choices, and social policies.

The second option is premised on agro-biodiversity. Small-scale farmers already provide over 70 percent of the food consumed by the local populations, produced largely by relying on traditional methods of farming, and reinforced by agroecology. This alternative path goes beyond productivity, profit, and increasing yields. It respects local food production, promotes the human right to food, increases agricultural biodiversity, balances crops with livestock, improves health and nutrition, and most significantly, addresses climate change by minimizing greenhouse gas emissions. Agroecology treads lightly on the Earth.

There is still scepticism about whether these gentler, more traditional methods of farming can meet the world's food needs. Before addressing that concern, it is important to realize that the fossil fuel–intensive agro-industrial model is responsible for devastation of forests and desertification of pasture land through over-stocking;

it pollutes water and soils, destroys biodiversity through loss of habitat, increases pollinator losses, and uses vast amounts of chemicals for fertilizers and to kill unwanted insects and plants, and requires huge quantities of water for irrigation.

Worse still, many of the crops produced by the agro-business approach are not even destined to provide nourishment for humans, but to create biofuels for our cars, or – in the case of around a third of the world's edible crops – to be used as feed for animals, the majority of which are kept in cruel confinement on industrial farms. These animals are never allowed to tread on the Earth, but live out their lives indoors under wretched conditions. Industrial livestock farming depends heavily on selective breeding, and in some countries hormones, to achieve quick growth, and on antibiotics to prevent animal diseases. To lower costs and raise profits, live animals as well as meat travel around the world before coming to our table. This is a classic lose-lose situation. It is not good for human health, and it is a terrible way to treat animals. According to a recent report of the WHO, an unhealthy diet is one of the major causes of non-communicable diseases, which are globally responsible for 70 percent of the deaths of people under age seventy. Those victimized are mostly concentrated in low- and middle-income countries. Despite this, meat consumption is skyrocketing globally as the Westernized diet is being adopt by many among the 3 billion new members of the world's middle classes who are enjoying rising incomes.

Food systems are a major factor influencing what we eat, how we live, and how and when we die. Modern-day diets are largely based on supply-oriented industrial food systems. This reality is explained and justified as a response to population growth and rising standards of living, as well as urbanization and economic globalization. Nevertheless, the overall pattern is not beneficial for human health and is also not ecologically sustainable from the perspective of planetary viability. Current food systems, producing massive amounts of cheap, ultra-processed food, rely on monoculture agriculture, as well as on excessive use of chemicals from farm to supermarket to ensure long shelf life, and distribute foods by way of reliance on global supermarket chains.

While our health is in danger, our planet is too. Although the livestock sector is central to the development of food systems, accounting for around one-third of global agricultural GDP, it is the largest user of global land area (26 percent), and crops devoted to animal feed account for one-third of global arable land. There are profound adverse effects on the environment if we take into account the indirect land use changes and feed crop production. The livestock sector of agriculture is directly and indirectly responsible for 14.5 percent of GHG emissions.

Can we do better? This book sets forth a bleak picture, but it also encourages us to think of better ways to produce food. The text contains some big and crucial messages appropriate for policy makers, but it also challenges all of us to alter behaviour on a personal level. Governments must overcome their reluctance to address these issues and should learn to work with all relevant partners, including farmers, producers, and consumers so as to address effectively the environmental and health impacts of the overconsumption of meat. As individuals we can take action regarding our own consumption and become active participants in debates around climate change, food security, and the health of our planet. We have just this planet on which we – and future generations – will live. Let's do all we can to make it a planet rich in biodiversity, governed by principles of fairness for all, where healthy lives are the norm and all people can flourish without destroying the Earth, causing misery to animals, and failing to take advantage of the agroecological alternative to agro-industrial food systems.

Hilal Elver
United Nations Special Rapporteur
on the Right to Food

INTRODUCTION

Joyce D'Silva and John Webster

The first response to the title of this book could well be: 'What meat crisis?' Indeed supermarket shelves and butchers' shops are well stocked with every kind of meat. Special offers on packs of chicken legs abound. At one point a 1 kilo pack of chicken portions can cost the same in a leading UK supermarket as a pack of four cans of beer. In fact, in the developed world, meat has probably never been so cheap.

Alongside the abundance of meat in our shops, restaurants and fast food outlets has come the increase in consumption. Some people must be eating maybe ten times as much meat per year as their great-grandparents consumed, possibly much more. Meat is no longer the special occasion food, like the fatted calf of Biblical fame; we don't have roast chicken as an expensive Sunday lunch special any more. Those on average incomes can eat meat three times a day and feel no poorer for it.

The truth is – this *is* the meat crisis! Too much meat for our own good health, too much for the dwindling global resources of land and water, too much for the health of our planet's climate and environment and too much to enable the animals we eat to have decent lives before we devour them.

This book is not a vegetarian or vegan gospel, although the editors will have no problem if any reader, having read the facts we present, makes that choice. Rather, this book is a call to policy makers, academics, and citizens to take steps to reduce meat production and consumption to sustainable levels.

The authors whom we have engaged represent key expertise in their respective fields. They each create a compelling part of the picture, and an alarming picture it is. Global meat and milk consumption is expected to roughly double in the first half of the 21st century. That means, barring some increases in 'efficiency' of production, an approximate doubling of the number of farm animals we slaughter for our consumption each year – from around 70 billion in 2017 to maybe 120 billion by 2050.

A huge amount of epidemiological research is being amassed, showing connections between over-consumption of meat with, for example, colon cancer. The saturated fats so abundant in most meats are recognized as contributing to the growing global epidemic of obesity and its knock-on conditions such as Type-2 diabetes and heart disease. As Mike Rayner and Peter Scarborough (Chapter 14) point out, whilst recognizing the nutritional value of some meat constituents in the diet and its contribution, in small amounts, to raising nutritional levels in the malnourished, it is its over-consumption, so easily achieved in our cheap-meat era, which concerns the health experts – and should concern all consumers. We should also not forget the associated threat to human health posed by diseases from livestock being passed to humans, a scenario ably addressed by Michael Greger in Chapter 12.

In a thought-provoking new chapter (13), Cóilín Nunan exposes the massive threat to human – and animal – health posed by the over-use of antibiotics in intensive farming.

As Tara Garnett shows in Chapter 3, livestock production is responsible for a large amount of the greenhouse gas emissions that result from human activity – more than equalling the emissions from transport globally. In fact most of us could do more for the climate by cutting our meat and dairy consumption rather than our car and plane journeys – although the editors would advocate choosing to do both!

We know that the Earth's forests help keep our planet in good health – and support an astonishing range of wild creatures and plants. Yet their devastation in South America has been mainly for cattle ranching and the growing of soya to feed primarily to farmed animals located in other parts of the world. Our best efforts to stop the destruction of our forests appear as yet to be no match for the bottomless pit of intensive livestock production.

With most global soya production destined not for tofu-eating vegans but for cattle, pigs, and poultry, and with nearly 40 per cent of cereals also destined for livestock consumption, we need only do the sums to see what an inefficient use of precious resources this is. Animals consume far more in calories than they can yield for our consumption. Meanwhile much of that land could be growing crops for direct human consumption. These issues around global crop resource use are discussed in a new chapter (4) by one of this book's editors, Joyce D'Silva. Already, the new trend for water- and land-scarce countries to buy up vast tracts of cheap land elsewhere in the world has been undertaken, not just to grow crops for their people, but to grow feed crops for their intensively farmed animals.

Water itself may become the crunch factor in the meat crisis – and the editors urge you to read Arjen Hoekstra's chapter (2), which should send alarm bells ringing in the corridors of power and policymaking.

Excreta from billions of farm animals has to go somewhere, and all too often it has leached into waterways, creating poisonous downstream pollution. Amazingly, in some countries farmers who pollute water courses are exempt from prosecution under environmental protection laws! Meanwhile the methane and nitrous oxide from animal slurry act as toxic greenhouse gases and the ammonia contributes to acid rain.

The predicted growth in farm animal numbers is unlikely to be achieved without industrial factory farming of animals. Webster, Weeks/Duncan, Butterworth, and Lawrence/Baxter (Chapters 7 to 10) spell out just what horrors this has meant for the animals incarcerated in such units. Truthfully we have, in many cases, selectively bred animals whose own bodies may be their worst enemy, susceptible to lameness and increasingly so vulnerable to disease that most would be unable to live out their 'natural' life span. To add insult to injury, we then confine them in cages, crates or concrete pens and sheds, where they are unable to act as their inheritance urges them: hens can no longer build nests, flap their wings fully or lay their eggs in privacy, pigs have no soil or other substrate to root in, many breeding sows may spend several weeks of each year unable even to turn round in their farrowing crates and natural grazers like cattle may be kept far from grassy fields, thus throwing their natural sleep-and-eat patterns into disarray and their overburdened digestive systems into uncomfortable acidic overload.

Are there solutions to the meat crisis? Of course there are, but their adoption and implementation will require vision, courage and, probably, financing in the initial stages.

The easiest solution may be for those in the developed world and middle-class consumers in rapidly developing transition countries like China and Brazil to radically cut their personal meat consumption. It should not be beyond the imagination of the advertising industry to develop great slogans to assist health and environmental authorities in achieving this cost-effective action. Government expenditure on many other areas of health could ease as a result.

Conservation measures and organic farming can help maintain precious soils and biodiversity and reduce application of artificial nitrogenous fertilizers and noxious pesticides, as Richard Young illustrates in his fascinating chapter (6). Animal manures can be returned to the soil in reasonable amounts to enrich it. Some can be treated in anaerobic digesters to become a local energy source.

Although the excessive demand for meat can lead to endemic over-grazing and deforestation, a more modest consumption of higher-value, higher-welfare meat could support the conservation and expansion of permanent grasslands that allowed cattle to graze (rather than consume soya and cereals). Permanent grasslands and especially silvo-pastoral systems where ruminants can graze and browse in comfort and security in an enriched environment of grasses, trees and shrubs have the potential to sequester carbon in the soil and offset the global warming effects of the methane belched by cattle and other ruminants as a natural consequence of rumen fermentation. In a fascinating new chapter (5), Alberto Bernués explores the potential of pasture-based farming.

Reducing meat production and over-grazing will lighten the burden on soils and waters and remove the *raison d'être* for much deforestation.

From the animal welfare viewpoint, smaller numbers of animals have the potential to be reared in more welfare-friendly conditions. Grazing land can not only sequester carbon, it can also provide a good environment for ruminants to live in, provided of course that they have shelter, supplementary feed when necessary and are managed well.

Lower animal numbers could give the remaining animals more space in their indoor accommodation and lead to the end of the close confinement cage and crate systems that have destroyed the life quality of so many animals and brought the phrases 'factory farming' and 'intensive farming' into justifiable disrepute. It is vital that we put into practice, not just the fine words in the Lisbon Treaty, which recognize animals as 'sentient beings', but that we actively promote husbandry systems and practices that enable the animals to enjoy their lives.

Colin Tudge and John Webster (Chapters 1 and 7) both remind us to not to forget the farmer, who produces our food and can play a vital role in achieving a truly greener countryside and maintaining it in a way that benefits local biodiversity too. The editors have no doubt that farmers want to take pride in their work. By reducing the numbers of animals they keep, by being helped to keep them in more welfare-friendly conditions and by diversifying where opportunity offers, we have no doubt that farmers' own emotional well-being will also be enhanced. For the few so-called farmers who have invested their lives in mass production with global agribusiness, we can only suggest they find an alternative way of farming, so that they can truly earn that honourable title of 'farmer'.

The first edition of this book focused on meat and dairy and concentrated on farmed mammals and birds. However, we are aware that many millions of people rely on eating fish as an important source of protein. As the oceans are increasingly depleted of wild fish stocks, aquaculture, including fish farming, is becoming more significant. We are delighted to add a new chapter (11) to this second edition where Steve Kestin discusses the implications of the growing fish farming industry on climate, resource consumption and biodiversity. As science confirms for us that fish can indeed feel pain, the health and welfare of fish are also issues that must be included in any discussion on the future direction of global food and farming.

We have not forgotten that culture, religion and personal ethical value systems may all play an important role in our lives and be invoked when making dietary decisions. Kate Rawles (Chapter 15) challenges us to develop ethical farming and food, and Martin Palmer (Chapter 17) ably spells out the reasoning behind some of these choices.

The greatest challenge is not to academics, who now have a wealth of research to hand, nor to individuals who are motivated to modify their diets, but to governments, global institutions, and policy makers, who have to find ways to achieve the desired levels of meat production and consumption. In two new chapters for this second edition, Peter Stevenson (in Chapter 16) discusses the politics and economics of animal welfare and sustainable agriculture, whilst Carol McKenna, (in Chapter 20) looks at how animal welfare standards are developing internationally in response to consumer and NGO pressure.

This is why we have included an important section on policy (Chapters 18 to 21), where leading thinkers like Stefan Wirsenius, Fredrik Hedenus, and David Bryngelsson; Tim Lang; Carol McKenna and Jonathan Porritt set out their recommendations, some of them truly radical, for the best way forward.

Finally we urge all our readers to be visionaries, to work at any level from personal to global to help bring about a greener and more compassionate world, where we can all access healthier food, where the planet's precious resources are nurtured, not devastated, where our carbon footprint is reduced and where the animals we farm for our food can have lives worth living. In this way we can have a level of meat and dairy production and consumption that is better for people, animals and our planet.

PART I

The impacts of animal farming on the planet

1

HOW TO RAISE LIVESTOCK – AND HOW NOT TO

Colin Tudge

Most shocking in the modern world is the contrast between what could be and what is. Biologically speaking, the human species should be near the beginning of its evolutionary run. Tsunamis and volcanoes happen, and asteroids are a constant threat, but the long history of the world suggests that with average luck our species should last for another million years – and then our descendants might draw breath and contemplate the following million. Experience and simple extrapolation suggest that if we manage the world well, it is perfectly capable of supporting all of us to a very high standard through all that time – the 7 billion or so who are with us now, and the 9.5 to 10 billion who will be with us within a few decades. Yet we are being warned from all sides – not simply, these days, by professional environmentalists but also by popes, archbishops, scientists, and some economists, that if we go on as we are, then the human species will be lucky to survive the present century in a tolerable or even in a recognizable form.

All too obviously, on all sides, the world is falling about our ears. The world's economies have not recovered from the collapse of the banks in 2008 – and, more to the point, it's clear to everyone who does not have a serious vested interest in the status quo that the prevailing, neoliberal economy, taking its lead from the "deregulated", maximally competitive global market, just will not do. In theory and demonstrably in practice it cannot deliver justice and security; yet all attempts to install alternatives are fiercely resisted. Worse still, the non-renewable resources on which we have come to depend – notably oil – are all too clearly finite, while those that theoretically are renewable or recyclable – fresh water, fertile soils, phosphorus – are dissipated far faster than they can be replenished. All the world's major habitats are compromised, down to and including the deep oceans. Half of all our fellow creatures are conservatively estimated to be in realistic danger of extinction within a century or so. A billion people – one in seven – are now undernourished. Another billion suffer "diseases of excess", or perhaps of covert deficiency: the world population of diet-related diabetics is now more than twice that of Russia. A billion live in urban slums – almost a third of all city-dwellers. Yet still the world's governments equate urbanization with progress.

Agriculture is at the heart of all these setbacks – affected directly by all of them, and a significant cause of most of them. And at the heart of all that is wrong with agriculture is livestock – again the victim and a principal cause of much that is awry with all the rest.

Nothing can be put right *ad hoc.* Everything depends on everything else. No individual mistake can be corrected without attending to all the others. We can't put agriculture on a secure and stable course unless we also create an economy that is sympathetic to sound farming, instead of one that, as now, makes it well-nigh impossible to farm sensibly without going bust. Farmers cannot produce good food by good means and sell it for what it is really worth unless people at large are prepared to pay for it – which means the world needs to restore its food cultures – and unless people are able to afford it – which brings us back to the economy. We cannot tackle any of the problems unless we give a damn, which is a matter of morality. It is very difficult, too, to make serious changes without the assistance or at least the compliance of governments – but the world's most powerful governments no longer seem to think it is their job to govern. They interfere with our lives but that is not the same thing at all. Certainly, Britain's governments since the 1970s have as a matter of policy handed over their traditional powers to the "the market", and to international agencies such as the World Trade Organization, which affect to oversee that market. As one professor of food policy has commented, Britain's food policy these past 30 years has been, "Leave it to Tesco".

Yet the world is still a wonderful place – extraordinarily productive and obliging, and far more resilient than we have a right to expect. Human beings are intelligent, skilful and despite appearances are steeped in what Adam Smith called "natural sympathy": not wanting their fellows or their fellow creatures to suffer, recognizing the debt that we all owe to each other. We have science, which gives us extraordinary insights, and ought to be one of the great assets of humankind, and technologies that give us extraordinary power, including "high" technologies – the kind that emerge from science. We should not be in a mess.

One essential – the *sine qua non* indeed – is to ensure good food for all, produced in ways that do not wreck the biosphere and wipe out our fellow creatures. But is this really possible?

Yes, is the answer – but not by the methods now advocated and foisted upon us by the ruling oligarchy of corporates and governments, and their chosen intellectual and expert advisers. We need to begin again from first principles.

How to feed everybody well and why livestock is crucial

Farming has to be productive of course, but it also has to be both sustainable and resilient: not wrecking the rest of the world as the decades pass, and able to change direction as conditions change – which is especially necessary as the climate shifts. But nature itself shows how all this can be achieved. Wild nature has been continuously productive through hugely turbulent changes of circumstance for 3.8 billion years. Farming is an artifice of course – a human creation – but if we want it to serve us well, and go on serving us, and not kill everything else, then we should seek to emulate nature. This is the principle of "agroecology".

So how does nature achieve its ends? In general, it is self-renewing – it taps in to renewable energy, which mainly (though not quite exclusively) is solar energy, and recycles the non-renewables: carbon, nitrogen, phosphorus, water, and all the rest. It manages all this with enviable efficiency because it is so diverse – millions of different species (we don't know how many, but perhaps around 8 million) acting in rivalry but also more importantly in concert; and it's because the system is so diverse that it is also so resilient. No one disaster can destroy everything – there have always been survivors through all the mass extinctions – and over time, all the creatures within the system, and the ecosystems as a whole, evolve, and adapt. The relationship between plants and animals, which are often perceived to be "dominant" because they are big and pro-active, is synergistic. The plants convert solar energy and minerals into carbohydrates, proteins, and the rest; and the animals plus the fungi, protozoans, and microbes (bacteria and archaeans) help to keep everything cycling.

Farming that emulated nature would be the same: deriving its inputs from renewables, wasting nothing, diverse, low-input – basically organic – balancing crops (plants) against livestock (animals). In principle this is simple. Natural.

In practice, in basic structure, this is how agriculture generally has been for the past 10,000 years. The emphasis in most traditional farming has been on crops, which must be grown on the prime land. The staples, mainly cereals, are grown by arable techniques (on the field scale), while most of the rest are raised by horticulture (on the garden scale). Traditional farmers everywhere commonly grew and grow many different crops – often a huge variety. Except in extreme circumstances (as in extensive grasslands and the highest altitudes and latitudes) livestock are kept mainly or exclusively to supplement the crops. They too are diverse – if not in species then certainly genetically. Overall, traditional farming is and was "polycultural".

In the West, it has been fashionable of late to argue that livestock are a drain on resources – and to suggest that they exacerbate global warming by producing methane gas as a by-product of rumination. In practice, in the modern world, both these criticisms are to some extent justified – but only because we do things badly: specifically, in general, because we have largely replaced traditional farming with industrial agribusiness.

Thus conceptually, and traditionally, livestock falls into two categories. On the one hand there are the specialist herbivores, both ruminants (cattle and sheep the main ones, with goats and deer as minor players) and hind-gut digesters such as horses and rabbits (which are important in some economies). Camels may be seen as "pseudo-ruminants", roughly similar to cattle in the way they deal with herbage, but differing in some details. In a state of nature the specialist herbivores derive most of their energy from cellulose – and this is an extraordinary trick to pull, and an extraordinarily valuable one, for cellulose is the most common organic polymer in nature. It is present and usually the prime component of every plant cell wall and so is common to all plants, growing in all circumstances. In nature at large there are megatonnes of it.

Human beings cannot derive significant quantities of energy from cellulose, but by raising specialist herbivores they gain vicarious access to the cornucopia that cellulose has to offer. Not every specialist herbivore can make use of every kind of leaf or stem – many plants are frankly toxic and/or protect themselves with thorns and whiskers and mucilage. But between them our domestic animals can derive nourishment from most common plants, which means that they can at least survive in most environments, and positively thrive in warm and rainy seasons when the plants are flourishing. So people who keep the right kinds of herbivores in the right proportions can survive in the most hostile landscapes. So it was that Job and his kin, in the Old Testament, lived very well in the desert (at least when he wasn't being assaulted by various plagues) with his mixed herd of cattle, sheep, goats, donkeys, and camels – the proportions spelled out in the Book of Job and still to be found in some African herds.

Even when the plants are dying and the livestock are hungry and losing weight, they still can be killed for meat. The food they supply doesn't even need to be stored and carried. Obligingly, it moves itself around. When the plants are growing, or are about to, the animals give birth – and then their owners live on their milk. Indeed, in well-run desert communities, the animals are killed for meat *only* in times of drought, when the vegetation languishes and they are liable to die anyway. Hence the Jewish edict in Leviticus: not to eat meat and drink milk at the same meal. (I was once told off in a Kosher restaurant for drinking milky tea with a salt beef sandwich.) The Masai drink the blood of their cattle, bleeding them at judicious intervals. Nor are livestock kept only for food. They are the source of textiles (wool) and leather, of fertility, of fuel (cow dung), and their bones are used to make tools and furniture and even sometimes for building. In much of the world animals are the chief transport and pull tractors and harvesters for good measure. This is no anachronism. In some parts of the world and some economies animal power is still the best. The sacred cows of India produced calves that were castrated to make oxen for draught power – and these were almost free because the cows traditionally were not fed: they fed themselves from wayside weeds and crop residues. In much of Africa cattle and sometimes goats are the principal currency; and currency in the form of cattle, unlike currency in the form of banknotes, or – as is the case nowadays – as figures in a computer, is real. In short, cattle and sheep may be a luxury in the middle-class West, but they are at the heart of some of the world's most venerable cultures (as clearly demonstrated throughout the Bible).

The second category of livestock is the omnivores – pigs and poultry. Both can derive some energy from cellulose – though opinions differ on this, and the ability seems to vary somewhat from breed to breed. On the whole, pigs and poultry eat the same kinds of things that humans eat. Yet their culinary standards are not high.

So they are traditionally raised on leftovers – food wastes and crop surpluses. Hence they supplement the overall economy. Furthermore, pigs in particular are great cultivators, eating weeds and digging up the soil and fertilizing it. Indeed, they have often been kept for this alone, with their meat as a bonus. Chickens traditionally were moppers-up of wastes who offered a more or less continuous supply of eggs. Typically the hens themselves were eaten primarily when their laying days were over, in casseroles and pot roasts, while the cockerels made *coq au vin* – but only as an occasional treat.

Traditionally, then, the best land was used for growing crops – arable and horticulture – with pigs and poultry used to clear up the loose ends and for cultivation; and the fields beyond the cultivated area, including the uplands, which were often too steep or too wet or too dry to grow crops, were used for the herbivores; although, of course, sheep and cattle also came on to the arable fields in periods of fallow, to allow the ground to rest and to add fertility. Overall, such a system is highly efficient – not necessarily in cash terms, within the modern economy, but in biological terms, which matters far more. Indeed, as Kenneth Mellanby pointed out in his classic book of 1973, *Can Britain Feed Itself?*, if we reinstalled such a structure in Britain then we could certainly be self-reliant in food. Nowadays we can add refinements too. Thus Martin Wolfe of the Organic Research Centre argues that all farming should be conceived as an exercise in agroforestry, and at Wakelyns Farm in Suffolk he demonstrates the principle of "alley-cropping": growing a variety of valuable trees in rows with arable or horticulture in between. He would like to keep livestock, too, but at present there are too few stockpeople on land to look after them. Aquaculture also has a big part to play (and fish are livestock too). Indeed, way back in 2008 I helped to organize a conference in Oxford on national self-reliance and concluded, as others did, that with an updated, Mellanby-style structure and with some modern varieties we could feed ourselves easily (Tudge, 2009).

The methane problem also is hugely diminished if we farm in this traditional, commonsensical way. Cattle do indeed exhale methane (it comes out the front end, not the back end), but if they are fed only on grass, then of course they can exhale only the carbon that the grass itself has acquired from the atmosphere by photosynthesis. So the excretion of methane could be viewed merely as a form of recycling. There is no net increase in atmospheric carbon. Furthermore, if the grazing is controlled, then much of the carbon dioxide that the grass fixes by photosynthesis finishes up in the roots rather than the leaves and remains uneaten, and as the roots die so the carbon content of the soil is increased, so that a well-grazed field can be a net carbon *sink* – the very thing the world needs. Thus, grazing livestock (in a controlled way) should be win–win. Livestock becomes a menace only when, as now, we feed half the world's cereal and most of the world's soya to animals that should be getting the bulk of their nutrient from grass and leftovers. We burn vast quantities of oil to grow that cereal and fell forest to grow the soya – and so contribute twice over, and prodigiously, to global warming. Yet the cereal and soya we feed to the animals need not be grown at all – or if it is, then we could be eating it ourselves. Again we find it is not the animals that are at fault but the system.

We can extend Kenneth Mellanby's principle. If all countries reinstalled the traditional structures, then almost all of them could be self-reliant – and without wrecking their own environments or the climate. Thus in November 2011 Professor Hans Herren, President of the Millennium Institute in Washington, DC, told a special meeting at London's House of Commons that the world already produces enough to provide food energy and protein for *14 billion* people – twice the present world population and 40% more than we should ever need.

The truth of this is evident from readily available statistics (as found on Google). Thus the world produces 2.5 billion tonnes per year of the major cereals: wheat, rice, and maize. One tonne of any of these provides enough food energy and protein to sustain three people – so 2.5 billion tonnes is enough for 7.5 billion. But the major cereals, important though they are, provide only half the world's food. The other half comes from minor cereals and other grains, pulses, nuts, fruits and vegetables, fungi, and all the products of animals including fish. In addition to energy and protein, vegetables, fruit, livestock, and the rest also provide all the vitamins, minerals, and cryptonutrients that we need. So the total adds up to *at least* 14 billion. Nowadays a billion people are hungry not because the world cannot produce enough food but because the food is not produced in the right places; crops are raised as commodities to be sold abroad for cash, rather than as food for the local population; and a huge amount is wasted. Indeed it is estimated that a third or more of crops in the Third World are lost in the field or in harvest, while in the rich world at third at least is thrown away after it reaches kitchen. We also feed about a third of our grain to livestock – which is mostly unnecessary. Finally, for good measure, perfectly wholesome crops are grown these days simply be burnt for "biofuel" which governments tell us is good for the planet but in truth is a giant scam. Crops grown specifically for animal feed or for fuel have nothing to do with real need and everything to do with short-term profit. In general, the more you can produce, the greater the possible return. So although we already have more than enough, the emphasis still is on more and more production.

In fact, the oligarchs who determine agricultural policy are still in thrall to the demographic theory of Thomas (known as "Bob") Malthus who in the late 18th and early 19th centuries predicted that the human population would be bound to outstrip its food supply and would grow and grow until it collapsed. His ideas inspired Ebenezer Scrooge in Charles Dickens's *A Christmas Carol* to speak of "the surplus population" (that was in 1843). Now we can see that Malthus was wrong. The UN demographers tell us that human numbers will level out of their own accord around 2050 to approximately 10 billion, and we already produce more than enough. But the experts continue to sing from the Malthusian hymn sheet because that is more profitable. It's surprising how much "modern" thinking, including modern science, is rooted in centuries-old ideas which, to a large extent, have long since been discredited. People, even intellectuals, or perhaps especially intellectuals, believe what they find convenient.

Now we come across a huge serendipity – or rather, two huge serendipities. To be sure, if we fed livestock only on grass or leftovers and (genuine) surpluses, then we would not produce as much meat as we do now. We might indeed produce far less, at least in some places. People in high places, keen to maximize profits by maximizing output, are wont to tell us therefore that if we did not grow many millions of hectares of soya and maize for cattle, pigs, and poultry, our diets would be intolerable – all lentils and garlic bakes. Again our rulers display their ignorance. They clearly know nothing about food. For the kind of farming that really could feed us all focuses on arable and horticulture with livestock in supporting roles and so produces "plenty of plants, not much meat and maximum variety": and these nine words – "plenty of plants, not much meat and maximum variety" – summarize all the most worthwhile nutritional theory of the past three decades.

Now for the second serendipity: these nine words also summarize the basic structure of all the world's greatest cuisines – of Provence, Italy, Turkey, Persia, Lebanon, Indonesia, India, China. All of them are plant-based, using meat and fish only sparingly – for flavour and texture, as a garnish, for stock, and eaten in bulk only on the occasional feast day. Even in normal climes, where the growing season is shorter, people traditionally fared well on relatively little meat. Britain traditionally made as much use as almost anyone of *all* parts of the animal (though we never quite got into chicken's feet as the Chinese did), the basis of endless root-rich stews, and is or was very strong on bakery – pies, puddings, cakes of all kinds, variations on a theme of flour. These cuisines are unsurpassed – the basis of all worthwhile *haute cuisine*. But they are not the cuisines of the elite. They are rooted in peasant cooking, devised by ordinary people from whatever grew around – which basically was what farmers found easiest to grow. It all works beautifully. To eat well and sustainably, we don't even have to be austere. We just have to grow what grows best and take cooking seriously. In truth, the future belongs to the gourmet.

So we should be heaving a great sigh of relief. Instead we are panicking, resorting to ever more exotic technologies – and are told from on high that we need to *double* food output by the end of the century or we will all starve, or at least a lot more people will, and that only high tech can save us (the flavour of the month is GMOs). As things are, we are practising agriculture that seems designed to do the precise opposite of what is required – and the oligarchs in charge are planning simply to do more of the same. It is all the grossest nonsense – and at the heart of this grossness, as always, is livestock. Livestock (like all of science) should be one of the great assets of humankind; but again (like science) it has become one of our principal threats.

What are we doing wrong?

Just about everything, is the short answer. "Modern" industrialized farming of the kind that is anomalously called "conventional" has rejected diversity in favour of monoculture. It does not recycle all inputs as traditional systems did and nature does. It relies on non-renewables – notably oil – as if there is no tomorrow, which indeed is becoming the case, and the manure that once was a prime reason for keeping livestock is routinely dumped (Kennedy, 2005).

In "modern" systems, livestock is not kept to balance and supplement the crops. Increasingly, animals have become the *raison d'être*. Ruminants are still fed on grass and browse of course, but they are also fed increasingly on concentrates, meaning cereals and soya. Animals raised in traditional ways – on grazing, browse, surpluses, and leftovers – add to our food supply; they augment and reinforce whatever the plants provide. Animals fed on staples that could be feeding us are not supplementing our diet. They are competing with us.

Meat output continues to increase so that by 2050, on present trends, livestock will be consuming enough of our own staple foods to feed 4 billion people. The additional 4 billion is roughly equivalent to the world population in the early 1970s when the United Nations held its first world conference to discuss what it saw as the global food crisis. At the same time, of course, the more livestock we raise the greater the problems they bring – excess greenhouses gases, destruction of forest, consumption of water. In such large numbers, in intensive units, they also become stewpots of infections, including several with the capacity to cause pandemic among human beings (see Greger, Chapter 12, this volume). Goodness me.

In short, if we are seriously interested in our own survival, and the future of the rest of the world, then the agriculture we have now is the grossest nonsense, ill-conceived and getting worse.

What's to be done?

Those now in power are wont to argue that the free market economy could still solve our problems, given time. After all, the market can succeed only by meeting the demands of its consumers: and consumers can change market practice by their spending patterns. Many consumers have objected to various forms of intensive livestock production and in response, some supermarkets are now seeking to improve animal welfare – buying only from farmers with high welfare standards. This is indeed encouraging, but there is cause to wonder how far this can be taken, and how quickly. Would it really be possible to reform the corporates who now control the world's food supply and the governments who support those corporates (because they are presumed to promote "economic growth"), just by exerting such consumer pressure?

No, is the short answer. If we are ever to solve the world's food problems, we – humanity – need to rethink farming from first principles: what it is for, how to do it, and who should be in charge. I have been thinking about all this for more than 40 years, ever since I attended the first ever World Food Conference in Rome in 1974 and saw how badly governments and big business handle the world's agriculture: how they fail to attack the obvious environmental, economic, and political problems head-on and instead do battle among themselves for power and wealth. The twin essentials of common morality and common sense sink beneath the politicking. But since that World Food Conference things have got worse. The immediate problem of mass famine has largely been solved (or at least it could have been) for which we should be grateful. But the political and economic framework has become less and less conducive to good and sensible farming that can feed us all well and go on doing so.

In fact, right now, two quite contrasting philosophies lie behind world agriculture. The first is that of "Enlightened Agriculture", an expression I coined in a 2004 book titled *So Shall We Reap*. "Enlightened Agriculture" is informally but adequately defined as:

> Farming that is expressly designed to provide everyone, everywhere, with food of the highest standard, without cruelty or injustice and without wrecking the rest of the world.

Since "Enlightened Agriculture" has a lot of syllables, it is sometimes shortened to "Real Farming". Either way, it's a simple, commonsensical idea, intended to achieve what governments claim they want to achieve. What else is farming for, if not to provide us all with good food and to look after the biosphere? And why should it not be kind, to people and to animals?

But this is not the prevailing view. In the 1970s I first heard people in high places say, "Farming is just a business like any other". Well, farms ought in general to be businesses – if we conceive business in the sense that many traditional businesspeople understood it: as the natural underpinning of democratic society. But all businesses are different, and as George Orwell said in a slightly different context, some are more different than others – and none is more different than farming. Farming stands at the heart of all the world's affairs, human and otherwise. We *have* to get it right. We cannot let it sink or swim in the way that we allow corner shops to sink or swim, or indeed entire factories (or indeed, in recent decades, entire industries). Agriculture can operate day to day according to the methods of business, but it isn't *just* a business.

But worse was to follow. In the 1980s the world's economy as a whole was overtaken by the Chicago-born philosophy of neoliberalism, officially adopted first by Margaret Thatcher in Britain and then by Ronald Reagan in the US. The whole global economy was reconceived as one great "de-regulated" market in which all traders of all kinds were invited or obliged to compete to maximize profit in the shortest time, and grab the biggest possible market share, or go to the wall. Agriculture was caught up in the melee, particularly in the neoliberal strongholds of Britain and the US. Now, despite a lot of high-flown rhetoric ("feed the world", "war on poverty", and all the rest) farmers the world over are encouraged or obliged not simply to make a profit (we all have to earn more than we spend somewhere along the line) but to compete ruthlessly to maximize their profits. That is a different mindset.

This different mindset requires farmers to do the very things that we and they should not be doing if we truly seek to provide everyone with good food, sustainably, in a rapidly changing world, and to provide good jobs which are among the keys to social justice, and take care of wild creatures, and ensure that whatever livestock we decide to keep live as well and comfortably as can be managed. The real task is not to maximize output but to acknowledge that enough's enough – and we already produce enough. When you think it through, you see that agriculture that really was designed to deliver all need and to go on delivering requires mixed farms, basically organic, with plenty of skilled farmers – all of which leads us to favour farms that are small to medium sized. But in the neoliberal economy farms are required to maximize production irrespective of need, at minimum cost. With the global price of oil adjusted to ensure that it undercuts all alternatives, and a mind-set geared to short-term profit, maximum output at minimum cost requires huge inputs of agrochemistry and heavy engineering, with minimum and preferably zero labour, and with simplified – monocultural – husbandry because machines can't handle complexity, all practised on the largest possible estates to achieve economies of scale (there are one-crop "farms" in the Ukraine and Brazil bigger than English counties). All this, the antithesis of what the world really needs, is called "progress".

With these thoughts in mind, my wife Ruth (West) and I, along with some good friends, set up our Campaign for Real Farming in 2008, and with it a website that has been a springboard for further activities. First of these was the Oxford Real Farming Conference (ORFC), which has met every January since 2010. It was conceived as an antidote to the Oxford Farming Conference which has been meeting for the past 60 years to extol the virtues of industrial farming and government policy. For the past several years Compassion in World Farming has partnered with us in mounting the ORFC programme.

At the 2012 ORFC we launched Funding Enlightened Agriculture (FEA), which helps farms and related businesses that are in line with enlightened thinking to get off the ground.

In 2016 we launched our College of Real Farming and Food Culture (CRFFC), which aims to bring together all the big ideas that are being developed worldwide to further the cause of Enlightened Agriculture.

The grand aim is to bring about an Agrarian Renaissance, an across-the-board shift in the practice, organization, and control of agriculture, and in the underlying science, and in our attitude towards it. Nothing less will do. Not the least of the requirements is to reintroduce the fundamental principle of morality, of which the principal component, so all the great religions agree, is compassion.

But the existing powers, the oligarchy of governments, corporates, banks, and their chosen intellectual and expert advisers, are wedded to the status quo. They will not lead the Agrarian Renaissance. Indeed they will oppose it. So we, people at large, the global regiment of Ordinary Joes, have got to make it happen for ourselves. The task is huge, but it's exciting, and millions of people worldwide are already on the case. There is scope for everyone to join in. The more who do, the greater the chances of rescuing the world.

References

Burnett, John (1966). *Plenty and Want.* Thomas Nelson, London.

Falk, Ben (2013). *The Resilient Farm and Homestead.* Chelsea Green Publishing, Vermont.

Gordon, Andrew M. and Steven M. Newman (1997). *Temperate Agroforestry Systems.* CAB International, Wallinford.
Hartley, Dorothy (1954). *Food in England.* Macdonald and Jane's, London.
Harvey, Graham (2008). *The Carbon Fields.* Grassroots, Bridgewater. Graham Harvey introduces the idea of mob grazing.
Kennedy, Jr., Robert F. (2005). *Crimes Against Nature.* Harper Collins, New York.
Large, Martin (2010). *Common Wealth.* Hawthorn Press, Stroud. Martin Large discusses the whole concept of the tripartite mixed economy, which surely is what Enlightened Agriculture really requires.
Lymbery, Philip and Isabel Oakeshott (2014). *Farmageddon.* Bloomsbury, London. On the general state of world agriculture with particular reference to animal welfare.
Mellanby, Kenneth (1973). *Can Britain Feed Itself?* Merlin Press, London.
Savory, Allan (2006). *Holistic Management Handbook.* Island Press, Washington. Allan Savory spells out the entire philosophy and practice of grassland management.
Tudge, Colin (1980). *Future Cook.* Mitchell Beazley, London (published in the US by Crown, New York, as *Future Food*). This is the only book I know that tries explicitly to show the direct relationship between food farming, sound nutrition, and great cooking.
Tudge, Colin (2004). *So Shall We Reap.* Penguin Books, London.
Tudge, Colin (2009). *Can Britain Feed Itself? Should Britain Feed Itself?* LandShare, Oxford.
Tudge, Colin (2016). *Six Steps Back to the Land.* UIT/Green Books, Cambridge, UK.

Reports

The following reports, available online, are also highly pertinent:

Agriculture at a Crossroads, produced in 2008 by an ad hoc international body known as IAASTD, co-chaired by Hans Herren and sponsored by the FAO, GEF, UNDP, UNEP, UNESCO, The World Bank, and WHO, and published by Island Press, Washington, in 2009. *Agriculture at the Crossroads* is as authoritative as it is possible to be (it involved 900 participants including world experts from 110 countries from all regions), and it emphasizes the key role of traditional farms and farming in providing the world's food and the need to support and build upon them: farms that in general are small, mixed, low-input, and skills-intensive, as advocated in this book.
Diversification practices reduce organic to conventional yield gap. Lauren C. Ponisio, Leithen K. M'Gonigle, Kevi C. Mace, Jenny Palomino, Perry de Valpine, Claire Kremen. Proceedings of the Royal Society of London B: Biological Sciences username. 2015 Volume: 282 Issue: 1800.
The Future of Food and Farming: Challenges and choices for global sustainability, (2011). *The Foresight report* claimed to be building on the IAASTD report of 2008 but in fact reversed its message. It acknowledged that traditional farms do have a role but continued to advocate high-tech industrial farming on the largest possible scale, geared to the neoliberal global market. The government's chief scientific adviser Sir John Beddington introduced the report with a warning that we cannot continue with "business as usual" – but then, with a few concessions here and there, recommended that we do just that. *The Future of Farming* has become the British government's (Defra's) standard reference. It says what the government wanted to hear.
Feeding the Future: "Small and Medium Scale Agroecological Farmers can address the Agricultural Challenges of the Twenty-First Century". The Land Workers' Alliance. November 2014.
Financing Community Food: Securing Money to Help Community Enterprises to Grow, Sustain, London, 2013.

Websites

The Campaign for Real Farming: www.campaignforrealfarming.org.
The College for Real Farming and Food Culture: http://collegeforrealfarming.org/.
Funding Enlightened Agriculture: www.feanetwork.org.
The Oxford Real Farming Conference: www.oxfordrealfarmingconference.org.

2

THE WATER FOOTPRINT OF ANIMAL PRODUCTS

Arjen Y. Hoekstra

Introduction

One single component in the total water footprint of humanity stands out: the water footprint related to the consumption of animal products. About 92 per cent of humanity's water footprint is related to the consumption of agricultural products; only 4.7 per cent relates to industrial products and 3.8 per cent to domestic water consumption (Hoekstra and Mekonnen, 2012). About 30 per cent of the water footprint related to global agriculture relates to livestock (Mekonnen and Hoekstra, 2012). Animal products generally have a much larger water footprint per kilogram or calorific value than crop products. This means that if people consider reducing their water footprint, they are advised to look critically at their diet rather than at their water use in the kitchen, bathroom and garden. Wasting water never makes sense, so saving water at home when possible is certainly advisable, but if we limit our actions to water reductions at home, many of the most severe water problems in the world will hardly be lessened. The water in the Murray-Darling basin in Australia is so scarce mostly because of water use for the production of various types of fruits, vegetables, cereals and cotton. The Ogallala Aquifer in the American Midwest is gradually being depleted because of water abstractions for the irrigation of crops like maize and wheat. Many of the grains cultivated in the world are not for human consumption but for animals. According to the Food and Agriculture Organization of the United Nations, around 35 per cent of the cereals produced in the world are used for animal feed. Animal products have a relatively large water footprint because of the water needed to grow their feed rather than the water volumes required for drinking. From a water-saving point of view it is obviously more efficient to eat the crops directly rather than indirectly by having them first processed into meat. Surprisingly, however, little attention is paid among scientists and policy makers to the relationship between meat consumption and water use (Hoekstra, 2014).

Consumers can reduce their direct water footprint – in other words, their home water use – by installing water-saving toilets, applying a water-saving showerhead, etc. For reducing their indirect water footprint – that is the water consumption behind the production of food and other consumer products – they have two options. One option is to substitute a consumer product that has a large water footprint with a different type of product that has a smaller water footprint. Eating less meat or becoming vegetarian is one example, but one can also think of drinking tea instead of coffee, or, even better, plain water. Wearing artificial fibre rather than cotton clothes also saves a lot of water. But this approach of substitution has limitations because many people do not easily shift from meat to being vegetarian and people like their coffee and cotton. A second option is that people stick to the same consumption pattern but select the beef, coffee or cotton that has a relatively low water footprint or that has its footprint in an area that does not have high water scarcity. This means, however, that consumers need proper information to make that choice. Since this sort of information is generally not available, this in turn asks for an effort from businesses to create product transparency and an effort from governments to install the necessary regulations. Currently we are far removed from a situation in which we have relevant information about the environmental impact of one piece of beef compared to another piece. The water footprint of beef, however, greatly varies across production systems and countries and strongly depends on feed composition. The same holds for other animal products.

In this chapter, I will start by comparing the water footprints of a number of animal products with the water footprints of crops. Second, I will compare the water footprints of a meat-based and a vegetarian diet. Then I will show that understanding the relation between food consumption and the use of freshwater resources is no longer a local issue. Water has become a global resource, whereby – due to international trade – food consumption in one place often affects the water demand in another place. Finally, I will argue for product transparency in the food sector, which would allow us to better link individual food products to associated water impacts, which in turn can drive efforts to reduce those impacts.

The water footprint of animal products

The water footprint concept is an indicator of water use in relation to consumer goods (Hoekstra, 2013). The concept is an analogue to the ecological and the carbon footprint but indicates water use instead of land or fossil energy use. The water footprint of a product is the volume of fresh water used to produce the product, measured over the various steps of the production chain. Water use is measured in terms of water volumes consumed (evaporated) or polluted. The water footprint is a geographically explicit indicator that not only shows volumes of water use and pollution but also the locations. A water footprint generally breaks down into three components: the blue, green and grey water footprint. The blue water footprint is the volume of fresh water that is evaporated from the global blue water resources (surface water and groundwater). The green water footprint is the volume of water evaporated from the global green water resources (rainwater stored in the soil). The grey water footprint is the volume of polluted water, which is quantified as the volume of water that is required to assimilate pollutants, such that the quality of the ambient water remains above agreed water quality standards (Hoekstra et al., 2011).

In order to understand better the water footprint of an animal product, we had better start by explaining the water footprint of feed crops. The water footprint (m^3/ton) of a crop when harvested from the field is equal to the total evapotranspiration from the crop field during the growing period (m^3/ha) divided by the crop yield (ton/ha). The crop water use depends on the crop water requirement on the one hand and the actual soil water available on the other hand. Soil water is replenished either naturally through rainwater or artificially through irrigation water. The crop water requirement is the total water needed for evapotranspiration under ideal growth conditions, measured from planting to harvest. It obviously depends on the type of crop and climate. Actual water use by the crop is equal to the crop water requirement if rainwater is sufficient or if shortages are supplemented through irrigation. In the case of rainwater deficiency and the absence of irrigation, actual crop water use is equal to effective rainfall. The green water footprint refers to the part of the crop water requirement met through rainfall; the blue water footprint is the part of the crop water requirement met through irrigation. The grey water footprint of a crop is calculated as the load of pollutants (fertilizers, pesticides) that leach from the field to the groundwater or run off from the field to nearby streams (kg/ha) divided by the difference between the maximum allowable and natural concentration for the chemical considered (g/l) and divided by the crop yield (ton/ha).

The water footprint of an animal at slaughter can be calculated based on the water footprint of all feed consumed during its lifetime and the volumes of water consumed for drinking and, for example, cleaning the sheds. One will have to know the age of the animal when slaughtered and the diet of the animal during its various stages of life. The water footprint of the animal as a whole is allocated to the different products that are derived from the animal. This allocation is done on the basis of the relative value of the various animal products, avoids double counting and assigns the largest shares of the total water input to the high-value products and smaller shares to the low-value products.

Table 2.1 shows the global average water footprint for a range of crop and animal products, expressed in terms of litres per kg, as well as per caloric value, per gram of protein and per gram of fat. These averages show that, as expected, animal products are more water-intensive than food crops. For every animal product one can find a crop product with equivalent nutritional value that has a smaller water footprint (Mekonnen and Hoekstra, 2012). One litre of soy milk, for instance, has a three times smaller water footprint than cow milk, and a soy burger has a fifteen times smaller water footprint than a beef burger (Ercin et al., 2012). The global average numbers hide the fact that there is a huge variation of the water footprint for each specific product because production circumstances vary widely. In the case of animal products, for instance, the composition and origin of the feed are important factors (Hoekstra, 2012).

TABLE 2.1 The water footprint of crops and animal products

Food item	*Global average water footprint*			
	litre per kg	*litre per kcal*	*litre per g protein*	*litre per g fat*
Crops				
Sugar crops	200	0.69	—	—
Vegetables	320	1.3	26	150
Starchy roots	390	0.47	31	230
Fruits	960	2.1	180	350
Cereals	1600	0.51	21	110
Oil crops	2400	0.81	16	11
Pulses	4100	1.2	19	180
Nuts	9100	3.6	140	47
Animal products				
Milk	1000	1.8	31	33
Eggs	3300	2.3	29	33
Chicken meat	4300	3.0	34	43
Butter	5600	0.72	—	6.4
Pig meat	6000	2.2	57	23
Sheep/goat meat	8800	4.3	63	54
Beef	15000	10	110	150

Source: Mekonnen and Hoekstra (2012)

Let us consider the example of beef from an industrial production system where it takes three years before the animal is slaughtered to produce 200kg of boneless beef (Hoekstra and Chapagain, 2008). Suppose that the animal has consumed 1300kg of grains (wheat, oats, barley, corn, dry peas, soybean meal and other small grains), 7200kg of roughages (pasture, dry hay, silage and other roughages), 24 cubic metres of water for drinking and 7 cubic metres of water for cleaning sheds, etc. This means that to produce 1kg of boneless beef, we have used about 6.5kg of grain, 36kg of roughages and 155 litres of water (only for drinking and servicing). Producing the volume of feed has cost about 15,300 litres of water. The water footprint of 1kg of beef thus adds up in this case to nearly 15,500 litres of water. This still excludes the volume of polluted water that may result from leaching of fertilizers in the feed crop field or from surplus manure reaching the water system. The example given here can be considered as more or less a global average case. The water footprint of beef will vary strongly, however, depending on the production region, feed composition and origin of the feed ingredients. In a grazing system, cows will eat more grass and roughage and less grains. When slaughtered after three years, they will have gained less weight and provide less meat. In terms of total volume, the water footprint of beef from an industrial system will thus be lower than for a grazing system, but maybe more important is that the water footprints are completely different in terms of where the water is sourced. The water footprint of beef from an industrial system may partly refer to irrigation water (blue water) to grow feed in an area remote from where the cow is raised. This can be an area where water is abundantly available, but it may also be an area where water is scarce and where minimum environmental flow requirements are not met due to overdraft. The water footprint of beef from a grazing system will mostly refer to green water used in nearby pastures. If the pastures used are either dry- or wetlands that cannot be used for crop cultivation, the green water flow turned into meat could not have been used to produce food crops instead. If, however, the pastures can be substituted by cropland, the green water allocated to meat production is no longer available for food-crop production. This explains why the water footprint is to be seen as a multidimensional indicator. One should not only look at the total water footprint as a volumetric value, but one should also consider the green, blue and grey components separately and look at where each of the water footprint components are located. The social and ecological impacts of water use at a certain location depend on the scarcity and alternative uses of water at that location.

Water consumption in relation to diet

Since food consumption gives the most important contribution to the water footprints of people, even in industrialized countries, dietary habits greatly influence the associated water footprint (Vanham et al., 2013a, 2013b; Jalava et al., 2014). A vegetarian diet can save a lot of water compared to a meat-based diet. In industrialized countries the average consumption is about 3400kcal per day; roughly 30 per cent of that comes from animal products. When we assume that the average daily portion of animal products is a reasonable mix of beef, pork, poultry, fish, eggs and dairy products, we can estimate that 1kcal of animal product requires on average roughly 2.5 litres of water. Products of vegetable origin, on the other hand, require roughly 0.5 litres of water per kcal, this time assuming a reasonable mix of cereals, pulses, roots, fruit and vegetables. Under these circumstances, producing the food for one day costs 3600 litres of water (see Table 2.2). In developing countries the average consumption is lower: about 2700kcal per day per person, only 13 per cent of which is of animal origin. Such a diet costs 2050 litres of water per day. These numbers are averages over averages, because, firstly, total caloric intakes and meat fractions assumed vary between and within nations and, second, the water requirements actually vary across production regions and production systems. For a rough comparison between the water footprints of a meat-based and a vegetarian diet, however, a consideration of global averages suffices. For the vegetarian diet we assume that a smaller fraction is of animal origin (not zero because of dairy products still consumed), but keep all other factors equal. In the example for the industrialized countries this reduces the food-related water footprint by 36 per cent

TABLE 2.2 The water footprint of two different diets for industrialized and developing countries

	Meat diet	*kcal/ day*	*litre/ kcal*[a]	*litre/ day*	*Vegetarian diet*	*kcal/ day*[b]	*litre/ kcal*[a]	*litre/ day*
Industrialized countries	Animal origin	950	2.5	2375	Animal origin	300	2.5	750
	Vegetable origin	2450	0.5	1225	Vegetable origin	3100	0.5	1550
	Total	3400		3600	Total	3400		2300
Developing countries	Animal origin	350	2.5	875	Animal origin	200	2.5	500
	Vegetable origin	2350	0.5	1175	Vegetable origin	2500	0.5	1250
	Total	2700		2050	Total	2700		1750

Notes:

[a] Estimates based on the weighted average of the water footprints (litre/kg) of the various products within a food category (from Hoekstra and Chapagain, 2008) divided by their respective caloric values (kcal/kg); the estimate for food from vegetable origin coincides with the estimate by Falkenmark and Rockström (2004); for food from animal origin, the latter use a higher value of 4 litres/kcal.

[b] This example assumes that the vegetarian diet still contains dairy products.

(see Table 2.2). In the case of developing countries the switch to vegetarian diet saves 15 per cent of water. Keeping in mind that for the 'meat eater' we had taken the average diet of a whole population and that meat consumption varies within a population, larger water savings can be achieved by individuals who eat more meat than the average person.

From the above figures it is obvious that consumers can reduce their water footprint by reducing the volume of their meat consumption. Alternatively, however, or in addition, consumers can reduce their water footprint by being more selective in the choice of which piece of meat they pick. Chickens are less water-intensive than cows, and beef from one production system cannot be compared in terms of associated water impacts to beef from another production system.

The relation between food consumption and water use: a global issue

Protecting freshwater resources can no longer be regarded as an issue for individual countries or river basins. Let us take Europe as an example. The water footprint of Europe – the total volume of water used for producing all commodities consumed by European citizens – has been significantly externalized to other parts of the world. About 40 per cent of the water footprint of European consumers lies outside Europe. The region is a large importer of crops like sugar and cotton, two of the thirstiest crops. Europe also imports large volumes of feed, like soybean from Brazil. As a result of international trade in food and feed, all countries import and export water in virtual form, virtually embedded in the traded agricultural commodities. Within Europe, all countries have net virtual water import: they use some water for making export products, but more water is used elsewhere to produce the commodities that are imported. Europe as a whole is a net importer of virtual water, which means that Europe's water security strongly depends on external water resources. How is Europe going to secure its future water supply? In many of Europe's source regions, water is being overexploited already, which means that the status quo cannot be maintained. A substantial proportion of existing problems of water depletion and pollution in the world relates to export to Europe. China and India are still largely water self-sufficient, but with rising food demand and growing water scarcity within these two major developing countries, one will have to expect a larger demand for food imports and thus external water demand. Given the increasing freshwater scarcity worldwide and the increasing number of countries seeking to externalize their water footprint, Europe will have to give up its position of the world's largest net virtual water importer. Instead, Europe will need to move to greater food self-sufficiency and a greater reliance on its own land and water resources.

About one quarter of the water use in the world is for making export products for the world market. It has been estimated that 76 per cent of international virtual water trade in the world relates to trade in food and feed crops, 12 per cent to trade in industrial products, and 12 per cent to trade in farm animal products (Hoekstra and Mekonnen, 2012). Countries like Australia, Canada, the United States, Brazil and Argentina have a net export of water in virtual form because of trade in animal products. Other countries, like Japan, China, Italy and Russia, have a net import. Total international virtual water flows related to global trade in animal products add up to 270 billion m^3/yr, a volume equivalent to about half the annual Mississippi runoff. How much water is virtually traded on the world market because of trade in feed is difficult to know because trade statistics are specified by type of crop but do not show the intended application of the traded crops. This becomes problematic because crops are grown and traded for different purposes, including food, feed and bioenergy. For informing trade policy and public policy on food, water and energy security, it is highly relevant to know for what purposes domestic natural resources are used and how national security relies on external natural resources.

Even now water is still mostly considered as a local or regional resource, to be managed preferably at catchment or river basin level. However, this approach obscures the fact that many water problems are related to remote consumption elsewhere. Water problems are an intrinsic part of the world's economic structure in which water scarcity is not translated into costs to either producers or consumers; as a result there are many places where water resources are depleted or polluted, with producers and consumers along the supply chain benefiting at the cost of local communities and ecosystems. It is unlikely that consumption and trade are sustainable if they are accompanied by water depletion or pollution somewhere along the supply chain. Typical products that can often be associated with remote water depletion and pollution are cotton and sugar products. For animal products it is much more difficult to tell whether they relate to such problems because animals are often fed with a variety of feed ingredients and feed supply chains are difficult to trace. So unless we have milk, cheese, eggs or meat from an animal that was raised locally and that grazed locally or was otherwise fed with locally grown feedstuffs, it is hard to say how and to which extent a product has affected the world's scarce freshwater resources. The increasing complexity of our food system in general and the animal product system in particular hides the existing links between the food we buy and the resource use and associated impacts that underlie it.

Product transparency in the food sector

In order to know what we eat, we need a form of product transparency that is currently completely lacking. It is reasonable that consumers (or consumer organizations on their behalf) have access to information about the history of a product. Since in this chapter we focus on the relation between food and water resources use and impacts, the most relevant question is: how water-intensive is a particular product that is for sale, and to what extent does it relate to water depletion and/or pollution? Establishing a mechanism that makes sure that such information is available is not an easy task. It requires a form of accounting along production and supply chains that accumulates relevant information all the way to the end point of a chain.

Figure 2.1 shows the various steps in the supply chain of an animal product. The chain starts with feed crop cultivation and ends with the consumer. In each step of the chain there is a direct water footprint, which refers to the water consumption in that step, but also an indirect water footprint, which refers to the water consumption in the previous steps. By far the biggest contribution to the total water footprint of all animal products comes from the first step: growing the feed. This step is the furthest removed from the consumer, which explains why consumers generally have little notion that animal products require a lot of water. Besides, the feed will often be grown in areas completely different from where the consumption of the final product takes place.

Governments interested in 'sustainable consumption' may translate this interest into their trade policy. The UK government, for example, given the fact that about

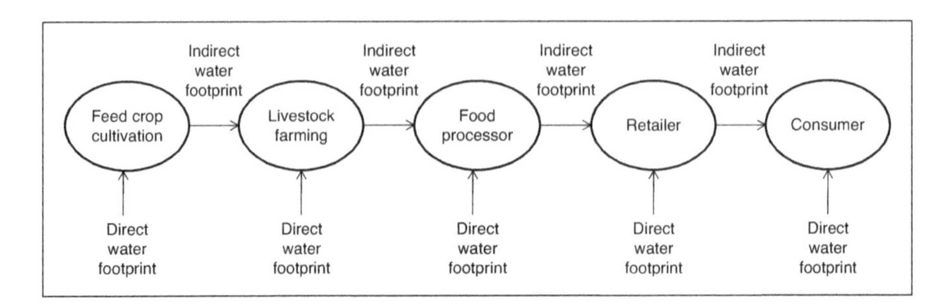

FIGURE 2.1 The direct and indirect water footprint in each stage of the supply chain of an animal product

75 per cent of the total water footprint of UK consumption lies outside the country (Hoekstra and Mekonnen, 2012), may strive towards more transparency about the water impacts of imported products. Achieving such a goal will obviously be much easier if there is international cooperation in this field. In cases where industrialized countries import feed from developing countries, the former can support the latter within the context of development cooperation policy in reducing the impacts on local water systems by helping to set up better systems of water governance.

Business can have a key role as well, particularly the large food processors and retailers. Since they form an intermediary between farmers and consumers, they are the ones that have to pass on key information about the products that they are trading. As big customers they can also put pressure on and support farmers to actually reduce their water footprint and require them to provide proper environmental accounts. If it comes to water accounting, there are currently several parallel processes going on in the business world. First of all, there is an increasing interest in the water use in supply chains, on top of the traditional interest in their own operational water use. Second, several companies, including for instance Unilever, have started to explore how water footprint accounting can be practically implemented. Some businesses think about extending their annual environmental report with a paragraph on the water footprint of their business. Others speak about water labelling of products (either on the product itself or through information available online), and yet others explore the idea of water certification for companies. The interest in water footprint assessment comes from various business sectors, ranging from the food and beverage industry to the apparel and paper industries, but within the food industry there is still little interest to consider the most water-intensive form of food: animal products.

Conclusion

Remarkably little is known about the relation between animal products and water resources protection. There is no national water plan in the world that even addresses the issue that meat and dairy products are among the most water-intensive consumer products, let alone that water policies somehow involve consumers or the food industry in this respect. Water policies are often focused on 'sustainable production', but they seldom address 'sustainable consumption'. One can find an endless number of publications on 'water and agriculture' and 'water for food', but they generally address the issue of water-use efficiency within agriculture (more crop per drop), hardly ever the issue of water-use efficiency in the food system as a whole (more kcal per drop).

Wise water governance is a shared responsibility of consumers, governments, businesses and investors (Hoekstra, 2013). As follows from the previous sections, each of those players has a different role. Consumers (or consumer and environmental organizations) can urge businesses and governments to create greater product transparency for animal products, so that they are better informed about associated water resources use and impacts. The advantage of involving consumers is that enormous leverage can be created to establish change. Consumers can further choose to consume fewer animal products and – when still consuming those products – they can choose, whenever proper information allows, from the meat, eggs and dairy products that have a relatively small water footprint or for which this water footprint has no negative environmental impacts. National governments can – preferably in the context of an international agreement – put regulations in place that urge businesses along the supply chain of animal products to cooperate in creating product transparency. Furthermore, governments can tune their trade and development cooperation policies towards their wish to promote consumption of and trade in sustainable products. Businesses, particularly big food processors and retailers, can use their power in the supply chain to effect product transparency of animal products. Businesses can also cooperate in water labelling, certification and benchmarking schemes and produce annual water accounts that include a report of the supply-chain water footprints and associated impacts of their products. Finally, investors like banks, pension funds and insurance companies can start including sustainable water-use criteria in their investment decisions.

References

Ercin, A.E., Aldaya, M.M. and Hoekstra, A.Y. (2012) The water footprint of soy milk and soy burger and equivalent animal products, *Ecological Indicators*, 18: 392–402.

Falkenmark, M. and Rockström, J. (2004) Balancing Water for Humans and Nature: The New Approach in Ecohydrology, Earthscan, London.

Hoekstra, A.Y. (2012) The hidden water resource use behind meat and dairy, *Animal Frontiers*, 2(2): 3–8.

Hoekstra, A.Y. (2013) The Water Footprint of Modern Consumer Society, Routledge, London.

Hoekstra, A.Y. (2014) Water for animal products: A blind spot in water policy, *Environmental Research Letters*, 9(9): 091003.

Hoekstra, A.Y. and Chapagain, A.K. (2008) *Globalization of Water: Sharing the Planet's Freshwater Resources*, Blackwell Publishing, Oxford.

Hoekstra, A.Y., Chapagain, A.K., Aldaya, M.M. and Mekonnen, M.M. (2011) *The Water Footprint Assessment Manual: Setting the Global Standard*, Earthscan, London.

Hoekstra, A.Y. and Mekonnen, M.M. (2012) The water footprint of humanity, *Proceedings of the National Academy of Sciences*, 109(9): 3232–3237.

Jalava, M., Kummu, M., Pokka, M., Siebert, S. and Varis, O. (2014) Diet change: A solution to reduce water use? *Environmental Research Letters*, 9: 074016.

Mekonnen, M.M. and Hoekstra, A.Y. (2012) A global assessment of the water footprint of farm animal products, *Ecosystems*, 15(3): 401–415.

Vanham, D., Hoekstra, A.Y. and Bidoglio, G. (2013a) Potential water saving through changes in European diets, *Environment International*, 61: 45–56.

Vanham, D., Mekonnen, M.M. and Hoekstra, A.Y. (2013b) The water footprint of the EU for different diets, *Ecological Indicators*, 32: 1–8.

3

LIVESTOCK AND CLIMATE CHANGE

Tara Garnett

The process of feeding ourselves has always had damaging consequences for our land (Diamond, 2005) and the animals we have reared. We have drained peatlands and chopped down forests to provide us with fertile agricultural soil, and we have used the animals in our care in often unspeakably cruel ways (Thomas, 1991).

Until now, though, we have always been able to expand our way out of the problem. There was always new land to use. The situation today is very different: there are more of us – but there are no more planets to exploit. By 2050 there will be 9–10 billion or more of us on this Earth and each one of us will need to eat. What we eat, and how we produce it, has a profound impact upon the long-term sustainability of the planet. Worryingly, however, the patterns of production and consumption that we in the developed world have adopted, and that the developing world is rapidly taking up, have potentially catastrophic consequences.

One of the major causes for concern is the rapid growth in the production and consumption of foods of animal origin. Apart from the potential welfare implications of how we actually rear these animals, the growth in livestock farming has damaging consequences for biological diversity, for water extraction and use, for soil and air pollution – and for climate change, which is the primary focus of this chapter.

We show that tackling climate changing emissions will require us to reduce the number of animals we rear and to change the way we rear them; and we will need to eat fewer foods of animal origin. This said, livestock production can also very much form a part of the solution – farm animals can help create a resilient, sustainable, biodiverse food system, if we rear them in the right way and at moderate scales.

Finally, the livestock-climate issue cannot and must not be seen as standing in opposition to development objectives, and in particular to the right of all people to food security. We need to develop strategies that explicitly link the goals of ensuring adequate access to nutritious food with that of achieving greenhouse gas (GHG) emission reductions from the agricultural and food sectors.

Climate change and international development: twin problems

The climate is changing and most of the change is caused by human activity. The latest report (2014) by the Intergovernmental Panel on Climate Change (IPCC) concludes that 'Warming of the climate system is unequivocal'; what is more, 'Anthropogenic greenhouse gas emissions have increased since the pre-industrial era. . . . Their effects, together with those of other anthropogenic drivers . . . are *extremely likely* to have been the dominant cause of the observed warming since the mid-20th century' (original emphasis) (IPCC, 2014).

The period 1880 to 2012 has seen a global rise in temperature of 0.85°C. Without serious action to address climate change, the global increase in temperature is likely to exceed 2°C by the end of the century and could be as high as 4.8°C (IPCC, 2014).

It is generally accepted that a rise of 2°C above pre-industrial levels, equivalent to a concentration of CO_2 equivalent (CO_2e) in the atmosphere above 450 parts per million (ppm), delivers the probability of 'dangerous climate change' (Schellnhuber et al., 2006). We could then experience major irreversible system disruption, with hypothetical examples including a sudden change in the Asian monsoon or disintegration of the west Antarctic ice sheet (Schneider et al., 2007). Note that even at 450ppm there is only a 50 per cent chance of keeping the temperature rise to 2°C or lower (Hadley Centre, 2005). What is more, even if the world stopped emitting any more GHGs as of now, we would still be 'committed', due to time lags in the Earth's climate mechanisms, to a rise of 1°C by the end of the century (or 0.1°C per decade). In short, we have very little room left for manoeuvre. While the global agreement signed in Paris at the end of 2015 marks a major step forward – governments across the world committed to "[h]olding the increase in the global average temperature to well below 2°C above pre-industrial levels and to pursue efforts to limit the temperature increase to 1.5 °C above pre-industrial levels" – the challenge ahead is to turn good intentions into effective actions. As discussed below, it is difficult to see how a 2°C – let alone a 1°C limit on temperature rise – is to be achieved without measure to curb emissions from the food and agricultural sector.

Compounding the problem is poverty. Around 2.4 billion people worldwide have no access to proper sanitation, more than a third of the world's growing urban population live in slums and over 800 million people live in absolute poverty (United Nations, 2015). Nearly 800 million people are malnourished and one in four children worldwide are stunted (IFPRI, 2015). While we in the developed world can afford to make drastic changes in our lifestyles (even if we may not want to) to tackle climate change, there is an urgent need for people in the developing world to *raise* their standard of living and – even if developed countries deliver on their promises on clean technology transfer and support – this will mean increases in GHG emissions.

The implications for the developed world are clear. If we are to limit climate change to 'safe' levels, *and* if the developing world economies are to achieve a reasonable standard of living, then rich countries, who contribute the bulk of present and historical greenhouse gas (GHG) emissions, need to reduce their emissions by 80 per cent or more (Committee on Climate Change, 2008). The IPCC's Fifth Assessment report suggests that to keep below a 2°C temperature increase absolute emission reductions of up to 70 per cent would be needed – while a 1.5°C limit would require reductions of up to 95 per cent (IPCC, 2014). Critically, we also need to be taking steps to reduce our emissions right now; the longer we put off taking action, the harder it will be to keep emissions beneath the 450ppm threshold (Stern, 2006).

Climate change and the role of food

The food chain contributes significantly to GHG emissions, both at national (UK) and international levels. Estimates vary, with ranges given from about 19 per cent (Garnett, 2008) of UK to 31 per cent (European Commission, 2006) of EU total emissions (reflecting, among other things, different methodological approaches), but clearly the impact is considerable.

Emissions arise at all stages in the food production cycle, from the farming process itself (and associated inputs) through manufacture, distribution and retailing, to the storing and cooking of food in the home or catering outlet. At the farming stage, the dominant GHGs are nitrous oxide (N_2O) from soil and livestock processes (faeces and urine) and methane (CH_4) from ruminant digestion and rice cultivation. Carbon dioxide (CO_2) emissions arise from the fossil fuel inputs used to power machinery and to manufacture synthetic fertilizers, albeit to a lesser degree. To these estimates should be added indirect emissions – those arising from agriculturally used land use change. However, in addition to these direct impacts there are also indirect emissions to consider: notably carbon dioxide emissions resulting from agriculturally induced changes in land use (such as deforestation, land degradation and the conversion of pasture to arable). These add considerably to direct farm stage impacts.

The IPCC estimates that emissions from the AFOLU sector (Agriculture, Forestry and Other Land Use) contribute to around 24 per cent of the emissions total. Around half of these are caused by direct agricultural emissions, while the remaining half arise from deforestation and other forms of land use change – the vast majority of which are agriculturally induced (Smith et al., 2014). Estimating future emissions is an undertaking inherently fraught with uncertainty, but assuming current developments both in technology and demand, emissions could increase by a further 17 per cent by 2050 (Bennetzen et al., 2016). As regards the UK, emissions associated with agriculture account for nearly half of the food chain's total impacts, or around 8.5 per cent of the UK's total GHG emissions (Garnett, 2008). If land use change emissions attributable to UK food consumption are included, the contribution of the UK food system to UK emissions rises from around 20 per cent to 30 per cent (Audsley et al., 2010).

Beyond the farm, the bulk of emissions are attributable to the fossil fuel used to process, transport and retail goods, for refrigeration and for cooking. Accurate global figures are lacking but one study estimates that emissions from these sources collectively contribute about 5–10 per cent of global GHG emissions.

In the UK, these beyond-the-farm-gate emissions collectively account for just over half of food's total impacts.

Greenhouse gas emissions and the contribution of the livestock sector

While the production and consumption of all foods contributes to GHG emissions, it is increasingly recognized that livestock's contribution to the food total is particularly significant. The vast majority of livestock's impacts occur at the farm stage, with subsequent processing, retailing and transport playing more minor roles (Berlin, 2002; Foster et al., 2006). A report by the Food and Agriculture Organization (FAO) estimates that, globally, the livestock system accounts for 14.5 per cent of GHG emissions – a figure that includes land use change impacts (Gerber et al., 2013) – and there is a large and growing literature on the GHG emissions associated with livestock rearing (Cederberg and Mattson, 2000; Cederberg and Stadig, 2003; Casey and Holden, 2005, 2006; Basset-Mens and van der Werf, 2005; Lovett et al., 2006; Garnett, 2009; EBLEX, 2009).

At the European level, an EU-commissioned report puts the contribution of meat and dairy products at about half of food's total impacts (European Commission, 2006). For the UK, it has been estimated (Garnett, 2008) that the meat and dairy products we consume (including the embedded emissions in imported products) give rise to around 60 million tonnes of CO_2e, equivalent to approximately 8 per cent[1] of the UK's total consumption attributable GHG emissions, or 38 per cent of all food's impacts. Importantly, the figure does not include land use change impacts associated with the production of feedstuffs overseas destined for UK livestock. Livestock account for the bulk of the UK's total agricultural impacts through the methane that ruminants emit, and through the nitrous oxide emitted both directly by livestock and indirectly during the cultivation of feed crops. According to the FAO, by 2050 the demand for meat and milk could increase by 73 and 58 per cent respectively on 2005/2007 levels (FAO, 2011). This clearly has implications for GHG emissions.

Life cycle analysis shows that ruminant animals, such as cattle and sheep, appear to be far more GHG intensive than monogastrics, such as pigs and poultry (see Table 3.1). This is because the former emit methane during the process of digesting their food. Methane is not only a potent GHG, but its production also leads to energy losses, which means that the feed conversion energy of ruminants is lower than that of monogastrics. As a result, the amount of feed energy needed to produce

TABLE 3.1 GHG intensity of livestock types in the UK

Livestock type	*Tonnes CO_2e/tonne*
(per tonne of carcass weight, per 20,000 eggs (about 1 tonne) or per 10m³ milk (about 1 tonne dry matter equivalent)	
Beef	16.0
Pig (pork and bacon)	6.4
Poultry	4.6
Sheep	17.0
Eggs	5.5
Milk and dairy products	10.6

Source: Williams et al. (2006).

a kilo of beef or of milk solids is greater than that required to produce an equivalent quantity of chicken, pork or eggs. Since the bulk of the anticipated increase in production and consumption will be met by increases in pig and poultry production, with much smaller increases in ruminant production, this is seen to act as a modifying influence in the growth of livestock-related GHG emissions (Steinfeld et al., 2006).

However, the apparent GHG superiority of white meat to red, and the implications for trends in emissions, is complicated by the possibility, suggested by some studies, that grazing livestock in some systems may have a role in sequestering soil carbon, meaning that their overall net GHG emissions may be low or even negative. This contested and under-researched issue is discussed further later in this chapter. Also necessary to consider are the differential benefits arising from different livestock types or systems.

The GHG benefits of livestock production

While livestock production contributes significantly to food-related GHG emissions, to conclude that a vegan agricultural and food system would be preferable is far too simplistic. Livestock farming has been practiced for millennia for good reason – livestock yield multiple benefits, and some of these are environmental. Table 3.2 briefly summarizes the potential benefits of livestock production and sets them against some of the disbenefits.

For a start it is worth pointing out the obvious: eating will always carry with it an environmental 'cost', although plant-based foods, on the whole, generate fewer GHG emissions. Meat and dairy products are an excellent source of nutrition, providing, in concentrated form, a range of essential nutrients, including energy, protein, iron, zinc, calcium, vitamin B12 and fat. This said, these nutrients can also be obtained from plant-based foods (or, in the case of vitamin B12, by fortification) (Appleby

TABLE 3.2 Potential benefits and disbenefits of livestock production

	Benefits	*Disbenefits*	*Comment*
Nutrition	Excellent for protein, calcium, iron, zinc, vitamin B12	Excessive fat; protein can be supplied in excess of requirements	Animal foods not essential, plants can substitute at lower GHG cost
Non-food benefits	Leather, wool, manure, rendered products	Manure can be a pollutant; leather production is a chemical-intensive activity	Is supply excess to demand?
Carbon storage	Pasture land stores carbon and (according to some studies) well-managed grazing practices can promote carbon sequestration although the evidence here is contested	Excessive grazing releases carbon; deforestation for pasture land or feed production releases carbon	Land use change from pasture to crops releases CO_2
Resource efficiency	Livestock can consume by-products	Grains and cereals feature very heavily in intensive systems	Some by-products could be used as a feedstock for anaerobic digestion or combusted for heat
Geography	Some land not suitable for cropping	Arable land used to grow cereals and oilseeds for livestock	Uplands and marginal lands could potentially be used for biomass production; agroforestry schemes could incorporate livestock

et al., 1999; Key et al., 1999; Sanders, 1999; Millward, 1999) and the importance of meat and dairy products in supplying these nutrients very much depends on where you are in the world, how rich you are and how much of them you are consuming.

On the one hand, in rich societies suffering from the health burdens of over-nutrition, the superabundance particularly of excessive fat and energy in animal products can be actively deleterious, while a diverse and nutritionally adequate range of plant-based foods are widely available. For these people, plant-based foods can provide adequate nutrition at lower GHG 'cost'.

Among poor societies, however, where meals are largely grain or tuber based, where access to a nutritionally varied selection of foods is limited and where there are serious problems of mal- and under-nutrition, keeping a goat, a pig or a few chickens can make a critical difference to the adequacy of the diet (Neumann et al., 2002). Moreover in many communities, livestock play valuable cultural and economic functions; they can be bought or sold as need arises, acting in effect as a form of mobile banking service and so contributing to the food and economic security of the household (Aklilu et al., 2008). Here the benefits of animal source foods may be considerable.

It is also important to note that animals provide us not only with nutrition but with non-food goods such as leather, manure (which improves soil quality and reduces the need for synthetic fertilizers), traction power and wool. If people did not obtain these goods from livestock, they would need to be produced by some other means and this would almost inevitably incur an environmental cost.

Perhaps most importantly, some livestock systems actively contribute to the avoidance of GHG emissions in two ways. At the right stocking density (and this is critical), grazing animals have an important role to play in maintaining, and perhaps in certain defined contexts, building carbon stocks in the soil (Allard et al., 2007) – although the evidence on sequestration is mixed. Ploughing this land for arable production would lead to the release of GHG emissions. It is also the case that much of the land used by grazing ruminants is not suited to other forms of food production (for example the Welsh uplands, or the Mongolian steppes). By eating animals that are reared on land unsuited to other food-producing purposes, we avoid the need to plough up alternative land to grow food elsewhere. Note that these potential carbon-sequestering, land utilization benefits are obtained from ruminant livestock systems and not from pigs and poultry – a benefit that is not captured by life cycle analysis or in the figures presented in Table 3.1, earlier in the chapter. Livestock can also play a vital role in mixed crop rotations; by consuming the clover planted to fertilize the soil, they give value (through the milk they provide) to what would otherwise be an economically unproductive part of the rotation. Their manure also helps fertilize and improve the structure of the soil. Livestock farming has another potential GHG-avoiding role in that livestock consume by-products that we cannot or will not eat. We, by eating animals who have themselves been fed on food and agricultural by-products, are consuming 'waste' made edible, and in so doing we avoid the need to grow food on alternative land – a process that could give rise to land use change emissions and require fossil fuel–based inputs. The feeding of some by-products to livestock is now limited in the EU by legislation; for example, there has been a ban on feeding pigs catering waste, or swill, of mixed plant and animal origin since 2003 (this ban was introduced in 2001 in the UK), following the outbreak of foot and mouth disease. And of course caution is needed: the feeding of certain by-products to animals can (as in the case of BSE) be catastrophic; in many developing world countries pig farming in peri-urban areas, where the pigs are fed on sewage, can give rise to food safety problems.

Moreover, when considering the benefits of livestock for soil carbon sequestration and resource utilization, it should be borne in mind that the gains are highly dependent on the type of system within which the livestock are reared and the scale of the demand for livestock products. At the extremes both of extensive and intensive livestock systems, the benefits tend to be outweighed by the disbenefits.

In extensive systems (such as those found in many parts of the developing world) that do not use additional feed inputs, there can also be soil carbon losses that result from overgrazing (Abril and Bucher, 2001) – that is, when the number of cattle being reared is greater than the land's carrying capacity. This is a significant concern in the developing world and it has been estimated that 52 per cent of agricultural land worldwide is moderately or severely degraded (United Nations, n.d.). Note that the UK is implicated in overgrazing-related carbon losses overseas when our demand for major agricultural commodities (often grown to feed intensively reared British livestock), pushes poor livestock farmers on to increasingly marginal and vulnerable pasture lands where soils are quickly degraded. Moreover, extensive cattle farming systems, such as Brazilian ranching, have a highly damaging effect because they trigger a shift from a very high carbon-sequestering form of land use (forest) to one that sequesters less carbon (pasture) – quite aside from the catastrophic impacts on biodiversity. Hence the potential carbon-sequestering role of livestock depends on good land management, the maintenance of appropriate stocking densities and – critically – on constraining expansion. In extensive systems where the farm animals are reared in climatically or geologically extreme conditions and receive no supplementation at all, they may also suffer from welfare problems.

Intensive systems, such as those found in the UK, present a different set of problems. For a start, while ruminants do graze on grasslands, these grasslands are not always a 'free' resource. In all, some 60 per cent of the grassland area in the UK receives nitrogen fertilizer applications (Defra, 2014a), and these give rise to N_2O emissions. While sheep and some cattle are indeed left for much of their lives to graze on the uplands, they are usually finished on fertilized lowland grass, perhaps supplemented with concentrates – without this extra input, the meat yield would be too low to be economically viable. Moreover, livestock of all types in intensive systems not only consume by-products but also large quantities of cereals that, arguably, could have been eaten directly and more efficiently by humans. Measured in terms of land area or GHG emissions per unit of protein or calories, it is less efficient to feed grain to animals that we then eat than it is for us to eat the grain directly. Globally, livestock have been estimated to consume about 35 per cent world cereal output (FAO, 2015) and the proportion is higher still in the UK (Defra, 2014b). The use of land to produce cereals for livestock ultimately leads to land use change either directly, by colonizing new land, or indirectly, by pushing existing activities (such as pastoral grazing) into new land.

The negative impacts of soy, a major input to intensive systems, are particularly striking. While soy-oil has its uses in industrial food manufacture and increasingly as a biofuel, the cake is produced in larger quantities and as such accounts for most of the crop's economic value (FAO, 2009). In some years demand for meal can actually drive soy production. Soy cannot, then, accurately be called a 'by-product'.

Soy farming has major implications for GHG emissions because of its role in land use change and particularly in deforestation (WWF, 2004; Nepstad et al., 2006; McAlpine et al., 2009). While cattle ranching has historically been a major driver of deforestation in Brazilian Amazonia, accounting for the bulk of direct deforestation, the relationship between cattle ranching and other drivers, particularly soy, is both close and complex. Cattle ranches are often set up to secure land tenure and to maintain cleared land, allowing other more profitable enterprises such as soy to move in (McAlpine et al., 2009). In the decade up to 2004, industrial soybean farming doubled its area to 22,000km^2 and is now the largest arable land user in Brazil (Elferink et al., 2007). Moreover, soybean cultivation not only makes use of land in its own right but has also acted as an important 'push' factor for deforestation by other industries; it takes land away from other uses, such as smallholder cultivation and cattle rearing, and pushes these enterprises into the rainforest (Nepstad et al., 2006; Fearnside and Hall-Beyer, 2007). Additionally, it provides income to purchase land for other purposes, including logging. Hence while beef cattle are a major direct cause of Brazilian deforestation, the role of soy as a second-stage colonizer has also been significant. This said, recent trends suggest that Brazil has had some success in curbing soy- and cattle-related land use change (Gollnow and Lakes, 2014); given rising demand for soy from China, the stability of these changes into the future, however, remains to be seen.

As highlighted earlier, the bulk of the projected doubling in the production and consumption of livestock is due to increases in intensive pig and poultry production. Intensively reared pigs and poultry are major consumers of soy. For example China is now the world's leading importer of soy (FAOSTAT, 2013), and nearly 80 per cent of its imports are in the form of soymeal, used to feed its growing meat (and especially pork and poultry) sector (Gale et al., 2014). Moreover, while pigs and poultry in intensive systems may be efficient converters of feed into meat, they rely on cereals and soy – in fact they actively compete, through the demand for grains, with land needed to grow crops for humans. As such, farming them in this way is implicated in land use change. Unlike grazing animals, they do not provide the benefit of carbon storage services.

This said, if the projected increase in animal source foods were met by either increases in extensive or intensive ruminant farming, the problem could arguably be worse. The direct land needs of ruminant cattle are large and expansion into forest areas would lead to major soil carbon losses. As for intensive beef and dairy systems – again, set to grow – these require not only grazing land but also significant cereal and oilseed inputs, which, as noted, they consume less efficiently than do pigs and poultry. As such, high-volume, intensive ruminant production would represent the worst of both worlds. We would have a system that emits methane (as well as the nitrous oxide that all animals emit) and that is also dependent on cereals and soy – a double whammy. Expansion of extensive grass-fed systems does not, therefore, present a solution.

To conclude, ruminant livestock *can* yield carbon storage and resource efficiency benefits, but this only takes place in certain extensive systems at certain stocking densities. Once the numbers of livestock are greater than the ability of the land to support them, the disbenefits, in the form of land degradation (and lower animal welfare) rise to the fore. Similarly, while livestock farming of all types can represent a form of resource efficiency, the volume of by-products available cannot alone feed the sheer numbers of animals that we appear to want to eat. Growth in demand is what turns a sustainable system into an unsustainable system.

Hence what emerges when discussing the benefits and disbenefits of livestock systems is that two factors are critical: the *type* of livestock system and the *scale* of livestock production and associated consumption. The right type of system at the right scale is needed to ensure that the benefits outweigh the disbenefits.

Reducing livestock-related GHG emissions: what can be done?

Policy makers in the developed world are increasingly aware of the need to tackle livestock-related emissions. There is now a very considerable and growing body of research examining how GHG emissions from agriculture in general, and from livestock more specifically, might be reduced (Clark et al., 2001; Committee on Climate Change, 2008; Garnett, 2008; Smith et al., 2014).

Broadly speaking, the focus is on efficiency: an approach that takes as its starting point the need to meet growing demand at lowest GHG cost. As highlighted, the key word here is demand. It is projected – and accepted – that demand for meat and dairy products will double by 2050, and while the consumption issue is starting to receive some attention in the developed world, growth in the developing world is taken to be inevitable.

Efficiency is taken to mean the production of as much meat, milk and associated products for as little GHG and land use 'cost' as possible. We explore the extent to which intensive production achieves its goals and highlight the implications for animal welfare, biodiversity and human health, before setting out an alternative approach.

The efficiency approach

The research literature on livestock GHG mitigation tends to focus on four main categories of action: improving the efficiency of breeding and feeding strategies; managing soils to sequester carbon; managing manure to reduce methane, nitrous oxide and ammonia emissions and (through anaerobic digestion) to produce energy; and decarbonizing energy inputs. Table 3.3 sets these out in more detail.

Approaches b and c relate to agriculture in general. Approach a is specifically livestock related and encompasses a range of strategies. A key element is to manage the feeding regime to achieve an 'optimal' balance between carbohydrate and protein – this is to ensure that the food is used by the animal to produce milk or meat rather than being 'wasted' in the form of methane or nitrogen losses. Note that the emphasis is very much on the use of cereal and protein inputs; ruminants fed a mixed diet of cereals and proteins emit fewer methane emissions per unit of milk or meat than grass-fed cattle (since there is less roughage) and breeding strategies are designed to maximize the capacity of the animal to be productive on a diet of concentrates. Similarly poultry and pig systems based on the rearing of fast-growing animals fed on energy- and protein-intensive concentrates reach slaughter weight rapidly. Emissions are therefore lower, since fewer days need to

TABLE 3.3 GHG mitigation – an efficiency approach

Approach	*Goals*	*Example measures*
a **Efficient husbandry**	More milk or meat per kg of GHG emissions	Optimizing feed conversion ratio through use of cereals and oilseeds in the right proportions to maximize yields at minimum GHG cost. Breeding for better partitioning of feed into milk (dairy); for better muscle tone (beef); for rapid growth (pigs and poultry) Methane inhibitors, feed supplements (e.g. oils), bovine somatotropin, genetic modification (all still at experimental stage); breeding for fertility and longevity (dairy cows)
b **Soil carbon management**	Retain or increase carbon in the soil	Improve pasture quality; restore degraded lands; minimum and no-till arable farming (feed and food crops)
c **Manure management**	Reduce methane, nitrous oxide and ammonia emissions; create biogas as a substitute for fossil fuels	Anaerobic digestion to produce biogas to substitute for fossil energy and an anaerobic digestate as a substitute for fossil fuel–based fertilizer inputs; compost manure to stabilize and improve its quality
d **Energy decarbonization**	Reduce CO_2 from fossil energy inputs	Anaerobic digestion as on farm energy source; more efficient energy management; renewables; reduced use of synthetic fertilizers

be spent heating and lighting their housing, and the feed conversion efficiency is higher.

The feed-optimization approach can be combined, in the case of dairy cows, with breeding strategies to increase productivity (by increasing that portion of feed intakes that is partitioned, through metabolic processes into milk) and fertility. To date there has been a strong emphasis on breeding for increased productivity, at the cost of reduced fertility, but there are signs now of greater focus on extending fertility. The fertility issue is relevant from a GHG, as well as from an animal welfare perspective because a rapid turnover of milkers due to early death or infertility means that energy inputs and greenhouse gas outputs are 'wasted' in the process of rearing heifers before they reach their first pregnancy and lactation. Once she has reached maturity, it is important to keep the cow milking for as long as possible after this period so that the investment in growth and development pays off and to keep the replacement rate as low as possible.

Parallel strategies for feed production include increasing the productivity of feed crops so that more crops can be grown on a given area of land, again through breeding and fertilizer strategies. Biomass production could form part of the efficiency picture. As rearing livestock on uplands becomes increasingly unprofitable, livestock farmers are leaving the hills. An alternative use for the uplands might be biomass production, an approach that contributes to carbon sequestration and also generates a fuel source. Under an efficiency scenario, most of the growth in livestock products will come from more profitable pigs and poultry, with their higher feed conversion efficiencies.

Note that these feeding and breeding approaches, while 'efficient', are inherently dependent on cereals and oilseeds. More grains to feed more animals will mean changes in land use.

Some attempts have been made to quantify the potential GHG savings achievable through a combination of approaches a–d. Most estimates consider the agricultural sector as a whole, as it is difficult to separate out livestock farming given its interconnectedness with the arable sector. However, since livestock contribute to the bulk of agricultural emissions (either through their direct emissions or through emissions generated by the production of feed crops for their consumption), these estimates are indicative of what might be possible for livestock systems too.

As regards global estimates, the IPCC (2014) provides a range of estimates based on different carbon prices (i.e. the higher the price of carbon, the greater the mitigation potential). At very high carbon prices, measures could in principle offset all of today's emissions. However, there are not only important practical limitations but also mixed impacts on other aspects of environmental concern (negatives as well as positives) and potentially damaging consequences for food security – for instance peatlands historically and currently used for agriculture would be reflooded. It is also important to note that the majority of the emission reductions modelled come from soil carbon management and that these practices are time limited – once soils have reached their maximum capacity to accumulate carbon, no further sequestration arises. Hence, if one assumed action now, by 2050, there will be far less to be gained from the soil carbon management approach. As such, it becomes increasingly important to tackle nitrous oxide and methane emissions, and given the anticipated growth in the livestock sector, their relative importance is set to grow.

As for livestock, the FAO (Gerber et al., 2013) estimates that reductions in the emissions intensity of animal products of about 30 per cent is possible, but warns that: "On a global scale, it is unlikely that the emission intensity gains, based on the deployment of current technology, will entirely offset the inflation of emissions related to the sector's growth".

The general picture that emerges, amidst enormous uncertainty, is that technical and managerial approaches are unlikely to be enough, or could have unwanted side effects. The reduction in emissions per unit of meat or milk will be offset by the doubling in demand. We need, however, to reduce emissions absolutely by 70–90 per cent by 2050. If the food chain does not play its part in contributing to the emissions reduction, then other sectors of society (housing, transport, energy supply and so forth) will have to reduce their emissions even more to compensate; and these sectors, given a growing global population, face exactly the same sort of challenges as does the food chain.

Since technology is unlikely to get us where we need to be, we need to look at changing the balance of foods we consume. This will include reducing our consumption of meat and dairy products – an approach that the IPCC's (2014) report reviewed. It found that the technical mitigation could be high, although the feasibility of implementing the necessary measures to achieve shifts in consumption is as yet under-researched and untested.

Leaving aside the (major) question of feasibility for the moment, what level of consumption shift might be needed? Meat and dairy intakes are particularly high in the developed world, and historically the developed world is responsible for the bulk of GHG emissions. One equitable approach to consider would be to examine what might happen if people in rich societies were to reduce their consumption of animal products. One possible option would be for the world's population to converge on consuming what in 2050 the global population on average is expected to consume: about 40kg of meat and 80kg of milk annually (as shown in Table 3.4).

This represents an increase on average meat and milk consumption in developing countries today, although this average masks very wide inequities in distribution:

TABLE 3.4 Global total and per capita consumption in 2006 and 2050 (projected)

MEAT						
	Population 2006 (bn)	*Population 2050 (bn)*	*Per capita consumption 2006 (T/person/yr)*	*Per capita consumption 2050 (T/person/yr)*	*Total consumption 2006 (Mt)*	*Total consumption 2050 (Mt)*
Developed countries	1.35	1.44	0.08	0.09	108.00	131.04
Developing countries	5.22	7.67	0.03	0.04	156.60	322.14
World	***6.60***	***9.15***	***0.04***	***0.05***	***264.00***	***448.35***
MILK						
Developed countries	1.35	1.44	0.20	0.22	270.00	319.68
Developing countries	5.22	7.67	0.05	0.08	261.00	582.92
World	***6.60***	***9.15***	***0.08***	***0.10***	***528.00***	***905.85***

Source: Alexandratos, N. and Bruinsma, J. (2012) 'World agriculture towards 2030/2050: the 2012 revision'. ESA Working paper No. 12–03. FAO, Rome.

average per capita annual meat and milk consumption in Sub-Saharan Africa, for example, is 10kg and 31kg respectively (Alexandratos and Bruinsma, 2012). For people in the developed world, however, consuming at this level would entail a very substantial change in habits. It would mean that we in the UK would halve the amount of meat we typically eat today, and reduce our milk consumption by an even more drastic two-thirds.

Unfortunately, however, action by the developed world alone will not be sufficient simply because the bulk of the projected increase in demand is set to come from the developing world. If we multiply reductions in per capita consumption by the number of people who are projected to be living in the developed and transition countries, and subtract this figure from the overall *anticipated* demand for meat and dairy products, there is still an absolute global increase in consumption – of about 30 per cent for meat and 50 per cent for milk. In other words, because of the disparities in population sizes, overall global volumes will still be higher in absolute terms than what they are today.

Clearly, reductions at this level are not sufficient. Another approach is to ask how much would be available to each individual in 2050 if we keep meat and dairy production at 2000 levels, so as to avoid a rise in livestock-related GHG emissions. A very simple calculation finds that in the context of 9 billion people in 2050, per capita consumption of meat and milk would need to be as low as 29kg and 58kg a year, respectively. Assuming a world population of 10 billion (as increasingly seems likely), the per capita availability falls further to 26kg and 53kg, respectively. This is approximately the average level of consumption of people in the developing world *today* and equates to around half a kilo of meat and a litre of milk per person per week.

These figures are strikingly low – they imply drastic declines for the rich and allow for no increase by the poor. Diets low in animal products can be nutritionally adequate, but – as highlighted – much depends on what else there is to eat and how equitably it is distributed. Policy makers need to think about developing food and agricultural strategies based on combining food and climate change policies – of prioritizing food security at minimum greenhouse gas cost.

The efficiency mindset as characterized by approach a, above, is not only unlikely to meet our emission goals but it also considers animals and their emissions simplistically as a problem to be managed in order to meet demand. Issues such as animal welfare, the health implications of increased meat and dairy consumption for the 2 billion of the world's population who are overweight or obese (IFPRI, 2015) and biodiversity losses are to be addressed by other means. Examples include marketing niche higher welfare systems for 'premium' customers who demand it, developing (for obesity) low-fat food formulations, functional foods, nutraceuticals and exercise programmes and intensifying production on agricultural land so as to create biodiversity havens, or ghettos on the land that remains.

There is an alternative way of thinking, however, which could be characterized by the phrase 'livestock on leftovers'. Such an approach seeks to work with what animals are good at – making use of marginal land and feeding on by-products that we cannot eat. It considers what the land and available by-products can sustainably support – and then assesses, on that basis, how much is available for us to eat (Garnett, 2009). It takes land and the biodiversity that it supports as its starting point, and as its ultimate constraint. This mindset considers demand to be negotiable and challengeable.

With this approach livestock can be integrated into a landscape so that they help store carbon in the soil, enhance the biodiversity of local ecosystems and make use of the leftovers from other food and agricultural processes. There will be a need to focus research on breeding programmes that emphasize robustness and flexibility and that improve the ability of ruminants to survive on marginal lands and of all livestock types to respond well to a variable supply of different foods – to cope well with a less nutritionally precise environment, as it were. We need also to consider how livestock can be reintegrated into arable farming systems in the developed world, as part of a mixed livestock – crop rotations and livestock – agroforestry systems.

A 'livestock on leftovers' approach need not, and should not, be purist. For example, in many developing-world countries, 'intensification' may include actions to ensure that cows have something better to eat than plastic bags – and there will be welfare as well as productivity gains from so doing. Options b, c and d outlined in Table 3.3 above will still be key to overall agricultural mitigation.

This 'livestock on leftovers' approach is likely to provide us with far lower quantities of meat and dairy than that afforded by intensification – but the system actively helps deal with the problem of climate change, while the efficiency approach is simply geared towards minimizing the damage that livestock cause. A livestock on leftovers approach would form part of an agricultural strategy that takes as its starting point the need to meet nutritional needs, while mitigating agricultural emissions.

A short note on fish

This chapter has focused on only on terrestrial animal source foods and as such has omitted a very significant contributor to human protein intakes: fish. While the volume of fish from capture fisheries has remained fairly stable, aquaculture has been growing at about 6 per cent a year in the last decade and now accounts for over 40 per cent of all fish harvested (FAO, 2014). There is the likelihood that if people reduce their consumption of meat and dairy products, they will increase the amount of fish they eat.

There is wide variation in the relative intensities of different fish species. For example a review by Nijdam et al. (2012) finds that emissions from wild fish vary by nearly an order of magnitude (from 1kg CO_2 eq/kg fish to 89kg CO_2 eq/kg fish). A study by Tyedmers into fuel use in fishing reported a range of fuel inputs to fisheries of 20–2000 litres of fuel per tonne of fish landed, largely because of differences in the intensity of fuel use by fishing vessels (Tyedmers, 2004). There are also substantial (although lesser) differences in aquaculture; the variation in carbon and in energy intensity here depends in part on the feed source (particularly the amount of fuel used in the fishing of the wild fish that go to feed the farmed fish) and partly on the inherent feed conversion efficiency of the farmed fish themselves (Pelletier and Tyedmers, 2010; Nijdam et al., 2012).

It is also very important to emphasize that a simplistic carbon accounting assessment risks ignoring the very serious broader environmental and ecosystemic issues associated with the fish and aquaculture sectors. In the case of wild fish, over 60 per cent of all stocks that have been monitored are now fully exploited; nearly 30 per cent are overfished (FAO, 2014).

As regards aquaculture, the issues here are complex. The sector has historically been associated in some parts of the world with significant environmental problems, including coastal pollution, the destruction of mangrove swamps and the escape of farmed fish into the seas, spreading disease. Carnivorous fish, such as salmon, trout and tuna, and omnivores like shrimps that are often reared on a carnivorous diet, are fed wild fish from stocks that may themselves be depleted – and these kinds of fish are the species that have grown most rapidly in popularity.

On the other hand, many forms of aquaculture – including all plant (such as seaweed) and mollusc cultivation, polyculture systems that incorporate these species and many forms of extensive to semi-intensive freshwater finfish production – rely little on marine inputs such as fish meal and could potentially make a significant and sustainable contribution to global food protein supplies (Tyedmers et al., 2007). (See Kestin's chapter in this book.) There is in particular, as yet, unexplored scope for increasing the use of algae and seaweeds, both as feedstuffs and for consumption in their own right.

In short, the picture currently presented by aquaculture is mixed, but there is great potential for improving the sustainability of the aquaculture sector (in particular in reducing its dependence on wild fish as a feed-source) and, in so doing, providing an alternative to livestock consumption and production.

Conclusions

Our food system faces enormous and difficult challenges. We need to reduce food and agricultural emissions by 70–95 per cent by 2050 while feeding a global population that will be a third higher than it is today. We also need to meet these goals within the constraints of what are essentially ethical 'non-negotiables': the safeguarding of biodiversity and a decent quality of life for the animals that we rear and eat. We are bound, of course, by the ultimate constraint – land.

The projected doubling in demand for meat and dairy products presents a possibly insuperable obstacle. At present technological improvements will not allow us to meet this demand and at the same time reduce emissions to the degree needed. It may conceivably be that we achieve a technological breakthrough, enabling us to meet demand while also reducing emissions – but it is likely that this will come at the expense of animal welfare and of biodiversity. There is, moreover, no guarantee that by producing enough food we achieve food security. Distribution and access are socio-economic, not just biological, challenges. One might argue that a more redistributive approach to meeting the food needs of the most vulnerable will be mindful of the environmental impacts – since it is the poorest who have to live most directly with the consequences of climate change.

By contrast, a business-as-usual approach continues the global trend towards further dependence on energy- and GHG-intensive lifestyles, and the challenge of trying to meet these demands will continue. By 2050, on current projections, the developing world will still, on average, be eating less than half as much meat as people do in the rich world, and only a third of the milk. There is a long way to go before they catch up with developed-world levels. Do we assume that ultimately they will want to eat as much meat and milk as we do, and do markets therefore seek to supply these volumes? When is enough enough? Who decides at what level justifiable wants turn into unsustainable greed? We need to start questioning the unquestionable – demand.

Time is running out. We have little time left to avert the worst impacts of climate change. We need to start tackling the problems we face – food security, climate change, animal welfare, biodiversity – in an integrated way rather than through the separate, sometimes conflicting strategies that we have today. The vision should be to achieve good nutrition for all at minimum environmental cost, and global policy makers will need to develop fiscal, regulatory and other measures to make this happen. Farm animals can play an important part in achieving this vision, but to do so, the livestock sector needs to understand and work with the strengths and limits of the land and its resources.

Note

1 Note that the figure is almost the same as the total attributable to agriculture. This results from different methods of quantifying agricultural and livestock emissions and different data sources and different boundaries. However, what is clear (and this is also evident from the UK GHG inventory) is that livestock account for the bulk of agricultural GHG emissions.

References

Abril, A. and Bucher, E. H. (2001) 'Overgrazing and soil carbon dynamics in the western Chaco of Argentina', *Applied Soil Ecology*, vol 16, no 3, pp. 243–249.

Aklilu, H. A., Udo, H. M. J., Almekinders, C. J. M. and Van der Zijpp, A. J. (2008) 'How resource poor households value and access poultry: Village poultry keeping in Tigray, Ethiopia', *Agricultural Systems*, vol 96, pp. 175–183.

Alexandratos, N. and Bruinsma, J. (2012) 'World agriculture towards 2030/2050: the 2012 revision'. ESA Working paper No. 12–03. FAO, Rome.

Allard, V., Soussana, J.-F., Falcimagne, R., Berbigier, P., Bonnefond, J. M., Ceschia, E., D'hour, P., Hénault, C., Laville, P., Martin, C. and Pinarès-Patino, C. (2007) 'The role of grazing management for the net biome productivity and greenhouse gas budget (CO_2, N_2O and CH_4) of semi-natural grassland', *Agriculture, Ecosystems and Environment*, vol 121, pp. 47–58.

Appleby, P. N., Thorogood, M., Mann, J. I. and Key, T. J. (1999) 'The Oxford Vegetarian Study: An overview', *American Journal of Clinical Nutrition*, vol. 70 (Supplement 3), pp. 525S–531S.

Audsley, E., Brander, M., Chatterton, J., Murphy-Bokern, D., Webster, C. and Williams, A. (2010) *How Low Can We Go? An Assessment of Greenhouse Gas Emissions From the UK Food System and the Scope to Reduce Them by 2050*, WWF-UK, Godalming.

Basset-Mens, C. and Werf, H. M. G. van der (2005) 'Scenario-based environmental assessment of farming systems: The case of pig production in France', *Agriculture, Ecosystems and Environment*, vol 105, pp. 127–144.

Bennetzen, E. H., Smith, P. and Porter, J. R. (2016) 'Decoupling of greenhouse gas emissions from global agricultural production: 1970–2050', *Global Change Biology*, vol 22, pp. 763–781, DOI: 10.1111/gcb.13120

Berlin, J. (2002) 'Environmental life cycle assessment (LCA) of Swedish semi-hard cheese', *International Dairy Journal*, vol 12, pp. 939–953.

Casey, J. W. and Holden, N. M. (2005) 'The relationship between greenhouse gas emissions and the intensity of milk production in Ireland', *Journal of Environmental Quality*, vol 34, pp. 429–436.

Casey, J. W. and Holden, N. M. (2006) 'Quantification of greenhouse gas emissions from suckler-beef production in Ireland', *Agricultural Systems*, vol 90, pp. 79–98.

Cederberg, C. and Mattson, B. (2000) 'Life cycle assessment of milk production: A comparison of conventional and organic farming', *Journal of Cleaner Production*, vol 8, pp. 49–60.

Cederberg, C. and Stadig, M. (2003) 'System expansion and allocation in life cycle assessment of milk and beef production', *International Journal of Lifecycle Assessment*, vol 8, no 6, pp. 350–356.

Clark, H., Klein, C. de and Newton, P. (2001) 'Potential management practices and technologies to reduce nitrous oxide, methane and carbon dioxide emissions from New Zealand agriculture', Prepared for Ministry of Agriculture and Forestry, New Zealand, September 2001.

Committee on Climate Change (2008) 'Building a low-carbon economy – the UK's contribution to tackling climate change', The First Report of the Committee on Climate Change, The Stationery Office, London, UK.

Defra (2014a) Table B.10, 'The British survey of fertiliser practice: Fertiliser use on farm crops for crop year 2014', Department for the Environment, Food and Rural Affairs, London, UK.

Defra (2014b) 'Agriculture in the United Kingdom', Department for the Environment, Food and Rural Affairs, London, UK

Diamond, J. (2005) *Collapse*, Penguin, London.

Druckman, A., Bradley, P. and Papathanasopoulou, E. (2008) 'Measuring progress towards carbon reduction in the UK', *Ecological Economics*, vol 66, pp. 594–604.

Elferink, E. V., Nonhebel, S. and Schoot Uiterkamp, A. J. M. (2007) 'Does the Amazon suffer from BSE prevention?' *Agriculture, Ecosystems and Environment*, vol 120, pp. 467–469.

English Beef and Lamb Executive (EBLEX) (2009) *Change in the Air: The English Sheep and Beef Production Roadmap – Phase One*, EBLEX, Warwickshire, UK.

European Commission (2006) 'Environmental impact of products (EIPRO): Analysis of the life cycle environmental impacts related to the total final consumption of the EU25', European Commission Technical Report EUR 22284 EN, May 2006. http://ec.europa.eu/environment/ipp/pdf/eipro_report.pdf.

FAO (2009) 'Monthly international prices for oilseeds, vegetable oils, and oilmeals/cakes', Food and Agriculture Organization, Rome. www.fao.org/economic/est/est-commodities/oilcrops/en/.

FAO (2011) World Livestock 2011 – Livestock in Food Security, Food and Agriculture Organization, Rome.

FAO (2014) *The State of World Fisheries and Aquaculture 2008*, Food and Agriculture Organization, Rome.

FAO (2015) *Food Outlook 2015*, Food and Agriculture Organization, Rome.

FAOSTAT (2013) http://faostat3.fao.org/browse/T/TP/E, last accessed 13 April 2016.

Fearnside, P. and Hall-Beyer, M. (2007) 'Deforestation in Amazonia', in Cleveland, C. (ed.) *Encyclopedia of Earth*, Environmental Information Coalition, National Council for Science and the Environment, Washington, DC (first published in the *Encyclopedia of Earth* 15 March 2007; last revised 30 March 2007), available at www.eoearth.org/article/Deforestation_in_Amazonia

Foster, C., Green, K., Bleda, M., Dewick, P., Evans, B., Flynn, A. and Mylan, J. (2006) 'Environmental impacts of food production and consumption', Report Produced for the Department for Environment, Food and Rural Affairs, United Kingdom.

Gale, F., Hansen, J. and Jewison, M. (February 2014) *China's Growing Demand for Agricultural Imports*, EIB-136, U.S. Department of Agriculture, Economic Research Service, United States of America.

Garnett, T. (2008) *Cooking Up a Storm: Food, Greenhouse Gas Emissions and Our Changing Climate*, Food Climate Research Network, Centre for Environmental Strategy, University of Surrey, Guildford, UK.

Garnett, T. (2009) 'Livestock-related greenhouse gas emissions: Impacts and options for policy makers', *Environmental Science and Policy*, vol 12, pp. 491–503.

Gerber, P. J., Steinfeld, H., Henderson, B., Mottet, A., Opio, C., Dijkman, J., Falcucci, A. and Tempio, G. (2013) *Tackling Climate Change Through Livestock – A Global Assessment of Emissions and Mitigation Opportunities*, Food and Agriculture Organization of the United Nations (FAO), Rome.

Gollnow, F. and Lakes, T. (2014) 'Policy change, land use, and agriculture: The case of soy production and cattle ranching in Brazil', *Applied Geography*, vol 55, pp. 203e211.

Hadley Centre (2005) 'Avoiding dangerous climate change', International Symposium on the Stabilisation of Greenhouse Gas Concentrations, Met Office, Exeter, UK, 1–3 February 2005.

International Food Policy Research Institute (2015) *Global Nutrition Report 2015: Actions and Accountability to Advance Nutrition and Sustainable Development*, Washington, DC, available at http://globalnutritionreport.org/

IPCC (2014) Climate Change 2014: Synthesis Report: Contribution of Working Groups I, II and III to the Fifth Assessment Report of the Intergovernmental Panel on Climate Change [Core Writing Team, R. K. Pachauri and L.A. Meyer (eds.)]. IPCC, Geneva, Switzerland, p. 151.

Key, T. J., Davey, G.K. and Appleby, P.N. (1999) 'Health benefits of a vegetarian diet', *Proceedings of the Nutrition Society*, vol 58, pp. 271–275.

Lovett, D. K., Shalloo, L., Dillon, P. and O'Mara, F. P. (2006) 'A systems approach to quantify greenhouse gas fluxes from pastoral dairy production as affected by management regime', *Agricultural Systems*, vol 88, no 2–3, pp. 156–179.

McAlpine, C. A., Etter, A., Fearnside, P. M., Seabrook, L. and Laurance, W. F. (2009) 'Increasing world consumption of beef as a driver of regional and global change: A call for policy action based on evidence from Queensland (Australia), Colombia and Brazil', *Global Environmental Change*, vol 19, pp. 21–33.

Millward, D. J. (1999) 'The nutritional value of plant based diets in relation to human amino acid and protein requirements', *Proceedings of the Nutrition Society*, vol 58, pp. 249–260.

Nepstad, D. C., Stickler, C. M. and Almeida, O. T. (2006) 'Globalization of the Amazon soy and beef industries: Opportunities for conservation', *Conservation Biology*, vol 20, no 6, pp. 1595–1603.

Neumann, C., Harris, D. M. and Rogers, L. M. (2002) 'Contribution of animal source foods in improving diet quality and function in children in the developing world', *Nutrition Research*, vol 22, no 1–2, pp. 193–220.

Nijdam, D., Rood, T. and Westhoek, H. (2012) 'The price of protein: Review of land use and carbon footprints from life cycle assessments of animal food products and their substitutes', *Food Policy*, vol 37, no 6, pp. 760–770.

Pelletier, N. and Tyedmers, P. (2010) 'A life cycle assessment of frozen Indonesian tilapia fillets from lake and pond-based production systems', *Journal of Industrial Ecology*, vol 14, no 3, pp. 467–481.

Sanders, T. A. (1999) 'The nutritional adequacy of plant-based diets', *Proceedings of the Nutrition Society*, vol 58, pp. 265–269.

Schellnhuber, H. J., Cramer, W., Nakicenovic, N., Wigley, T. and Yohe, G. (2006) *Avoiding Dangerous Climate Change*, Cambridge University Press, Cambridge.

Schneider, S. H., Semenov, S., Patwardhan, A., Burton, I., Magadza, C. H. D., Oppenheimer, M., Pittock, A. B., Rahman, A., Smith, J. B., Suarez, A. and Yamin, F. (2007) 'Assessing key vulnerabilities and the risk from climate change', in Parry, M. L., Canziani, O. F., Palutikof, J. P., Linden, P. J. van der and Hanson, C. E. (eds.) *Climate Change 2007: Impacts, Adaptation and Vulnerability: Contribution of Working Group II to the Fourth Assessment Report of the Intergovernmental Panel on Climate Change*, Cambridge University Press, Cambridge, pp. 779–810.

Smith, P., Bustamante, M., Ahammad, H., Clark, H., Dong, H., Elsiddig, E. A., Haberl, H., Harper, R., House, J., Jafari, M., Masera, O., Mbow, C., Ravindranath, N. H., Rice, C. W., Robledo Abad, C., Romanovskaya, A., Sperling, F. and Tubiello, F. (2014) 'Agriculture, Forestry and Other Land Use (AFOLU)', in Edenhofer, O., Pichs-Madruga, R., Sokona, Y., Farahani, E., Kadner, S., Seyboth, K., Adler, A., Baum, I., Brunner, S., Eickemeier, P., Kriemann, B., Savolainen, J., Schlömer, S., Stechow, C. von, Zwickel, T. and Minx, J. C. (eds.) *Climate Change 2014: Mitigation of Climate Change. Contribution of Working Group III to the Fifth Assessment Report of the Intergovernmental Panel on Climate Change*, Cambridge University Press, Cambridge, United Kingdom and New York, pp. 811–922.

Smith, P., Martino, D., Cai, Z., Gwary, D., Janzen, H. H., Kumar, P., McCarl, B., Ogle, S., O'Mara, F., Rice, C., Scholes, R. J., Sirotenko, O., Howden, M., McAllister, T., Pan, G., Romanenkov, V., Schneider, U., Towprayoon, S., Wattenbach, M. and Smith, J. U. (2008) 'Greenhouse gas mitigation in agriculture', *Philosophical Transactions of the Royal Society*, vol 262, pp. 780–813.

Steinfeld, H., Gerber, P., Wassenaar, T., Castel, V., Rosales, M. and Haan, C. de (2006) *Livestock's Long Shadow: Environmental Issues and Options*, Food and Agriculture Organization, Rome.

Stern, N. (2006) *The Economics of Climate Change: The Stern Review*, Cambridge University Press, Cambridge (Although the Stern review takes as its threshold the higher CO_2e level of 550ppm, the adequacy of this figure has been increasingly called into question and is currently the subject of UK Government scrutiny).

Thomas, K. (1991) *Man and the Natural World: Changing Attitudes in England 1500–1800*, Penguin, London.

Tyedmers, P. (2004) 'Fisheries and energy use', in Cleveland, C. (ed.) *Encyclopedia of Energy*, vol 2, Elsevier, Amsterdam, pp. 683–693.

Tyedmers, P., Pelletier, N. and Ayer, N. (2007) 'Biophysical sustainability and approaches to marine aquaculture: Development policy in the United States', Report to the Marine Aquaculture Task Force, available at www.whoi.edu/sites/marineaquataskforce, last accessed 24 May 2010.

United Nations (2015) *The Millennium Development Goals Report 2015*, United Nations, New York.

United Nations (n.d.) World Day to Combat Desertification 17 June, available at www.un.org/en/events/desertificationday/background.shtml

Williams, A. G., Audsley, E. and Sandars, D. L. (2006) 'Determining the environmental burdens and resource use in the production of agricultural and horticultural commodities', Main Report, Defra Research Project ISO205, Bedford, Cranfield University and Defra.

WWF (2004) 'ISTA Mielke', Oil World Annual 2004, Hamburg, May 2004 cited in Jan Maarten Dros, *Managing the Soy Boom: Two Scenarios of Soy Production Expansion in South America*, available at www.panda.org/downloads/forests/managingthesoyboomenglish_nbvt.pdf, last accessed 24 May 2010.

4

GOLDEN FIELDS, BURNING FORESTS AND HUNGRY PEOPLE

How corn and soy are impacting us all

Joyce D'Silva

Not many of us have seen with our own eyes the golden cornfields of the US, stretching away to the horizon, nor have we seen the endless green fields of soya, perhaps edging up to a distant line of as-yet-unscathed forest in Brazil. In themselves, these scenes could be breathtaking and one could pause to wonder at the capacity of modern farming to grow such splendid and abundant crops, which must surely be helping to feed the world. Do not be fooled!

The vast majority of those crops are not being grown to feed people directly – they are being grown for animal feed. As the global population increases and countries like China develop a more affluent urban middle class, the demand for animal products is soaring. The Food and Agriculture Organisation of the United Nations, (the FAO), has estimated roughly a doubling of demand for meat from 2000–2050 (Steinfeld et al., 2006). More animals will necessarily be farmed to meet the demand and most of those animals will inevitably be reared in indoor intensive farms or muddy feedlots, divorced from their natural food sources of grasses, leaves or roots. They will instead be fed on corn, soymeal and other crops grown specifically as feed crops. The world has not fully appreciated the massive negative impacts of this use of land, fertiliser and chemicals on the Earth, on the animals – and on us.

Land, trees and people

Agriculture already occupies 30% of the global land area (UNEP, 2014). The area used for growing crops increased by around 11% between 1961 and 2007 (UNEP, 2014) and has already encroached into precious forests and other areas of special ecological diversity, such as the Cerrado in Brazil. Over the last five decades, deforestation has occurred at a rate of around 13 Mha per year on average (UNEP, 2014).

The two main global drivers of deforestation appear to be the spread of palm oil plantations, particularly in Indonesia and other parts of southeast Asia, the cultivation of feed crops (such as soya beans, especially in Brazil) and the growth of pastures for cattle grazing (Stern, 2007). Palm oil is now ubiquitous in "Western" processed foods, although the palm kernel meal is increasingly being used as an ingredient in animal feed. The European Union (EU) alone imported around 2 million tonnes of it in 2012 (Index Mundi, 2016). China is another big importer.

The USDA predicts that as crop yield growth is tailing off, land use expansion will increase to meet the growing demand, with much of this expansion likely to be in South America, the former Soviet Union, and Sub-Saharan Africa. This land is likely to be taken from former pasture or forested areas (Westcott, 2012). In 2014 Brazil's crop bureau, Companhia Nacional de Abastecimento (CONAB) estimated that Brazil would see an increase in sowings in the following year of more than 2.3m hectares (Agrimoney Investment Forum, 2014).

This raises the issue of so-called "land grabbing", where local people are unable to provide documentary evidence of their land ownership and are removed, sometimes, although not always, with compensation. Their small plots are ploughed over and commodity crops are planted over vast areas.

Who is eating soya?

Around 85% of the global soybean crop is crushed to produce meal and oil, with about 78.5% resulting in soy meal and about 19% oil, with the remaining 2.5% lost in processing (The Nature Conservancy, 2012). This soybean meal is primarily used as animal feed, and is currently the largest source of protein feed in the world (The Nature Conservancy, 2012). In fact 98% of global soybean meal is used as animal feed (Soyatech, 2015). Soy contains around 38% protein – twice as much as pork, three times more than eggs, and 12 times more than milk (WWF, 2016a). The obvious thought here is: what a great protein source for humanity! Yet people mainly consume soya indirectly through their consumption of meat, dairy products, eggs and fish! Just a small amount of soya is processed to make soya flour, or products like tofu and soya milk, soya-based meat substitutes and soy sauces, and it is an ingredient in some household products. So it's not the tofu-eating and soya milk–consuming vegetarians and vegans who should be blamed for deforestation!

The oil is used for cooking and in a range of food and other household products, although it is increasingly being used for biodiesel. There is a strange irony in producing a so-called "ethical" fuel to replace a fossil fuel, yet at the same time driving environmental degradation. Both soy meal and oil are traded on the futures markets.

Soy is grown primarily in the United States and certain South American countries, such as Brazil, Argentina and Paraguay, where "land grabbing" is a huge cause of social unrest. It is also grown in China, which used to export soy products. Due to the rapid growth of meat consumption and intensive farming in China, the country has now become a major importer of soy from Brazil and the US, in order to feed its growing numbers of pigs, poultry and cattle.

Falling water tables in the north of China have made soy production – and any reliable arable farming – difficult. As it takes 1,500 tons of water to produce 1 ton of soybeans this is another factor contributing to China's growing demand for soy (The Nature Conservancy, 2012). Dry conditions can affect soy-growing areas of Brazil too, but expansion of the soy crop into areas such as the northeastern Mato Grosso and the northeast region of Mapitoba (an acronym of the first two letters of Maranhão, Piauí, Tocantins and Bahia states) is forecast (Agrimoney Investment Forum, 2014). The Cerrado is a huge area of dry grassland, woodland, forests and wetlands with great bird and plant biodiversity and is also an important source of water. It is rapidly turning into a soy-producing region.

The Chinese case is fascinating. Way back in 1995, Lester Brown published a prophetic book, *Who Will Feed China?* (Brown, 1995). He foresaw that China would turn from a soy-exporting country to a major soy (and grain) importer due to the growth in meat consumption. For some years after the book he became *persona non grata* in China, but more recently has been fêted there and was awarded and made an advisor to the International Fund for China's Environment (personal communication). The Worldwatch Institute summarises one of his book's main arguments: "China's dependence on massive imports, like the collapse of the world's fisheries, will be a wake-up call that we are colliding with the earth's capacity to feed us. It could well lead us to redefine national security away from military preparedness and toward maintaining adequate food supplies" (Worldwatch Institute, 2016).

Lester was right. China's soy imports went from 0.8 million tonnes in 1995 (the year Lester's book was published) to 69 million tons in 2013 (Earth Policy Institute, 2014). It has been estimated that by 2020, China will be importing 75%–90% of Brazil's soya exports (The Nature Conservancy, 2012).

Whilst imports of soya to China and other Asian countries is growing, it is estimated that imports of soya to the EU may decline and become a specialised trade in non-GM soya, as European consumers have shown themselves opposed to GM food products. The EU imports around 35 million tonnes of soybeans/meal every year, whereas by 2020 China's imports are predicted to reach 110 million metric tonnes (WWF, 2016b).

The US uses much of its soy production for its own large industrial animal farming industry but still exports about a third of its soy, mostly to China (over 24 million tonnes in 2010/11) with much smaller amounts to Mexico (over 3 million tonnes) and the EU (2 million tonnes) (USDA, 2016).

Corn, cattle and cars

Corn (maize) is the most widely produced feed grain in the United States, with around 36% of the crop providing the main energy ingredient in livestock feed (Westcott, 2012; Foley, 2013).

Again with corn, we see the huge influence that China is having – and will have in the future – on agricultural markets. China's imports of corn are projected to rise steeply and account for almost half the overall growth in world corn trade over the next 10 years (Westcott, 2012). With its own growing demand for meat, Mexico is second only to China in projected growth for corn imports over the next 10 years (Westcott, 2012).

However, US corn exports are not expected to rise hugely, as more and more home-grown corn, standing now at about 40%, is being used as feedstock for ethanol production (Foley, 2013). The corn that reaches citizens directly is often in the form of high-fructose corn syrup, hardly a contributor to a healthy diet (Foley, 2013). As Jonathan Foley, Director of the Institute on the Environment at the University of Minnesota, says: "In short, the corn crop is highly productive, but the corn system is aligned to feed cars and animals instead of feeding people" (Foley, 2013).

Between 1995 and 2010, US crop subsidies to corn totalled around $90 billion – not including ethanol subsidies and mandates (Foley, 2013). Those fields are golden in more ways than one!

Another issue in the US is that around 90% of both soy and corn crops are now genetically engineered (referred to as GM or GE) varieties. However, there is a growing market for non-GM products in the US, including a burgeoning organic food market, so some production is non-GM.

In spite of efforts to increase crop yields, it seems that a plateau has been reached and we no longer see the huge increases of the last 40 years or so. One factor in this is the difficulty of obtaining sufficient water for crop growth, with irrigation wells having to be dug deeper and deeper. The unfortunate result of this is that the agricultural sector will likely look more to land-use expansion to meet increasing demand in the future.

Overall it is predicted that more soya and corn will be grown in the coming years in developed and emerging economies, primarily targeted at the animal feed industry (Heffer and Prud'homme, 2015).

Soils

Another factor affecting crop yields is soil degradation. The FAO reports that globally approximately 33% of soils are facing moderate to severe degradation (FAO, 2015). The FAO stresses: "the current rate of soil degradation threatens the capacity to meet the needs of future generations, unless we reverse this trend through a concerted effort towards the sustainable management of soils". The FAO estimates that worldwide 75 billion tonnes of soil are lost every year, costing approximately US $400 billion per year (Steinfeld et al., 2006). Brazil, for example, loses 55 million tons of topsoil every year due to erosion from soy production (WWF, 2006).

Traditional enrichment of soils with animal manures, as one finds in mixed farming and organic systems, has been replaced with the use of commercially produced fertilisers. These increase crop yields in the short term, but appear to reduce natural fertility over the longer term. In addition, the kind of mono-cropping as seen in industrial agriculture uses not just fertilisers, but chemicals such as herbicides and pesticides which kill weeds and harmful crop-eating insects, but also damage beneficial insects and the below-soil life of the tiny creatures who live there and who enrich the composition of the soil.

The FAO estimates that one-third of global arable land has been lost though erosion in the past 50 years, with ongoing losses of an estimated 10 million ha each year (FAO, 2011b). The loss of this degraded land results in further expansion of crops into grassland, woodland and forests, leading to further loss of biodiversity.

Fertilisers, fossil fuels

Fertiliser use for corn is massive. The Fertilizer Institute says that in the fiscal year 2008, a total of 54.9 million tons of fertiliser material were used in the United States. As the Institute suggests that corn needs 1.5–2 pounds (nearly 1 kilo) of fertiliser nutrients per bushel and soya needs 1.00 to 1.5 pounds, this may not be surprising (Fertilizer Institute, 2016). Some would disagree with using nitrogen on soya beans as the crop fixes nitrogen via natural processes. Others argue that as soya yields are pushed ever higher, extra nitrogen needs to be applied. Globally the figure for 2009 stands at over 92 million tonnes of nitrogen fertiliser (FAOSTAT, 2016).

Nitrogen fertilisers are made from ammonia (NH_3), which is produced by the energy-intensive Haber-Bosch process, using natural gas and nitrogen from the air. This ammonia is used as the basis for all other nitrogen fertilisers, such as anhydrous ammonium nitrate and urea. As the Haber-Bosch process allows industrial-scale production of ammonia, and the resulting fertiliser has led to huge increases in crop yields over the years, some reckon that the process itself has enabled the population explosion (Smil, 1999). The Haber process now produces 450 million tonnes of nitrogen fertiliser every year (Smil, 2004).

EIA's 2010 Manufacturing Energy Consumption Survey estimates that the US nitrogenous fertiliser industry consumed more than 200 trillion Btu (British Thermal Units) of natural gas as feedstock in 2010 and another 152 trillion Btu for heat and power (Hicks, 2010). In some countries, such as China, coal is used instead of natural gas. Other types of fertiliser production also rely on fossil fuels (Union of Concerned Scientists, 2008).

Altogether, nitrogen fertiliser production alone is responsible for about 50% of the fossil fuel used in agricultural production (Foresight Report et al., 2011) and uses about 5% of global natural gas supplies. In addition, significant amounts of methane (CH_4) can be emitted during the production of nitrate (FAO, 2011b).

The other main fertilisers are phosphorous and potassium, both of which are mined and processed, so fuel undoubtedly makes up a significant portion of their direct and indirect costs (Heath, 2014). Spreading fertilisers on the crops requires significant amounts of fuel.

Humans and other animals need phosphorus in their diets and phosphorus is an essential nutrient for crop growth. The mineral phosphorus is mined from rock phosphate mines. The world's largest source of phosphate rock is in and around Morocco, with smaller amounts found in the Middle East, China and the US. Reserves in the latter two countries may last only around another 50 years, so the world may become dependent on sources in West Africa, which some predict could last for around 300 years (Vaccari, 2009). Sadly, yet more fossil fuels are needed to transport approximately 30 million tonnes of phosphate rock and fertilisers around the world annually (Cho, 2013).

In 2009 the world used over 32 million tonnes of phosphate fertiliser (FAOSTAT, 2016). The process of converting phosphate rock into fertiliser is considered inefficient and in need of improvement; 40–60% of the phosphate is reportedly lost in the process (Gilbert, 2009).

The use of phosphate fertilisers to produce meat is highly inefficient compared to its use to produce plant crops. So although phosphorus (P) is an essential nutrient for livestock, its efficiency of utilization is below 40% (Kebreab et al., 2012). Ten times as much P goes into the production of meat as is delivered by dietary P in the meat; only four times as much P goes into the production of vegetables as is delivered by dietary P in the vegetables. If rock phosphate becomes scarce or prohibitively costly, it will no longer be viable or ethical to waste it on feed for intensive livestock production (Soil Association, 2010).

As animals excrete around half the phosphorus they consume via feed crops or dietary supplements, manure is also a useful fertiliser in itself. Organic farms aim to rely mainly on animal manure as a source of phosphorus although they are allowed to supplement this with external sources if the soil indicates that extra P is required.

Sadly the modern landscape of mono-cropping reveals a different picture, with animal manures replaced with mined P fertilisers.

Polluted waters

Massive fertiliser use not only increases crop growth – it is leading to the growth of runoff into rivers and seas, leading to water pollution.

With such a huge proportion of global cereals and soya being grown for animal feed, it is not surprising that the United Nations (UN) concludes that "Intensive livestock production is probably the largest sector-specific source of water pollution" (United Nations, 2011).

A recent paper by US and Canadian scientists says, "The planetary boundary for freshwater eutrophication has been crossed while potential boundaries for ocean anoxic events and depletion of phosphate rock reserves loom in the future" (Carpenter and Bennett, 2011).

In Europe the livestock sector accounts for 23%–47% of the nitrogen river load to coastal waters and 17%–26% of the phosphorus river loads (Liep, 2015).

Unabsorbed nitrogen and phosphorus from fertilisers and chemicals from pesticides together with large amounts of soil wash into lakes, rivers and coastal waters, polluting waters and damaging ecosystems along the way, causing eutrophication. Algal blooms develop, the water is deprived of oxygen and fish and other creatures in the water gradually die off. The growing dead zone in the Gulf of Mexico is mainly a result of such runoff. Even the US government's own agency lays the blame squarely at the door of the fertilisers used on the corn and soy growing areas upstream in the Mississippi and Atchafalaya rivers, with 1.6 million metric tonnes p.a. of total nitrogen in the form of nitrate ending up in the Gulf (NOAA, 2016).

But it's not just the Gulf of Mexico. The FAO estimates that, through eutrophication, fertiliser use has adversely impacted many marine and riverine ecosystems, producing over 400 aquatic "dead zones" worldwide, covering an area of 245,000 sq.km (FAO, 2011a).

The European Nitrogen Assessment (ENA) reports that 75% of industrial production of reactive nitrogen (Nr) in Europe is used for fertiliser (2008 figure) (ENA, 2011). The ENA points out that the primary use of Nr in crops in Europe is not directly to feed people but to provide feeds to support livestock.

The ENA estimates that environmental damage related to Nr effects from agriculture in the EU-27 is €20–€150 billion per year. A cost-benefit analysis shows that this outweighs the benefit of N-fertiliser for farmers of €10–€100 billion per year (ENA, 2011).

It's not only waterways that are polluted from fertiliser production and use – greenhouse gas levels also rise. The greenhouse gases carbon dioxide, methane and nitrous oxide are produced during the manufacture of nitrogen fertilisers (Wood and Cowie, 2004). In addition, nitrogen fertilisers can be converted by soil bacteria to that highly toxic greenhouse gas, nitrous oxide. Approximately 79%–88% of total EU agriculture's nitrogen emissions (in which ammonia plays a part) are due to livestock production (Westhoek et al., 2015).

Pesticides and herbicides

Of course crops like corn and soybeans are also subject to spraying with both pesticides and herbicides to kill crop-eating insects and weeds. Corn is frequently sprayed with atrazine, a herbicide developed in 1958. After glyphosate, it is the most common herbicide used in the US and is also widely used in Australia. However, the European Union banned its use in 2004 after levels in groundwater went above the permitted maximum (European Commission, 2004).

It has also been problematic in the US, with high levels found in groundwater, and the US Environmental Protection Agency (EPA) has expressed concern about this (EPA, 2007). Some studies in animals have shown atrazine to be an endocrine disruptor (EPA, 2007); however, the EPA has not been convinced of this, although it reviews the research evidence every 15 years. Meanwhile atrazine continues to be used on corn as well as several other crops such as sugarcane and sorghum. Syngenta, which makes atrazine, claims that it saves up to 85 million tonnes of soil erosion every year by supporting conservation tillage and no-till farming (Syngenta, 2016). What is certain is that atrazine does persist in both soil and water for a significant time. In 2012 Syngenta agreed to pay $105 million to water companies in the US Midwest for contamination of their water with atrazine (Findlaw, 2016).

Most soy produced in South America or the US is now GM, with the crop resistant to the herbicide glyphosate, which can be sprayed on several times during the growing season. Already some tolerance to glyphosate has been occurring, and new GM varieties are being created to be resistant to other herbicides. Recently, the

WHO's International Agency for Research on Cancer (IARC) has listed glyphosate as "probably carcinogenic to humans" (IARC, 2015).

It's an anomaly that some of the foods which may be most fundamentally nutritious for humans, such as soy, corn and an array of vegetables and fruits, may be posing an actual threat to our health from the residues of chemicals they contain.

Biodiversity

According to WWF, between 1970 and 2010 populations of mammals, birds, reptiles, amphibians and fish around the globe dropped an astonishing 52% (WWF, 2014). WWF bases this figure on its living planet index, which is calculated using trends in 10,380 populations of over 3,038 vertebrate species (fishes, amphibians, reptiles, birds and mammals).

With soils degraded and waters polluted, it is not surprising that industrial mono-cropping, much of it for animal feed, is the major culprit in causing loss of biodiversity. Globally food production accounts for 60%–70% of total biodiversity loss (PBL Netherlands Environmental Assessment Agency, 2014). The European Commission states that the livestock sector may be the leading player in the reduction of global biodiversity through its demand on land (European Commission staff working paper, 2011). The contribution of livestock farming to the present global loss of biodiversity is estimated by a Dutch study to be around 30% (Westhoek et al., 2011). EU Member States have identified agriculture including intensification, as one of the main causes of wildlife loss and habitat degradation (European Commission, 2015).

As for pesticides, a row persists over the use of neonicotinoids. These pesticides are widely used on corn and also used to "treat" soyabean seeds and other crops. There is mounting evidence that both honeybees and bumblebees may be adversely affected by neonics, as they are commonly called. However, the manufacturers dispute this. In 2013 the European Union banned the use of three neonics which are commonly used to treat pant seeds (European Commission Implementing Regulation, 2013).

Way back in 1992 the Convention on Biological Diversity (CBD) affirmed that "the conservation of biological diversity is a common concern of humankind" (CBD, 1992). There were high hopes that governments would devote time, research, money and legislation to protect biodiversity. Over the years some action has been taken, but the fundamental problems associated with industrial arable and animal farming remain.

The CBD's 20 Aichi Biodiversity Targets aim at achieving a world without biodiversity loss or degradation of ecosystems by 2050. In 2010 the CBD published *Global Biodiversity Outlook*, which included an update on achievements regarding the targets set in the Aichi Biodiversity Targets. In several areas there had been progress, but four of the 20 targets were actually showing progress in the *wrong* direction. One of these targets not being achieved was "Pollution from excess nutrients has been brought to levels that are not detrimental to ecosystem function and biodiversity". In other words, pollution from agricultural fertilisers and other chemicals is getting worse, not better.

Is it all worth it?

Could all these detrimental impacts of industrial crop and animal farming be outweighed by the urgency of feeding a growing global population? After all, we are likely to be anthropocentrics at heart, with our major motivation being the health and well-being of ourselves and our descendants. Yet even those who are motivated by compassion for the hungry or concern for the planet's long-term viability may think these impacts are necessary – even if regrettable.

Sadly the sums just don't add up. Although 36% of the world's crop calories are fed to animals, three-quarters of this is wasted due to the low efficiency with which animals convert cereals to meat and milk. Studies show that for every 100 calories fed to animals in the form of human-edible crops, we receive on average just 17–30 calories in the form of meat and milk (Lundqvist et al., 2008; Nellemann et al., 2009).

A University of Minnesota paper indicates that the efficiency rates may be even lower for some animal products. It concludes that for every 100 calories of grain that we feed to animals, we get only about 40 new calories of milk, 22 calories of eggs, 12 of chicken, 10 of pork or 3 of beef (Cassidy, 2013). The paper also looks at protein conversion. It reports that for every 100 units of protein contained in grain fed to animals, we receive only about 43 units of protein from milk, 35 from eggs, 40 from chicken, 10 from pork or 5 from beef.

The same paper puts the argument a different way. It calculates that worldwide a hectare of cropland produces on average sufficient calories to feed 10.1 people. But the calories delivered for human consumption, after accounting for animal feed, biofuels and other industrial uses, only feed six people per hectare (Cassidy, 2013).

The FAO has said, "When livestock are raised in intensive systems, they convert carbohydrates and protein that might otherwise be eaten directly by humans and use them to produce a smaller quantity of energy and protein. In these situations, livestock can be said to reduce the food balance" (FAO, 2011a). A Chatham House paper concludes that the feeding of cereals to animals is "staggeringly inefficient" (Bailey, 2014). The paper points out that the "use of crops and arable land for livestock production indirectly places rich meat and dairy consumers in competition for calories with poor crop consumers". The International Institute for Environment and Development stresses that using cropland to produce corn, soybeans and other crops for animal feed rather than to grow food for direct human consumption is "a colossally inefficient" use of resources (IEED, 2015).

As indicated earlier, 36% of the world's crop calories are fed to animals, but, as we have seen, only 17%–30% of these calories are returned for human consumption as meat or milk (Cassidy, 2013). The effect of this is that 70%–83% of the 36% of the world's crop calories that are used as animal feed are wasted; they produce no food for humans. This means that 25%–30% (70%–83% of 36%) of the world's crop calories are being wasted by being fed to animals.

There is something inherently unbalanced – and possibly morally wrong – about a system which uses vast amounts of land to grow crops and fertilises them inefficiently and with polluting and energy-intensive materials, treats them with questionable chemicals, then feeds much of those crops to animals, creating further inefficiencies in their transformation to meat and milk, and then prices the resulting products so cheaply that many people eat too much of them, adversely affecting their own health in the process – and may end up needing state-supported health care as a consequence. (See Chapter 14 in this volume.)

For such a crazy system to be maintained – and even promoted – somebody somewhere must be making a handsome profit from it and have considerable power to fend off critics. Who could that be? The seed companies, with their patents on the new GM crop varieties? The corn barons? The soy companies? The fertiliser manufacturers? The agrochemicals companies? The fossil-fuel energy companies? The beef barons, the global chicken and pig breeder companies? The retail and fast food chains, which trade in the cheap meat?

We can surmise that it is not the advocates of organic or mixed agroecological farming, nor the soil specialists and biodiversity experts, nor the local councils often charged with environmental cleanup, nor is it the national health care services or the cancer or heart specialists, who tend to advocate healthy, low-meat-and-dairy diets to their patients.

Dear reader, I only ask the questions and hope that the answers become clear and help create an eagerness for change.

Paths for the future?

Meanwhile let's look at some of the possible ways forward. Farming, like so many other activities, needs to disengage from its dependence on fossil fuels. Solar energy and other alternative energy sources may be able to power the machinery and vehicles necessary for farming. Processed fertilisers can be largely replaced by animal and green manures, and soils will be enhanced at the same time. Soils can also be protected with no-till methods.

Governments need to act to protect remaining forests, wetlands and special environmentally sensitive areas. The spread of soy, corn and cattle grazing into biodiverse-rich or vulnerable areas must be halted.

There is a strong case to be made for raising farm animals on foods which do not compete with human needs, such as grasses, forages, crop and food wastes (appropriately handled). Poultry raised in African villages subsist for months by scavenging their own food – they are not in competition with humans. Silvo-pastoral systems are another good example – covered in more detail elsewhere in this book. (See Chapter 5 in this volume.)

Ultimately, governments, international agencies and individuals need to embrace dietary change alongside environmental protection. Without it, the environment, including biodiversity and the biosphere, will not be able to support humanity *ad infinitum*. Dietary change will also bring better health and quality of life to a population which is growing in numbers and girth, and it will reduce pressure on national health services. The experts are already pointing the way.

One of Europe's leading environmental scientists, Dr Henk Westhoek, says that halving the consumption of meat, dairy products and eggs in the EU would result in 23% per capita less use of cropland for food production (Westhoek et al., 2015). With so much phosphorus used for growing crops for animal feed (and thereby for meat production), the Soil Association has estimated that "[a] vegetarian diet [requires] 0.6 kg phosphorus a year (or 4.2 kg of phosphate rock), whilst a meat-based diet requires 1.6 kg phosphorus a year (or 11.8 kg of phosphate rock)" (Soil Association, 2010). The European Commission stresses that "animal protein production is much less efficient than that of vegetable protein". It points out that "to produce one kilogram of protein from cereals requires the use of 20 m^2 of land; for poultry meat and milk this is 35 m^2, for pork 60 m^2 and for beef over 100 m^2" (European Commission Consultation Paper, 2012).

A key study shows that business as usual will result in large increases in global cropland that take us beyond the safe operating space before 2050. In contrast to this, global cropland can be reduced by a 50% reduction in food waste and a significant reduction in global meat and dairy consumption. (Bajželj, 2014). A similar recommendation comes from the WWF Living Forest Report of 2011, which urges a 50% reduction in meat consumption in OECD countries by 2050. Only by doing this can WWF's goal of Zero Net Deforestation and Forest Degradation (ZNDD) be achieved (Taylor, 2011).

But can we really expect the Chinese for example to cut back on meat consumption, when their new urbanised middle classes have only recently been able to indulge in regular meat eating? We cannot be food imperialists. That kind of imperialism is likely to be no more productive than the colonial kind. It may sound unlikely, but the Chinese government is well aware of the environmental and health impacts of this move to a more carnivorous diet. A 2014 communication from China's National Program for Food and Nutrition (2014–2020) emphasises that they should aim for "rational food consumption with modern nutritional concept, to develop a nutrition-oriented modern food industry", including "inheriting a healthy dietary tradition of consuming mainly vegetable food and less animal food, protecting food with local characteristics, innovating and booming Chinese food culture" (China's National Program, 2014).

Personally, I listened to the world-famous Chinese pianist Lang Lang being interviewed on BBC Radio in early 2016. When asked how one could help students prepare for their piano examinations, he said – to my surprise – that they should eat more vegetables and fruit! This unexpected answer may well be based on a similar message from the Chinese authorities.

Sustainable development goals

There is a final important argument to be made here. The world's nations have committed to achieving the Sustainable Development Goals (SDGs). Without change in the way we farm intensively and in our feeding of nutritious crops to animals for poor conversion to meat, milk and eggs, it is hard to see how some of the SDGs can be achieved. For example the noble goal of ending hunger by 2030 (SDG 2) – if it's business as usual in using so much soy, corn and other cereals for feeding animals in intensive farms, how can this be achieved? The goal of ensuring availability and sustainable management of water and by 2020 protect and restore water-related ecosystems, including mountains, forests, wetlands, rivers, aquifers and lakes (SDG 6) is hardly likely to be achieved if the world's best arable land continues to be subjected to a torrent of nitrogen and other fertilisers, herbicides and pesticides.

Regarding the goal of ensuring sustainable production and consumption patterns (SDG 12) – well, if the issue of meat consumption is not addressed, it is hard to see how this worthy goal can be achieved. Sustainably managing forests and restoring biodiversity loss (SDG 15) are again worthy goals, but it is impossible to see how they can be achieved in such a short time frame (by 2020) without radical change to our food and farming systems.

As for taking urgent action to combat climate change (SDG 13), of relevance here is a systematic review of 14 papers on diet and GHG emissions by Elinor Hallström, which showed not only that the vegan diet had the greatest impact on reducing GHG emissions (around 55%), followed by vegetarian diets and healthier diets in which less meat is eaten, but that the same diets had a similar impact on reducing demand for agricultural land, with the vegan diet reducing demand on land by nearly 60% (Hallström, 2014). Similarly the research published in 2014 by Dr Peter Scarborough of the Department of Public Health at the University of Oxford showed that the diet-related GHG emissions in kilograms of carbon dioxide equivalents per day (kgCO2e/day) were lowest for those on a vegan (no animal products) diet, 2.89 kgCO2e/day, and highest for those eating most meat, 7.19 kgCO2e/day (Scarborough et al., 2014).

Surely a signpost for a more environmentally friendly dietary future?

References

Agrimoney Investment Forum, 2014, www.agrimoney.com/news/brazil-soy-crop-and-exports-to-soar-next-season-6894.html

Bailey, R., Froggat, A., and Wellesley, L., 2014, *Livestock – climate change's forgotten sector.* London: Chatham House.

Bajželj, B. Richards, K.S. Allwood, J.M. Smith, P., Dennis, J. S., Curmi, E., and Gilligan, C.A., 2014, *Importance of food-demand management for climate mitigation.* Nature Climate Change. www.nature.com/doifinder/10.1038/nclimate2353

Brown, L., 1995, *Worldwatch website.* www.worldwatch.org/bookstore/publication/who-will-feed-china-wake-call-small-planet, accessed 8/3/16.

Carpenter, S.R., and Bennett, E.M., 2011, Reconsideration of the planetary boundary for phosphorus. *Environmental Research Letters* 6(1), 014009. doi: 10.1088/1748-9326/6/1/014009

Cassidy, E.S., West, P. C., Gerber, J. S., and Foley, J. A., 2013, Redefining agricultural yields: From tonnes to people nourished per hectare: University of Minnesota. *Environmental Research Letters* 8(3), 034015.

CBD (Convention on Biological Diversity), 1992, www.cbd.int/doc/legal/cbd-en.pdf www.cbd.int/gbo/gbo4/publication/gbo4-en-hr.pdf

CBD (Convention on Biological Diversity), 2014, *Global biodiversity outlook 4*. www.cbd.int/gbo/gbo4/publication/gbo4-en-hr.pdf

China's National Program, 2014, www.chinadaily.com.cn/m/chinahealth/2014-05/16/content_17514010.htm

Cho, R., 2013, *Phosphorus: Essential to life – are we running out?* Columbia University Earth Institute. http://blogs.ei.columbia.edu/2013/04/01/phosphorus-essential-to-life-are-we-running-out/

Commission Implementing Regulation (EU) No 485/2013 of 24 May, 2013, Amending implementing regulation (EU) No 540/2011, as regards the conditions of approval of the active substances clothianidin, thiamethoxam and imidacloprid, and prohibiting the use and sale of seeds treated with plant protection products containing those active substances. http://eur-lex.europa.eu/LexUriServ/LexUriServ.do?uri=OJ:L:2013:139:0012:0026:EN:PDF

Earth Policy Institute, 2014, Compiled from U.S. department of agriculture, production, supply and distribution, electronic database. www.fas.usda.gov/psdonline, updated 10 February 2014.

EPA, 2007, *Atrazine: Chemical summary: Toxicity and exposure assessment for children's health* (PDF) (Report). U.S. Environmental Protection Agency. 2007–04–24. Washington, D.C.

European Commission, 2004, 2004/248/EC: Commission decision of 10 March 2004 concerning the non-inclusion of atrazine in Annex I to Council Directive 91/414/EEC and the withdrawal of authorisations for plant protection products containing this active substance (Text with EEA relevance) (notified under document number C(2004) 731.

European Commission, 2015, *The state of nature in the EU*. http://ec.europa.eu/environment/nature/pdf/state_of_nature_en.pdf

European Commission Consultation Paper, 2012, *Options for resource efficiency indicators*. http://ec.europa.eu/environment/consultations/pdf/consultation_resource.pdf

European Commission Staff Working Paper, 2011, Analysis associated with the roadmap to a resource efficient Europe Part II, SEC (2011) 1067 final. Brussels. http://ec.europa.eu/environment/resource_efficiency/pdf/working_paper_part2.pdf

European Nitrogen Assessment (ENA), 2011, www.nine-esf.org/ENA

European Union, 2013, http://eur-lex.europa.eu/LexUriServ/LexUriServ.do?uri=OJ:L:2013:139:0012:0026:EN:PDF

FAO, 2011a, *World livestock 2011: Livestock in food security*. Rome: UN Food and Agriculture Organization (FAO).

FAO, 2011b, *FAO in the 21st century, Ensuring food security in a changing world*. Rome: FAO.

FAO, 2015, *Healthy soils for a healthy life, 2015*. FAO. www.fao.org/soils-2015/faq/en/

FAOSTAT, 2016, http://faostat3.fao.org/browse/R/*/E, accessed 28/4/16.

Fertilizer Institute, 2016, www.tfi.org/statistics/statistics-faqs, accessed 10/3/16.

Heffer, P., and Prud'homme, M., 2015, *Fertilizer outlook, 2015–2019*. . Paris: International Fertlizer Industry Association.

Findlaw, http://injury.findlaw.com/product-liability/atrazine-lawsuit-overview.html, accessed 27/4/16.

Foley, J., 2013, Scientific American 5/3/2013. *It's time to rethink America's corn system*. www.scientificamerican.com/article/time-to-rethink-corn/

Foresight Report: The future of food and farming, 2011. London: The Government Office for Science. www.gov.uk/government/uploads/system/uploads/attachment_data/file/288329/11-546-future-of-food-and-farming-report.pdf

Gilbert, N., 2009, The disappearing nutrient. *Nature* 461, 716–718.

Hallström, E., Carlsson-Kanyama, A., and Börjesson, P., 2014, Environmental impact of dietary change: A systematic review. *Journal of Cleaner Production* 91, 1–11, Elsevier.

Heath, R.H., 2014, www.quora.com/How-are-fertilizer-prices-related-to-crude-oil

Hicks, S., and EIA, 2010, *Energy for growing and harvesting crops is a large component of farm operating costs.* EIA's 2010 Manufacturing Energy Consumption Survey, Energy Information Administration. Washington, D.C.

IARC Monographs, March 2015, *Volume 112: Evaluation of five organophosphate insecticides and herbicides.* www.iarc.fr/en/media-centre/iarcnews/pdf/MonographVolume112.pdf

IEED Briefing, March 2015, *Sustainable intensification revisited.* http://pubs.iied.org/17283IIED.html

Index Mundi, 2016, www.indexmundi.com/agriculture/?country=eu&commodity=palm-kernel-meal&graph=imports, accessed 9/4/16.

Kebreab, E., Hansen, A., and Strathe, A., December 2012, Animal production for efficient phosphate utilization: From optimized feed to high efficiency livestock. *Current Opinion in Biotechnology* 23(6), 872–877. doi: 10.1016/j.copbio.2012.06.001. Epub 2012 Jul 14.

Liep, A., Billen, G., Garnier, J., Grizzetti, B., Lassaletta, L., Reis, S., . . . Weiss, F., 2015, Impacts of European livestock production. *Environmental Research Letters* 10(11). http://iopscience.iop.org/article/10.1088/1748-9326/10/11/115004

Lundqvist, J., Fraiture, C. de, and Molden, D., 2008, *Saving water: From field to fork – curbing losses and wastage in the food chain.* SIWI Policy Brief. SIWI. www.siwi.org/documents/Resources/Policy_Briefs/PB_From_Filed_to_Fork_2008.pdf

The Nature Conservancy, 2012, *An overview of the Brazil-China soybean trade and its strategic implications for conservation.* www.nature.org/ourinitiatives/regions/southamerica/brazil/explore/brazil-china-soybean-trade.pdf.

Nellemann, C., MacDevette, M., Manders, T., Eickhout, B., Svihus, B., and Gerdien Prins, A., 2009, *The environmental food crisis – the environment's role in averting future food crises.* A UNEP Rapid Response Assessment. United Nations Environment Programme, GRID-Arendal. www.unep.org/pdf/foodcrisis_lores.pdf

NOAA, 2016, National Oceanic and Atmospheric Association (NOAA). *The Causes of Hypoxia in the Northern Gulf of Mexico.* http://service.ncddc.noaa.gov/rdn/www/media/documents/hypoxia/hypox_finalcauses.pdf, accessed 25/4/16.

PBL Netherlands Environmental Assessment Agency, (2014), *How sectors can contribute to sustainable use and conservation of biodiversity.* CBD Technical Series No. 79, cited in CBD (2014) Global Biodiversity Outlook 4, Montreal.

Scarborough, P., Appleby, P., Mizdrak, A., Briggs, A., Travis, R., Bradbury, K., and Key, T., July 2014, Dietary greenhouse gas emissions of meat-eaters, fish-eaters, vegetarians and vegans in the UK. *Climatic Change* 125(2) 179–192.

Smil, V., 1999, "Detonator of the population explosion" (PDF). *Nature* 400, 415. doi: 10.1038/22672.

Smil, V., 2004, *Enriching the Earth: Fritz Haber, Carl Bosch, and the transformation of world food production.* Cambridge, MA: MIT Press. ISBN 9780262693134.

Soil Association, 2010, *A Rock and a hard place: Peak phosphorus and the threat to our food security.* SA, Bristol, UK. www.susana.org/_resources/documents/default/2-1143-policyreport-2010peakphosphate1.pdf

Soyatech, 2015, www.soyatech.com/soy_facts.htm, accessed 29/7/15.

Steinfeld, H., Gerber, P., Wassenaar, T., and Castel, V., 2006, *Livestock's long shadow.* Rome: Food and Agriculture Organization of the UN.

Stern, N.H. et al., 2007, Great Britain, Treasury. *The economics of climate change: The Stern review*. Cambridge, UK; New York: Cambridge University Press.

Sustainable Development Goals SDGs, 2015, *United Nations*. www.un.org/sustainable development/sustainable-development-goals/

Syngenta, 2016, www.atrazine.com/atramain.aspx, accessed 27/4/16.

Taylor, R. (ed.), 2011, *WWF living forest report*. Gland, Switzerland: WWF.

UNEP, 2014, www.unep.org/Documents.Multilingual/Default.asp?DocumentID=2796&ArticleID=10993&l=en

Union of Concerned Scientists, 2008, *Hidden costs of industrial agriculture*. August 17, 2012. Ref below. www.ucsusa.org/food_and_agriculture/our-failing-food-system/industrial-agriculture/hidden-costs-of-industrial.html, accessed 27/4/16.

United Nations, 2011, *World economic and social survey 2011*. www.un.org/en/development/desa/policy/wess/wess_current/2011wess.pdf

USDA, *Economic research service*. www.ers.usda.gov/topics/crops/soybeans-oil-crops.aspx, accessed 27/4/16.

Vaccari, D.A., 2009, Phosphorus: A loomıng crisis. *Scientific American* 300(6), 54. http://web.mit.edu/12.000/www/m2016/pdf/scientificamerican0609-54.pdf

Westcott, P., 2012, *USDA agricultural projections to 2021, USDA, economic research service*, February 2012. www.ers.usda.gov/amber-waves/2012-september/long-term-prospects-for-agriculture.aspx#.VtR6zU0rG1s

Westhoek, H., Lesschen, J. P. Rood, T., Wagner, S., De Marco, A. Murphy, D., Leip, A., van Grinsven, H. Sutton, M.A., and Oenema, O. 2011, *The protein puzzle: The consumption and production of meat, dairy and fish in the European Union*. PBL Netherlands Environmental Assessment Agency.

Westhoek, H., Lesschen, J.P., Rood, T., Wagner, S., De Marco, A., Murphy-Bokern, D., . . . Oenema, O., May 2014, Food choices, health and environment: Effects of cutting Europe's meat and dairy intake. *Global Environmental Change* 26, 196–205. www.sciencedirect.com/science/article/pii/S0959378014000338

Westhoek, H., Lesschen, J.P., Leip, A., Rood, T., Wagner, S., De Marco, A., Murphy-Bokern, D., Pallière, C., Howard, C.M., Oenema, O., and Sutton, M.A., 2015, *Nitrogen on the table: The influence of food choices on nitrogen emissions and the European environment*. ENA Special Report on nitrogen and food. Edinburgh: Centre for Ecology & Hydrology.

Wood, S., and Cowie, A., (2004). *A review of greenhouse gas emission factors for fertiliser production*. Washington, DC: IEA Bioenergy.

Worldwatch Institute website, www.worldwatch.org/bookstore/publication/who-will-feed-china-wake-call-small-planet, accessed 8/3/16.

WWF, 2006, *Facts about soy production and the Basel criteria*. http://wwf.panda.org/wwf_news/?unewsid=73900

WWF, 2014, *Living planet report*. http://wwf.panda.org/about_our_earth/all_publications/living_planet_report/

WWF, 2016a, http://wwf.panda.org/what_we_do/footprint/agriculture/soy/facts/, accessed 26/2/16.

WWF, 2016b, http://wwf.panda.org/what_we_do/footprint/agriculture/soy/soyreport/the_continuing_rise_of_soy/the_market_for_soy_in_europe/

5

ANIMALS ON THE LAND

Ecosystem services and disservices of grazing livestock systems

Alberto Bernués

1. Introduction

How good or bad are livestock for the environment? Are domestic animals part of the problem or part of the solution when fighting, for example, climate change? There is not an easy (or correct) answer to these questions; it can be both – it very much depends on the way animals are reared, on the type of production systems. In other words, the key lies not so much with the animals themselves or their use as food, but with the ways animals are incorporated in agroecosystems and food systems (Gliessman, 2015).

This chapter attempts to shed some light on the controversial issue of grazing livestock and the environment, and to identify sustainable pathways of development that help to reconcile animal production, environmental preservation, and socio-cultural values that are important for society. The chapter is structured as follows. First, I shall discuss the wide diversity of livestock farming systems and their multiple (economic, socio-cultural, environmental) outcomes, briefly describe some contrasting trends in their recent evolution and introduce the concepts of multifunctionality and ecosystem services (ES) and disservices (EDS). The ES framework will be used to describe the main negative and positive outcomes and livestock grazing systems (sections 3 and 4, respectively) and the multiple conflicts (trade-offs) that can arise between them. Next, I shall illustrate with a case study how we can value public (nonmarket) goods provided by grazing agroecosystems, with special emphasis on socio-cultural and economic perspectives (section 5). Finally, I shall introduce some strategies to design more sustainable grazing livestock systems using the principles of agroecology, and point to some guidelines for policy design (section 6).

2. A wide diversity of livestock farming systems and their multiple outcomes

Today, livestock farming systems differ widely in the use of natural resources and inputs (imported grain feeds, agrochemicals, fossil energy) and outcomes obtained (production levels, or environmental, social and cultural outcomes). In addition, they are located in very diverse agroecological, socio-economic and market contexts all around the world. For example, there are very few similarities in the ways and motivations of Masai people to rear their animals in West Africa and the large industrial feedlots for beef production in the US. Hence, when analyzing any aspect of sustainability of animal production, it is key to discriminate among the different ways that livestock can be reared and its multiple purposes (Bernués et al., 2011).

This chapter will focus on "animals on the land", i.e. livestock farming systems that are based on grazing. The animals in these systems are predominantly ruminants (cattle, sheep and goats) because of their unique capacity to use fibrous plant-based diets that are not digestible for humans. Although I have used European conditions for many of the examples, I believe the main arguments are valid in many other places across the world.

Broadly speaking, we have observed a dual trend in the way animal agriculture, and grazing livestock production in particular, has evolved in the last decades: industrialization, specialization and enlargement in areas with favourable agroecological and market conditions; marginalization, or even abandonment, in remote, difficult-to-work areas (mountain areas, Mediterranean grasslands, steppes, arid and semi-arid zones, etc.). These areas, in which animal production was traditionally one of the very few economic options, still contribute important natural values, including cultural landscapes and biodiversity, and constitute the habitat for many endangered wild species. Both trends, intensification of agriculture and abandonment of marginal areas, have been pointed out as main drivers of biodiversity loss, for example, in the Biodiversity Strategy to 2020 of the European Union (European_Commission, 2011) or in the Global Biodiversity Outlook of the Convention of Biological Diversity (Secretariat of the Convention on Biological Diversity, 2010).

Interactions between the animal farming intensity and the environment are complex, often not unidirectional, and can originate multiple conflicts (trade-offs) between different outcomes and across spatial and temporal scales. In a very generic, therefore inaccurate, manner we can imagine these interactions to have an inverted-U shape (Box 5.1). So the question is, where is the right balance? In other words, how do we integrate animals in agroecosystems and in food systems? There is not an easy or unique answer to this question. It will depend on the particular biophysical characteristics of the agroecosystem, on the socio-economic context and, not least, on the policy objectives, which should respond to the relative importance that society assigns to the multiple outcomes derived from animal agriculture in particular, and the societal concerns about the model of agriculture and the food system in general.

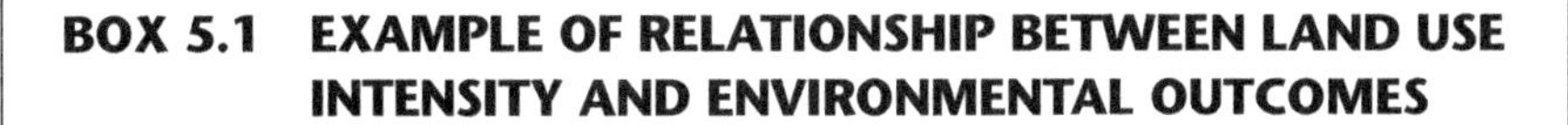

BOX 5.1 EXAMPLE OF RELATIONSHIP BETWEEN LAND USE INTENSITY AND ENVIRONMENTAL OUTCOMES

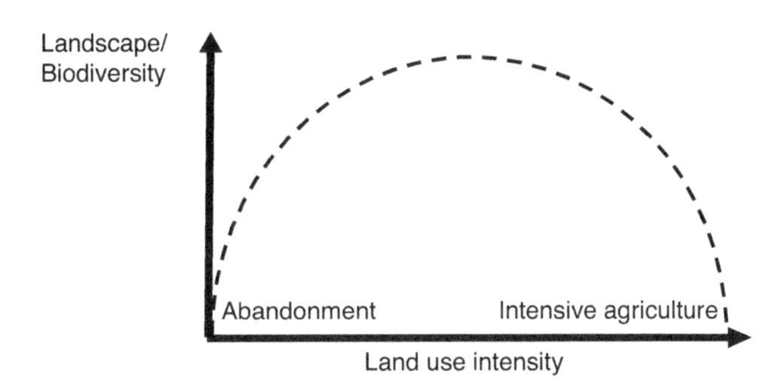

FIGURE 5.1 Graph showing the relationship between land use intensity and environmental outcomes

According to the intermediate disturbance hypothesis (Huston, 1979), an increase of land use intensity can improve the quality or amount of other outcomes delivered by the agroecosystem (agricultural landscape features, number of species, recreational values, etc.) to a maximal level, situated somewhere at an intermediate level in the extensification-intensification continuum, after which further increases of intensification reduces the quality or amount of these attributes – all this within a specific agroecosystem.

Due to their potential to deliver multiple outcomes, grazing livestock farming systems are considered representative examples of multifunctional agriculture. The concept of ***multifunctionality*** generically refers to the interconnectedness of agriculture's different roles and functions (IAASTD, 2009). It recognizes agriculture as a multi-output activity producing not only private (market) goods such as food, feed or fibre, but also public goods such as agricultural landscapes, farmland biodiversity, water quality, soil functionality, etc. There are three approaches to the analysis of multifunctional agriculture. The first is an economic approach that jointly considers the production of private and public goods, for which the concepts of positive and negative externalities and market failure are key (further developed later in the chapter). The second is a development approach that recognizes the many contributions of animal agriculture to livelihoods and development and includes aspects such as food security, capital savings, poverty alleviation, and cultural heritage. This is used mostly in developing countries. The third approach, which is Europe-centred, establishes multifunctional agriculture as the means to preserve the agricultural landscape and to sustain rural development, including tourism and recreation, and to preserve the production of quality products that are linked to specific areas (see Renting et al. (2009) for a comprehensive review).

The multidimensional nature of agriculture is further developed by the ***ecosystem services*** (ES) concept, launched by the Millennium Ecosystem Assessment, which has become prominent in the academia and policy debate. ES are defined as the direct and indirect benefits that people get from ecosystems, including agroecosystems. Formally, ecosystems services can be classified into four groups: *provisioning* ES are material or energy outputs including goods such as food, water, fuel, timber and fibre; *regulating* ES are biophysical processes providing benefits such as climate regulation, flood prevention, waste treatment and water purification; *cultural* ES are recreational, aesthetic and spiritual benefits provided by ecosystems; and *supporting* ES, such as soil formation, photosynthesis or nutrient cycling, are the various processes that are necessary for the production of all the other ES. The last three groups (regulating, supporting and cultural ES) can be also denominated as *nonprovisioning* ES and mostly constitute *public goods*: individuals cannot be excluded from their use, and their use by one individual does not reduce their availability to others (Cooper et al., 2009).

Within the ES framework, the negative outcomes or externalities derived from agriculture are called ecosystem disservices (EDS) (Zhang et al., 2007). EDS of animal agriculture are very large, including habitat loss, nutrient runoff and pesticide pollution. These are reviewed in detail in other chapters of this book.

An additional key characteristic of public goods or nonprovisioning ES (as well as EDS) is that they generally do not have a market price, therefore farmers have little or no economic incentive to produce (or internalize) them, so public intervention is required to achieve a desirable level of provision according to societal demands. Moreover, they are very difficult to measure and value, and so agri-environmental policies tend to ignore them. Before discussing how we can measure and value nonmarket functions of animal agriculture, I shall briefly describe the most relevant ecosystem services and disservices of grazing livestock systems.

3. Ecosystem disservices of grazing livestock systems

The multiple and significant negative externalities of livestock have been object of extensive debate in a large number of papers and reports since the FAO Livestock's Long Shadow report was issued (Steinfeld et al., 2006). This seminal report reviewed the impacts of the livestock sector on the environment in terms of: land degradation, atmosphere and climate, water and biodiversity at the global scale. However, as the report recognizes, the livestock sector is very heterogeneous: from only grazing (mostly ruminants), to mixed agriculture-livestock systems, and landless or industrial farming systems (mostly pigs and poultry), so global estimates can be misleading. Likewise, grazing systems themselves differ widely in terms use of natural resources, productivity level and outcomes obtained (Ripoll-Bosch et al., 2012). The boundary between the production of ES and EDS is not neat; the two are often provided in bundles, and many trade-offs do exist. My intention is not to provide a quantified inventory of negative externalities of grazing livestock but to critically analyze the most important ones.

3.1 Emission of greenhouse gases

Animal agriculture is responsible for a large share (18% according to Steinfeld et al. (2006)) of global greenhouse gas emissions to the atmosphere. In brief, these emissions come from carbon dioxide from deforestation and land conversion to pastures and feed crops, consumption of fossil fuels in industrial agriculture, methane production from enteric fermentation in ruminants and nitrous oxide from manure. Many studies quantifying the carbon footprint of animal products advocate an intensification of animal production to mitigate emission of greenhouse gases (GHG) (Steinfeld and Gerber, 2010), moving away from beef and sheep/goat meat to pork and poultry, and from rustic, traditional animals to specialized, highly productive ones. The main rationale behind this proposal is the so-called efficiency gain: i.e. more output with less input, and therefore less environmental impact per kg of product. However, the picture gets a bit more complicated when we consider not just animal production but farming systems as a whole, and examine in more detail the concept of efficiency itself.

Efficiency is expressed most simply as the ratio of output to input, at a certain time and place. This efficiency measure can change dramatically according to the units of input and output that we choose to consider. The carbon footprint of sheep farming systems in Mediterranean conditions (grazing system, mixed sheep-cereal system and zero-grazing [industrial system]) constitutes an illustrative example (Ripoll-Bosch et al., 2013).

The carbon footprint of lamb meat (when considered as the only output of the production system) decreases with the level of intensification (highest for the grazing system and lowest for the industrial system [Table 5.1]). However, in contrast to industrial systems, grazing and mixed (sheep-crops) systems are multifunctional and provide other outcomes (public goods such as biodiversity and landscape conservation). When allocating the carbon footprint to the diversity of outcomes, the carbon footprint of lamb meat is reversed: with lowest values for the grazing system and highest for zero-grazing system. The main GHG is methane, and its contribution

TABLE 5.1 GHG emissions (CO_2-eq/kg of lamb meat) with or without consideration of ES and contribution (%) of CO_2, CH_4 and N_2O to total GHGs

	Without ES allocation	*With ES allocation*	*Contribution*		
	Kg lamb meat	*Kg lamb meat*	CO_2	CH_4	N_2O
	(CO_2-eq/kg)	*(CO_2-eq/kg)*	*(%)*	*(%)*	*(%)*
Grazing	51.7	27.7	7.9	61.6	30.5
Mixed	47.9	35.4	21.0	57.6	21.4
Zero-grazing	39.0	39.0	29.1	59.4	11.5

Source: Ripoll-Bosch et al. (2013)

remains nearly steady across systems. The emission of CO_2 is proportional to the combustion of fossil fuels and increases with intensification. Emission of N_2O is higher in grazing systems because of direct manure deposition; however, the positive effect of manure on soil organic matter and fertility is well known, indicating a trade-off between GHG emissions and soil quality.

In the example above, we can see that the consideration of single or multiple outputs can have a drastic effect on efficiency, in this case measured as carbon footprint. Trade-offs among ES and EDS are ignored if we use analytical tools that cannot deal with multiple outcomes at the same time. For example, direct comparisons of the environmental impact of livestock using Life Cycle Analysis are difficult because of the key incidence on the results of:

- the functional unit (e.g. emissions per kg of product, per hectare of land, or per person) (Nguyen et al., 2012);
- the boundary of the system under analysis (e.g. inclusion of land use and land-use change issues (Nguyen et al., 2013) or the potential of carbon sequestration of grassland soils (Soussana et al., 2010); and
- the difficulty to include other environmental aspects such as biodiversity and landscape which operate at larger temporal and spatial scales (Vries et al., 2015).

Additionally, the different nature of inputs can also drastically change the results of the analysis, for example the consideration of renewable vs. non-renewable energy, or the competition for land between food for humans and feed for animals (Zanten et al., 2015).

I shall consider further the nature of inputs (human edible vs. non-edible) when reviewing the efficiency of grazing animals to deliver provisioning ES (meat and milk). However, it is already clear that a single efficiency ratio, or methodology for analysis of environmental impact, is not capable of addressing the multiple interrelations, nor the dynamic processes in which agricultural systems are increasingly operating.

3.2 Land degradation: deforestation and desertification

Environmental consequences of land degradation are multiple, including contribution to climate change (loss of biomass and organic matter in soils), biodiversity loss (habitat destruction), landscape modification (vegetation change and soil erosion), alteration of the water cycle, etc. (Steinfeld et al., 2006). These interrelated aspects often are related to industrial (zero-grazing) livestock systems and are covered in greater detail in other chapters of this book.

The two most important forms of land degradation caused, or influenced, by grazing livestock systems are deforestation and desertification. Deforestation caused by the long-term loss of natural vegetation is more evident in tropical and subtropical areas, mostly in Latin America and Asia. Desertification, caused by the deterioration of the physical, chemical and biological properties of soils that become eroded, occurs specially in arid and semi-arid environments, mostly in Africa.

According to Steinfeld et al. (2006), carbon released due to deforestation of large forest areas of Latin America and Asia is responsible for 34% of the total GHG emissions by livestock. In the Amazon, the number of cattle has increased dramatically from nearly 9 million in 1975 to 70 million in 2007 (Gerber, 2010). About 70% of deforested land is occupied by pasture, with feed crops (typically soybean) accounting for most of the remainder. Even if grazing livestock is not always the primary cause of deforestation (extraction of timber comes first), it is certainly a major contributor. However, forest is cleared not only for production of cheap abundant forage, but very often as the easiest way of land appropriation and speculation (Mertens et al., 2002). These authors conclude that deforestation in Brazil is driven by the consumption of livestock commodities and the development of new marketing chains. However, the socio-economic factors involved in deforestation are complex and interrelated, the process being fuelled by investments in infrastructure (roads, energy, etc.), macroeconomic policies for financial credit and subsidies and land tenure laws (Goers et al., 2012; Lambin et al., 2001).

However, livestock farming systems in tropical (and temperate) environments can be effectively adapted to use land more efficiently, enhance the nutrient cycles, improve animal welfare, increase biodiversity and obtain a profitable production by diversifying the resource base with shrubs and trees. Silvopastoral systems (a type of agroforestry systems) that intentionally combine trees, shrubs and forages in an integrated manner to enhance productivity and other ecosystem services, notably biodiversity and capture of carbon, are a good example of this (Broom et al., 2013). This author reviews the results of research carried out in Africa, Spain and especially Latin America.

Livestock overgrazing, i.e. above the natural carrying capacity of the ecosystem, is usually identified as the main cause of desertification of large arid and semi-arid rangelands around the world, particularly in Africa, where around 73% of dry lands are degraded (Steinfeld et al., 2006). However, a number of reviews on the issue conclude that this is an oversimplification of the evidence and does not support this deduction (Dodd, 1994; Weber and Horst, 2011). Arid and semi-arid rangelands change dramatically within and between years and, therefore, are considered as non-equilibrium ecosystems where temporary and permanent changes, mainly driven by abiotic factors (climatic variability), are difficult to identify. Ignoring this, agricultural development policies in many African countries have tried to replace the traditional pastoralism with sedentarization (that precipitates urban migration) and conversion of better rangelands to croplands. Local overstocking and degradation occur in the remaining areas and, in severe drought periods, both agricultural and pastoral areas cannot provide food. It is in this agro-pastoral frontier where land degradation is concentrated. Instead, evidence indicates that, rather than being inherently destructive, grazing livestock, when managed in an ecologically sound manner, are necessary for the maintenance of arid and semi-arid rangelands (Lambin et al., 2001) and may be the only activity consistent with long-term sustainable food production in these areas (Dodd, 1994).

We may conclude that negative environmental impacts (EDS) of grazing livestock systems can be significant, with great variation across regions and farming systems. Nevertheless, despite the increasing amount of available data and sophistication of analytical tools, many fundamental questions remain relating e.g. to the functional units of analysis, system boundaries, spatial and temporal scales and the metrics chosen for efficiency. Changing the perspective in any of these dimensions obliges us to consider the multiple trade-offs that will certainly appear. Most work is devoted today to examine the room for technical improvements. However, the economic and socio-cultural context in which livestock farms operate is generally ignored (Herrero et al., 2015). As expressed by Lambin et al. (2001), we need to move beyond identifying global driving forces of land use change and analyze the responses of the people to local economic opportunities and mediating institutional factors. This is crucial not only to understand how farmers and other stakeholders make decisions (e.g. uptake of innovations), but also to set priorities for research, agricultural and rural development policies in different areas of the world.

4. Ecosystem services of grazing livestock systems

Grazing livestock systems also have the potential to provide multiple ES. For example, a study about sheep drove roads in Spain identified 34 different ES within three categories: provisioning (10), regulating (regulation of ecosystem processes) (12) and cultural (12) (Oteros-Rozas et al., 2013). A recent revision of literature on ES provided by grazing livestock systems in Europe documented that the main focus of research has been on biodiversity, landscape and carbon sequestration (Rodríguez-Ortega et al., 2014). It is worth mentioning that the first two categories of ES (provisioning and regulating) are intrinsically dependent on the existence of grazing livestock farming systems. They include the reduction of risk of forest fires, particularly in Mediterranean areas (Cooper et al., 2009). These three ES, together with the provision of quality foods linked to the territory (provisioning ES), are widely recognized by society in different countries (Bernués et al., 2015a; Bernués et al., 2014), showing in this case a good correspondence between social perception and scientific focus. We will now describe these ES.

4.1 Food provisioning and food quality

Within the current debate about the need to "feed the world", it is widely (and often self-interestedly) affirmed that intensive or industrial animal farming is more efficient than extensive or grazing-based farming and therefore essential to feed the increasing demand for meat, especially in emerging economies. However, in the search for increased efficiency for feed conversion into animal protein, diets have massively incorporated grains that can be directly used for human nutrition (Wilkinson, 2011). If efficiencies of energy and protein animal production are calculated on the basis of human-edible food, ruminants on pasture have great advantages over industrial systems (Table 5.2). Similar findings are demonstrated for land use efficiency if the suitability of land for cultivation of food crops (instead of feed for animals) is accounted for (Zanten et al., 2015).

TABLE 5.2 Feed conversion ratio (input per unit of output) of different species for total and edible inputs

	Total		*Edible*	
	Energy (MJ)	*Protein (Kg)*	*Energy (MJ)*	*Protein (Kg)*
Milk	4.5	5.6	0.47	0.71
Suckler beef (upland)	40.0	26.3	1.9	0.92
Lamb (lowland)	52.6	30.3	2.5	1.1
Pig meat	9.3	4.3	6.3	2.6
Poultry meat	4.5	3.0	3.3	2.1

Source: Wilkinson (2011)

Additionally, food production is not just a matter of quantity. Despite the decreasing consumption of red meat in Europe, the demand for high-value, local and traditional products is on the rise. Consumers give an increasing importance to intrinsic (product characteristics) and extrinsic (production process characteristics) quality attributes of meat. Regarding their intrinsic quality, grass-based animal products have a more favourable fatty acid profile in comparison to intensively produced meat, from a human health perspective (French et al., 2000). Regarding the extrinsic quality, attributes such as grass-fed, locally produced, respect for animal welfare, etc., are increasingly relevant in the consumer quality evaluation process in response to safety, health and "ethical" concerns of consumers (Figure 5.2) (Bernués et al., 2003). From a marketing perspective, meat producers and suppliers should understand consumers' tangible and intangible demands with respect to meat quality and then translate these into intrinsic or extrinsic characteristics to respond to these ethical demands.

4.2 Prevention of forest fires and other regulating services

The ecosystems that have sustained long-standing pastoral activities have reached their actual biological features through the co-evolution of human activities and nature, chiefly between grazing livestock and vegetation. The decline of traditional animal farming practices and the abandonment of land in large areas, for example High Nature Value (HNV) farmland areas in Europe, have generally led to undesirable environmental consequences, notably biodiversity loss (discussed later in the chapter) (EEA, 2004). In many Euro-Mediterranean regions, this process of abandonment has been particularly intense and continues today, in combination with a process of intensification that further reduces grazing pressure (Riedel et al., 2007). As a consequence, a general process of shrub invasion and afforestation is described in many geographical areas, especially in mountains; for example, Casasús et al. (2007) pointed out an increment of 528 kg DM ha^{-1} year^{-1} in shrub biomass in mountain areas excluded from grazing (Figure 5.3). Encroachment and afforestation threatens the traditional diverse mosaic landscapes, but also the future use of pastures by domestic or wild animals, for example birds and butterflies linked to open farmland areas. Another effect of

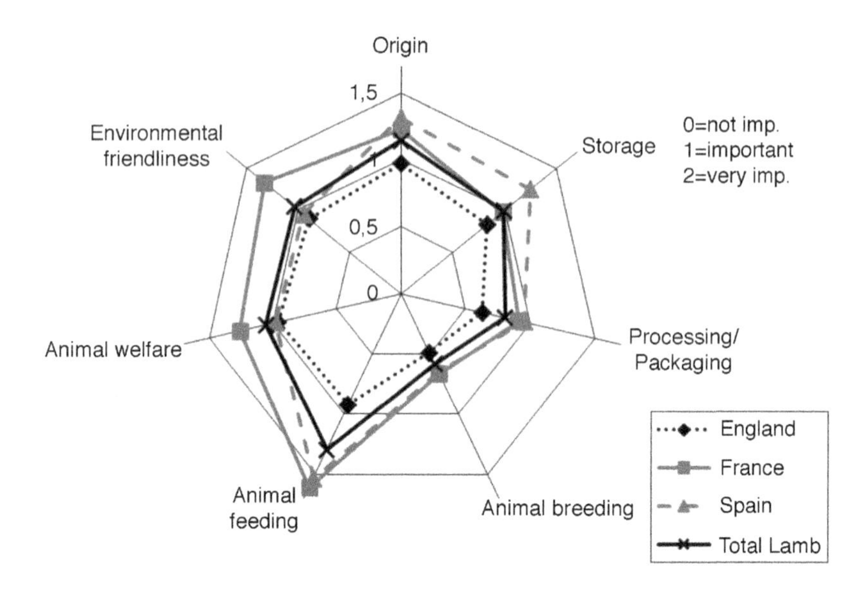

FIGURE 5.2 Relative importance of extrinsic quality attributes of lamb meat for consumers in several countries in Europe. A production process that guarantees animal feeding (based on pastures), the origin of the meat and ethical demands in terms of animal welfare and respect for the environment were highly appreciated by consumers.

Source: Modified from Bernués et al. (2003)

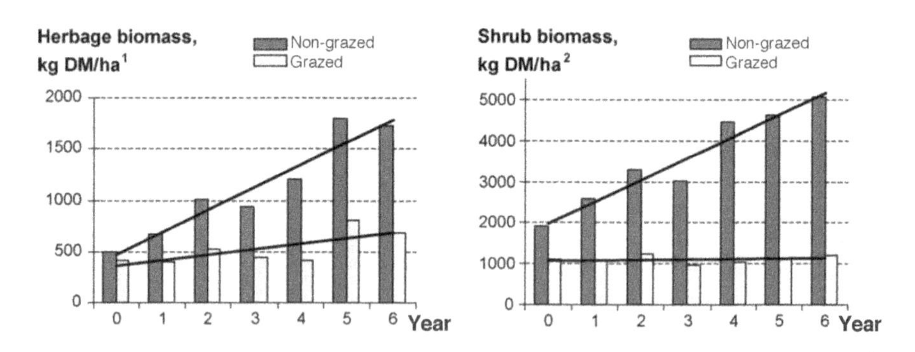

FIGURE 5.3 Changes in herbage and shrub biomass in grazed and non-grazed areas in six years in a forest pasture located in the Pyrenees (945–1400 m.a.s.l.). The effect of grazing by cattle on the herbaceous and shrub vegetation is represented. In the grazed areas, total herbage biomass was constant but herbage quality was much higher in grazed areas. Shrub biomass remained constant throughout the experiment, while it increased significantly in non-grazed areas at a rate of 528.3 kg DM/ha/year.

Source: (Casasús et al., 2007)

critical importance is the increased risk of environmental hazards, in particular forest fires, which in drier areas are can lead to erosion and ultimately desertification. For these reasons, in HNV farmland areas across Europe, livestock grazing is considered a tool that can modulate the vegetation dynamics and efficiently collaborate with other initiatives in the prevention of wildfires, accumulation of soil organic matter, regulation of the water cycle, generation of suitable habitat for endangered species or the naturalization of simplified forest ecosystems.

4.3 Supporting services: biodiversity

The number of studies on the relationships between grazing livestock systems and biodiversity is increasing quickly in recent years (Rodríguez-Ortega et al., 2014). Biodiversity-related conflicts in Europe are caused by two main processes: intensification of agriculture linked to changing scale of operations and abandonment of HNV farmlands (Henle et al., 2008). The current process of encroachment of vegetation as consequence of a reduction in traditional extensive grazing is causing a decline in species with an unfavourable conservation status in Europe. For example, Fonderflick et al. (2010) establishes a clear relationship between landscape changes in Mediterranean upland pastoral systems and bird populations. In the case of spiders, rare or specialist species are often replaced by generalists or species associated to forested areas (Oxbrough et al., 2006). Additionally, the distribution of some scavenger species (vultures) shows a strong spatio-temporal link with pastoral areas, as there is a direct dependency on the carcasses of the grazing domestic animals they feed on (Olea and Mateo-Tomas, 2009). In summary, most studies agree on the general importance of grasslands agroecosystems for the conservation and management of biodiversity. However, relationships between grazing animals, pasture management and the richness of plant and animal species are complex and concern various spatial and temporal scales, so further research is needed.

4.4 Agricultural landscapes and cultural services

Since the domestication of animal species occurred some 10,000 years ago in the eastern Mediterranean there has been a continuous process of co-evolution of people, domestic animals and landscapes. For instance, the practice of transhumance (nomadism) to maximize the use of different natural resources in diverse periods of the year has intensified this relationship, together with other practices such as hay-making or wood collection. Today, livestock grazing systems are considered as the best representatives of multifunctional agriculture in Europe, as they have multiple non-market functions such as the preservation of agricultural landscapes, their contribution to rural development, including tourism and recreation, and the preservation of cultural heritage values, such as the production of traditional food products referred earlier (Bernués et al., 2015a). The evolution of agriculture, in particular animal agriculture, has a direct influence on the cultural landscape we can find today (Box 5.2). Landscape is analyzed from different perspectives: vegetation dynamics (referred to previously), landscape heterogeneity or aesthetic quality.

Although aesthetic preferences are inherently subjective and incorporate social constructs, some features such as the presence of forb flowers (more abundant in grazed areas), the diversity of land types and uses (diversified mosaic) and even the presence of animals on the landscape contribute to explain its attractiveness. Other cultural ES, commonly defined as the non-material benefits that people obtain from ecosystems, include spiritual enrichment, cognitive development, recreation or the aforementioned aesthetic experience. These ES are normally enjoyed in bundles and are very difficult to quantify and value (Plieninger et al., 2015).

BOX 5.2 MULTIFUNCTIONAL LANDSCAPES

Research has shown that the cultural services, particularly the aesthetic and recreational values of the landscape, are clearly recognized by society at large. When presenting different agroenvironmental policy scenarios to people, the majority prefer a policy that targeted the provision of ecosystem services, which are better guaranteed by grazing livestock systems. In the image, the current agricultural landscape evolves differently according to the policy that is implemented. The liberalization of policy scenario means a further increment of bushes and trees, reduction of meadows and further closure of the landscape. The targeted support policy results in a light decrement of bushes and trees, with some increment of meadows, resulting in a diversified mosaic landscape. People are willing to pay for a policy that promotes the sustainability of sheep and goat farms and the ecosystem services they provided. (For more information see Bernués et al., 2015a.)

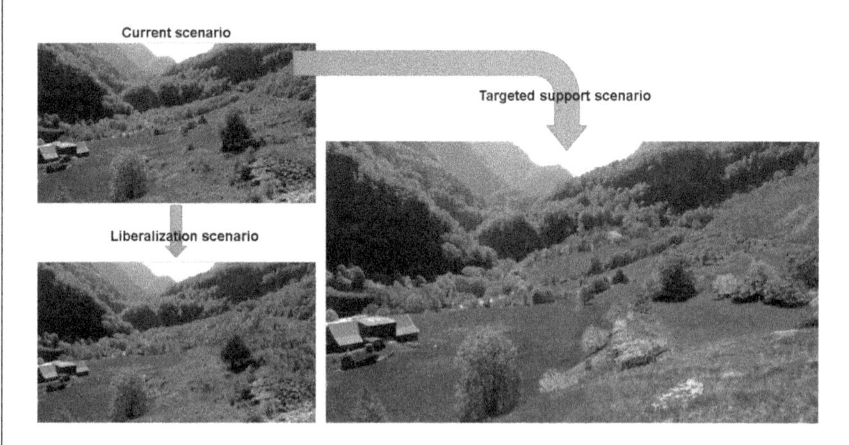

FIGURE 5.4 Multifunctional landscapes. The relative importance of ecosystem services delivered by Mediterranean grazing agroecosystems according to the number of times they were mentioned during the FG with farmers and non-farmers.

Source: Bernués et al. (2014)

5. Valuing public goods of grazing agroecosystems: a case study in Mediterranean Europe

Most ES described in the previous section constitute public goods that do not have a market price (non-market goods) and are therefore very often ignored in the evaluation of animal production systems and in policy design. Farmers, in consequence, do not get appropriate incentives to provide them, nor do they benefit from indirect economic benefits derived from certain ES they deliver, e.g. cultural services such as recreation and tourism attraction. This is why current agricultural policies stress, at least in their spirit, the need to account for agroenvironmental indicators in order to quantify the impacts of agriculture on the environment and to shift the emphasis towards payments based on environmental goods. The question that follows is: how do we measure the importance of ecosystems services for society, so we can establish concrete policy targets and, eventually, compensate farmers in an equitable way for the public goods they deliver?

Some ES of functions of agriculture, specially the cultural ones, are considered by many as incommensurable and therefore impossible to reduce to a single unique measure of value. This is why the literature recommends using a combination of biophysical, socio-cultural and economic perspectives (Rodríguez-Ortega et al., 2014).

The following case study aims to quantify in an objective and precise manner the multifunctional (socio-cultural and economic) valuation of livestock and mixed livestock-crops farming systems of Mediterranean mountain agriculture. Deliberative methods (focus groups with farmers and with non-farmers) form the basis for the selection of ES relevant for society. A survey-based stated preference method was used to rank these ES and obtain their economic value according to the willingness to pay of i) the local residents of the study area, and ii) the general population in the region where the study area was located. Respondents were presented with different policy scenarios that produced various levels of ES provision, defined in sound biophysical terms. A full explanation of the methodology, results obtained and implications can be obtained from Bernués et al. (2014). This study was used to create a conceptual framework for market-driven development of value chains for animal food products through the ecosystem service concept.

5.1 Mediterranean mountain agriculture

Traditional agricultural activities have suffered a notorious recession in recent decades in many Euro-Mediterranean regions. This recession has originated changes in the type and intensity of land utilization such as intensification of the management system, reduction of grazing and abandonment of remote rangeland areas. Consequently, a general process of vegetation encroachment and landscape closure is happening. The Sierra y Cañones de Guara Natural Park (SCGNP) is a protected mountain area located in Northeast Spain that constitutes a representative example Mediterranean mountain agroecosystem. The park constitutes a Special Protected Area (EU Birds Directive) that includes three Sites of Community Importance (EU Habitats Directive). Originally created to protect scavengers, which are highly dependent on carcasses of domestic animals for feeding, the park attracts many visitors due to its rich geological (canyons, caves, etc.), cultural (prehistoric and megalithic art, traditional buildings, villages) and natural (endangered species, diversity of landscapes, scavengers and other birds of prey, etc.) heritage. Today, about 50% of the park is private and communal shrub rangelands and the main agricultural activity is grazing livestock (32,651 meat sheep, 700 goats, 1,199 beef cattle and 259 mares), with some agriculture (mostly olive trees and cereals) in more favourable areas. The degree of integration between animals, natural resources and crops is very high, with animals using a wide diversity of resources throughout the year (Box 5.3).

BOX 5.3 GRAZING CALENDAR OF A REPRESENTATIVE MIXED SHEEP-CEREAL FARM IN SIERRA Y CAÑONES DE GUARA NATURAL PARK

A wide variety of resources is used throughout the year by the flock, depending on requirements of animals with different physiological status (lactating, gestating, etc.) and availability of pastures, forages and crops. Livestock and agriculture practices are closely interconnected: e.g. manure is the main fertilizer of crops, the cultivation of sorghum and forage turnips provides animal feed when other resources are scarce and helps to control weeds without using pesticides in crop rotations. This integration has major implications in terms of management, labour demand and organization (sometimes in competition with tourism activities) and production, with a wide diversity of specific quality products linked to the territory (lamb meat, cheese, olive oil, etc.) that are highly valued.

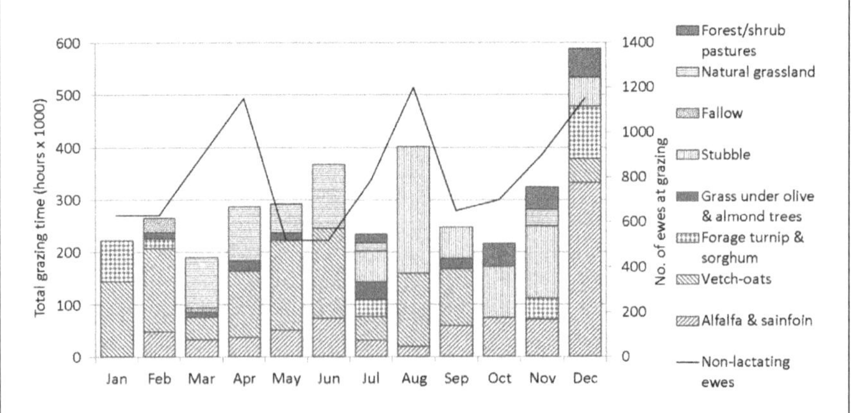

FIGURE 5.5 Grazing calendar of a representative mixed sheep-cereal farm in Sierra y Cañones de Guara Natural Park Choice experiment. The actual choice sets presented to respondents used different combinations of ES levels in the liberalization and targeted support scenarios.

Source: Bernués et al. (2014)

5.2 Socio-cultural and economic valuation of ecosystem services

The deliberative research approach showed that the most important ES in SCGNP were (in descending order): aesthetic value (landscape/vegetation), provision of food (mainly discussed in terms of quality and safety of products), gene pool protection (biodiversity maintenance), life cycle maintenance (nutrient cycling, photosynthesis), provision of raw materials (mainly forage and firewood), disturbance prevention (forest fires), water purification/waste management (with water pollution attached to industrial livestock systems as opposed to grazing ones), soil fertility/erosion prevention and other cultural ES such as spiritual experience, recreation and culture (Figure 5.6). There were some differences between the perceptions of farmers and those of urban citizens. Farmers gave more importance to regulating ES, such as disturbance prevention (forest fires) and soil fertility/erosion prevention, the provision of raw materials and supporting ES. These ES were directly related to their own farming activity or to local circumstances and interests. Urban citizens showed more general concerns and gave more importance to all cultural ES, in particular opportunities for recreation, spiritual and cultural experiences and to the provision of food, mainly relating to quality and safety issues.

In a second stage, local and general population respondents were asked to choose their most preferred policy scenario to deliver ES among three alternatives. The status quo scenario corresponded to the current policy applied in the area of study with the actual level of ES previously identified, whereas the liberalization

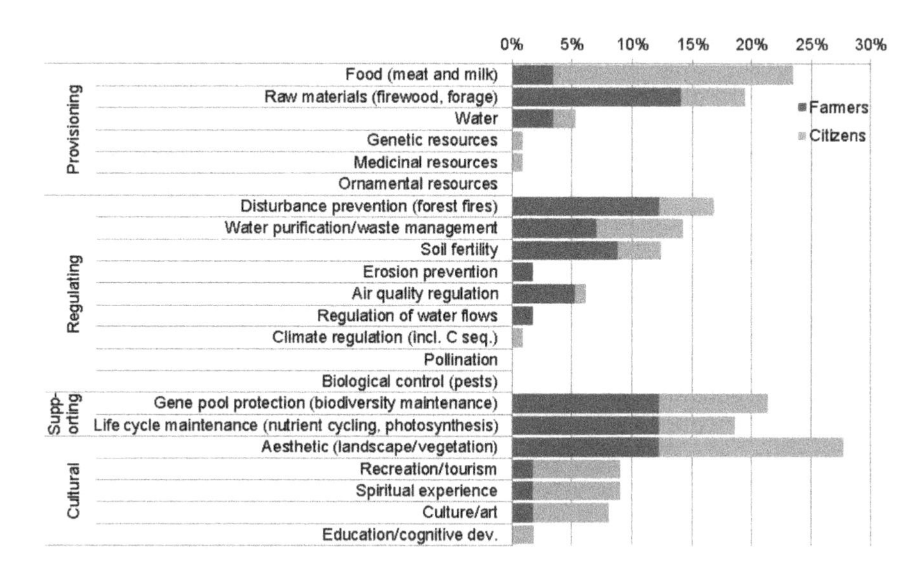

FIGURE 5.6 Relative importance of ecosystem services delivered by Mediterranean grazing agroecosystems according to the number of times they were mentioned during the FG with farmers and non-farmers

Source: Bernués et al. (2014)

TABLE 5.3 Choice experiment. The actual choice sets presented to respondents used different combination ES levels in the liberalization and targeted support scenarios (adapted from Bernués et al., 2014).

Choice	*Liberalization*	*Targeted support*	*Current policy*
Landscape			
Bushes	+++	+	+
Meadows and crops	+	+	No change
Wildlife (bearded vulture)	7 pairs	15 pairs	11 pairs
Forest fires/year	6	2	4
Quality products linked to territory	2	6	4
	Sheep cheese	Sheep cheese	Sheep cheese
	Lamb meat	Lamb meat	Lamb meat
		Organic lamb	Pasture pork
		Pasture pork	Olive oil
		Pasture beef	
		Olive oil	
Annual cost €	15	75	45

(reduction of agroenvironmental support) and targeted support (additional funding to agroenvironmental schemes) scenarios represented lower and higher levels of ES delivery respectively (see Table 5.3).

From analysis of responses we obtained a ranking of ecosystem services and the willingness of society to pay for their delivery. The prevention of forest fires (≈50% of total willingness to pay) was valued by the general population as a key ecosystem service delivered by mountain agroecosystems, followed by the production of specific quality products linked to the territory (≈20%), biodiversity (≈20%) and cultural landscapes (≈10%). The value given by local residents to the last two ecosystem services differed considerably (≈10% and 25% for biodiversity and cultural landscape, respectively). The comparatively low importance assigned to these ES could be because their consequences for human well-being are not immediate or not easily perceived. From the analysis of data we estimated the Total Economic Value[1] of Mediterranean mountain agroecosystems to be ≈120€ per person per year, three times the current level of support of agroenvironmental schemes (Table 5.4).

Clearly there has to be an element of subjectivity in the estimation of TEV. Nevertheless we believe that we are justified in concluding from this study:

1 There has been a large underestimation of the socio-cultural and economic values of ecosystem services of Mediterranean grazing agroecosystems, the welfare loss linked to further abandonment in these areas and the cost of inaction;

TABLE 5.4 Willingness to pay (WTP) (€ person^{-1} year^{-1}) and composition of Total Economic Value (TEV). Source: Bernués et al. (2014).

ES	*Value component of TEV*	*General population*			*Local population*		
		WTP	*%*	*Rank*	*WTP*	*%*	*Rank*
Landscape	Non-extractive direct use	10.0	8.2	4	49.5	25.2	3
Biodiversity	Non-use existence	22.2	18.3	3	17.4	8.8	4
Forest fires	Indirect use	64.4	53.2	1	79.3	40.3	1
Product quality	Extractive direct use	24.5	20.2	2	50.6	25.7	2
TEV		121.2	100.0		196.8	100.0	

2 The willingness of the population (both local and general) to pay for the provision of ES derived from Mediterranean mountain animal agriculture clearly exceeds the current level of public support in Europe; and
3 There is room to enlarge the economic resources dedicated to agroenvironmental schemes that currently support farmers in a horizontal manner, and to better target environmental objectives, allowing these schemes to become Payments for Ecosystem Services.

Finally, it is important to note that the ES that are relevant for people can vary across regions, socio-economic and policy contexts, and cultural backgrounds (Randall, 2002). The valuation exercise explained above is context specific and generalization should be approached with caution. However, the study has been replicated under the contrasting conditions of Nordic countries with similar results (Bernués et al., 2015a).

5.3 Value chains based on ecosystem services: "from landscape to fork"

Apart from public intervention through government-based agroenvironmental policies, the market could also contribute to maintaining grazing livestock and grassland agroecosystems with further development of differentiated value chains. This could be done by linking agricultural landscapes (grazing agroecosystems) with consumers and citizens. I present now a conceptual "from landscape to fork" framework for novel food-value chains. The concept moves beyond the classic "from farm to fork" approach by placing the farm (or the food system) as in intermediary between agroecosystems and society. These three main components can be affected by markets, policies and other general drivers (Figure 5.7).

The first component of our framework is the agricultural landscape – in our case the grassland agroecosystems that provide a wide variety of ES to farmers (e.g. forage) and society in general (explained in previous sections). The second

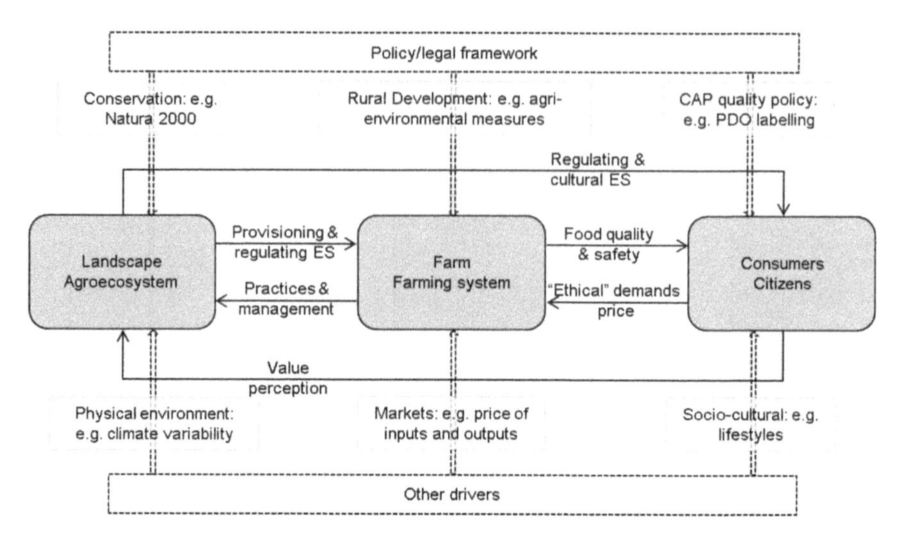

FIGURE 5.7 Scheme of the "landscape to fork" approach

Source: (Bernués et al., 2015b)

component is the farmer and his or her farm that benefits from provisioning and non-provisioning (regulating, supporting) services from the agroecosystem and, at the same time, affects the agroecosystem with particular agricultural practices (e.g. transhumance, extended grazing periods, crop rotation). The farm provides specific quality products that can be linked to the particular agricultural landscape or agroecosystem in which it is located. The third component is the consumer, and more generally society at large, which increasingly shows "ethical" concerns about the model of agriculture and the food chain. Consumers' demands for differentiated quality food products has been widely discussed in the literature. In meat, the increasing importance of extrinsic quality attributes (related to health and safety concerns of consumers or the growing interest in personal "stories" linked to food and consumption experiences) and concerns for the animals' welfare and the environment constitute two of the main future trends with regard to meat consumption (Grunert, 2006). This opens up an opportunity for extensive livestock farmers willing to move from the standard bulk production of meat to differentiated, value-added products, capable of exploiting the possibilities of alternative ways of producing food in a way that adds to consumer well-being.

6. Towards sustainable animal agriculture

Today, ***sustainable intensification*** of animal production, understood as increasing food production from existing farmland while minimizing pressure on the environment, is perceived by many as the main, if not the only, pathway to feed an increasing world population. Sustainable intensification relies on increasing input efficiency and (bio-)technological innovation. Under this pathway, further industrialization and enlargement of operations can be expected. However, sustainability is not just a matter of production; by definition, sustainable development must embrace economic, environmental and social aspects at the farm and food chain levels. Even if sustainable intensification could also be understood as an increase of environmental services per hectare (Buckwell et al., 2014), social sustainability issues are normally ignored. Therefore, a broader view suggests that sustainable intensification cannot be a meaningful goal without regard for who intensifies, where and who benefits from the changes (Hanspach et al., 2013).

There is also a general consensus on the need to reduce food waste in our food system and, in developed economies, to modify human diets by reducing the consumption of meat (especially from ruminants) to increase the sustainability of the whole food system. However, as we have mentioned, performance of animal agriculture in terms of sustainability will depend on the metrics we use to measure efficiency of the food system. Due to the increasing scarcity of fossil fuels and the imperative need to reduce their use, the amount of renewable or non-renewable energy that has been used to generate a particular agricultural product or service constitutes a key indicator. Emergy analysis (Odum, 1996) refers to the energy memory or embodied energy of a product or process. It computes the different qualities of energies involved in the processes of production in one type of energy unit (usually solar energy), allowing for comparison across production systems. An application of energy accounting to dairy systems with different levels of intensity can be obtained from Vigne et al. (2013).

An alternative approach to analyze sustainability is to move from kg of meat produced per animal to number of nourished people per ha – in other words, move the role of animals in the food system from a source of high-quality protein to uses or resources that cannot be otherwise be used for food production (Schader et al., 2015). These authors have recently shown that combining the change of consumption patterns and the reduction of feed components that compete with human nutrition to raise animals can constitute an alternative pathway to significantly reducing the environmental impacts of livestock production (GHG emission −18%, arable land occupation −26%, N surplus −46%, P surplus −40%, non-renewable energy use −36%, pesticide use −22%, fresh water use −21% and soil erosion potential −12%) while providing sufficient energy and protein for humans. This sustainability pathway would mean a significant increase of ruminants on grasslands and a drastic reduction of monogastrics, which would be fed with by-products and food waste. The study underlines the need to link the discussion of sustainable food production and ***sustainable food consumption***.

6.1 Designing novel grazing livestock systems

Many voices call for a change of paradigm in agriculture, moving away from the current one-size-fits-all linear model towards more localized, diversified, circular farming systems, based on renewable resources. Under this paradigm, agroecology then acquires a central role in the design of livestock systems, which are expected to provide not only food but also a wide range of other services and benefits to society.

Agroecology has been defined as a scientific discipline that applies ecological theory to the design and management of agroecosystems in order to enhance their sustainability (Altieri, 1987). Later, agroecology emerged as a social movement comprising a set of "sustainable" agricultural practices, and more recently the concept widened to encompass the whole food chain, from food production to distribution and consumption (Wezel et al., 2009). The integration of animals in agroecosystems can make the difference in realizing the long-term ecological sustainability and socio-economic viability goals of animal agriculture (Gliessman, 2015), which needs to be reconfigured to minimize its negative impacts, produce food and other ecosystem services and increase their adaptive capacity to face an increasingly uncertain future (markets volatility, climate variability, shifts in dietary preferences, food security) (Dumont and Bernués, 2014). To extend ecological thinking into animal production systems, Dumont et al. (2013) illustrated the five principles of agroecology, adapted to animal production systems. These principles are:

- Adopt management practices aiming to improve animal health;
- Decrease the external inputs needed for production;
- Decrease pollution by optimizing the metabolic functioning (i.e. key ecological processes) of farming systems;
- Enhance diversity within animal production systems to strengthen their resilience; and
- Preserve biological diversity in agroecosystems by adapting management practices.

Mixed integrated farms have the highest potential to enhance these agroecological principles at the farm and local levels. Animals and crops perform different functions and can produce beneficial synergies between them, due to the movement of energy, nutrients and cash between the two components (see Box 5.3 for an example). The different types of integrated systems that exist in the world and the beneficial roles of animals in these systems are explained in detail by Gliessman (2015) (Chapter 19). These roles include: production of protein-rich foods, utilization of crop residues and by-products, recycling of nutrients to soil and improve soil health, shaping of vegetation, reduction of pesticide use, provision of a wide diversity of ecosystem services. In socio-economic terms, mixed farming can reduce economic vulnerability by spreading the risk among activities and improve adaptive capacity towards uncertain market and climate conditions. Additionally, mixed crop-livestock systems constitute the backbone of smallholder agriculture around the world, producing about half of the world's food, contributing to poverty alleviation (Herrero et al., 2010). Recent studies propose the shift to mixed systems as the better adaptation strategy to climate change, reducing the pressure on tropical forests, increasing market orientation and improving rural livelihoods in the world's less developed regions (Weindl et al., 2015).

Feed self-sufficiency and diversification of feed resources are key factors for economic and environmental performance in real mixed animal-crop farms. Unless these are optimized, specialized farms are likely to be more efficient, as shown, for example, in Veysset et al. (2011) in beef systems in France. In this study, *organic farming* is described as a prototype of integrated livestock-crop agriculture that meets the core principles of agroecology. The economic and environmental advantages derived from input self-sufficiency (specially for feed) and diversity of resources have been demonstrated also in dairy cattle (Lebacq et al., 2015) and in sheep systems (Benoit et al., 2009).

Summing up, designing sustainable animal production systems able to adapt to varying types of disturbances (economic and biophysical) will demand a paradigm shift in scientific focus. We should quickly move towards holistic and interdisciplinary research methods, involving different disciplines, ecology, economics and social. The consideration of various temporal and spatial (beyond the farm) scales is required to understand the relationships between human activities (production and consumption) and the biophysical processes involved. However, it is at the farm level where the decision-making takes place and where most policies should be targeted in order to be effective. Therefore, a new approach for the whole research-development-innovation chain should be explored to bridge the gap between science and practice (Dumont and Bernués, 2014).

6.2 Implications for policy design

Policies trying to solve the agriculture-nature conflict can be organized around three approaches (Tanentzap et al., 2015): regulatory (e.g. limits on pesticide use); community-based (e.g. promoting partnerships between different stakeholders); and economic, which either compensates farmers for the public goods they deliver ("provider gets" principle) or internalizes environmental costs ("polluter pays" principle), for example establishing taxes. I shall briefly discuss the last two approaches, which could be considered two sides of the same coin, since resources to pay for ecosystem services delivered by certain farming systems could be obtained from taxes on negative externalities produced in other farming systems.

Payments for ecosystem services (PES) can be implemented to promote the delivery of public goods by farmers. For any PES system to be effective, non-provisioning ES (public goods) must be incorporated into decision making, and agricultural policies should not focus only on provisioning of food and other animal products. As many ES (e.g. spiritual values, cognitive development, and certain regulating and supporting services) cannot be readily translated into monetary values, or doing so can be undesirable, the socio-cultural values of ES need to be considered. Any PES system should be based on existing scientific evidence about the effects of agricultural practices and land management regimes on the environment, and prioritized across different agroecosystems and regions. However, the socio-cultural, economic and biophysical contexts across different sites strongly influence public perception on the value of ES (e.g. the prevention of forest fires is key in Mediterranean countries but not in northern Alpine areas) and therefore policy design needs to be flexible.

Research has shown that there is a large underestimation of the socio-cultural and economic values of ecosystem services of grassland agro-ecosystems, the welfare loss linked to further environmental degradation due to further abandonment of these areas, and the cost of inaction. By individualizing support, monitoring objective indicators for ecosystem services and targeting particular agricultural practices, the so-called "green" subsidies may truly become rewards for the delivery of public goods to society.

Internalization of animal production externalities requires the quantification of all direct and indirect (external) costs. There is an increasing acknowledgement of the limitations of the cost-benefit framework as a measure of sustainability (Bebbington et al., 2007) and alternative approaches, such as full-cost accounting, might correct these limitations, contributing to shifts in policy making. The effects of a diet with an excess of (processed) meat on the environment and on human health are widely reported; however, very few studies quantity the economic cost of the health care or the environmental burden derived from this excess of meat consumption in developed countries, and neither do they consider the widely divergent benefits and costs of industrial vs. grassland-based animal production systems. Because health and environmental costs are externalized, the price of meat produced in industrial (zero-grazing) systems is artificially low.

7. Conclusion

The role of meat and other animal products to satisfy the demands of society, and the consequences of different ways of production for the environment is, and will continue to be, a complicated and controversial matter. However, if we pose a simple question to the reader so he or she can contribute to more sustainable animal agriculture, this question could be: how do we behave as "concerned" consumers (and citizens)? In my view, the right answer is "eating less, better (pasture-based) meat".

Note

1 The Total Economic Value (TEV) refers to all aggregated values provided by a particular (agro)ecosystem. The TEV taxonomy includes different *use* and *non-use* values. Use values can be split into direct (extractive resources used directly such as fish, timber, etc.) and indirect (non-extractive services used indirectly such as recreation). Non-use values do not involve direct or indirect use of the ecosystem, but reflect value of future use or the satisfaction that individuals derive from its existence (e.g. intrinsic value of diversity of species) (Rodríguez-Ortega et al., 2014).

References

Altieri, M.A., 1987. *Agroecology: The scientific basis of alternative agriculture.* Westview Press, Boulder, CO.

Bebbington, J., Brown, J., Frame, B., 2007. Accounting technologies and sustainability assessment models. *Ecological Economics* 61, 224–236.

Benoit, M., Tournadre, H., Dulphy, J.P., Laignel, G., Prache, S., Cabaret, J., 2009. Is intensification of reproduction rhythm sustainable in an organic sheep production system? A 4-year interdisciplinary study. *Animal* 3, 753–763.

Bernués, A., Olaizola, A., Corcoran, K., 2003. Extrinsic attributes of red meat as indicators of quality in Europe: An application for market segmentation. *Food Quality and Preference* 14, 265–276.

Bernués, A., Rodríguez-Ortega, T., Alfnes, F., Clemetsen, M., Eik, L.O., 2015a. Quantifying the multifunctionality of fjord and mountain agriculture by means of sociocultural and economic valuation of ecosystem services. *Land Use Policy* 48, 170–178.

Bernués, A., Rodríguez-Ortega, T., Olaizola, A., 2015b. From landscape to fork: Value chains based on ecosystem services FAO-CIHEAM Network on Sheep and Goats (Joint seminar of the Productions Systems and Nutrition sub-networks). FAO-CIHEHAM, Montpellier, France, p. 10.

Bernués, A., Rodríguez-Ortega, T., Ripoll-Bosch, R., Alfnes, F., 2014. Socio-cultural and economic valuation of ecosystem services provided by Mediterranean mountain agroecosystems. *Plos One* 9, e102479.

Bernués, A., Ruiz, R., Olaizola, A., Villalba, D., Casasús, I., 2011. Sustainability of pasture-based livestock farming systems in the European Mediterranean context: Synergies and trade-offs. *Livestock Science* 139, 44–57.

Broom, D.M., Galindo, F.A., Murgueitio, E., 2013. Sustainable, efficient livestock production with high biodiversity and good welfare for animals. *Proceedings of the Royal Society B: Biological Sciences* 280: 20132025.

Buckwell, A., Heissenhuber, A., Blum, W., 2014. The sustainable intensification of European agriculture. A Review Sponsored by the RISE Foundation.

Casasús, I., Bernués, A., Sanz, A., Villalba, D., Riedel, J.L., Revilla, R., 2007. Vegetation dynamics in Mediterranean forest pastures as affected by beef cattle grazing. *Agriculture, Ecosystem, and Environment* 121, 365–370.

Cooper, T., Hart, K., Baldock, D., 2009. *Provision of public goods through agriculture in the European union.* Institute for European Environmental Policy, London.

Dodd, J.L., 1994. Desertification and degradation in sub-Saharan Africa: The role of livestock. *BioScience* 44, 28–34.

Dumont, B., Bernués, A., 2014. Editorial: Agroecology for producing goods and services in sustainable animal farming systems. *Animal* 8, 1201–1203.

Dumont, B., Fortun-Lamothe, L., Jouven, M., Thomas, M., Tichit, M., 2013. Prospects from agroecology and industrial ecology for animal production in the 21st century. *Animal* 7, 1028–1043.

EEA, 2004. *High nature value farmland: Characteristics, trends and policy challenges.* European Environmental Agency, Copenhagen, p. 27.

European_Commission, 2011. Our life insurance, our natural capital: An EU biodiversity strategy to 2020, Communication from the Commission to the European Parliament, the Council, the Economic and Social Committee and the Committee of the Regions, COM (2011) 244, p. 17.

Fonderflick, J., Caplat, P., Lovaty, F., Thévenot, M., Prodon, R., 2010. Avifauna trends following changes in a Mediterranean upland pastoral system. *Agriculture, Ecosystem and Environment* 137, 337–347.

French, P., Stanton, C., Lawless, F., O'Riordan, E.G., Monahan, F.J., Caffrey, P.J., Moloney, A.P., 2000. Fatty acid composition, including conjugated linoleic acid, of intramuscular fat from steers offered grazed grass, grass silage, or concentrate-based diets. *Journal of Animal Science* 78, 2849–2855.

Gerber, P., 2010. *Livestock in a changing landscape, volume 2: Experiences and regional perspectives.* Island Press, Washington, DC.

Gliessman, S.R., 2015. *Agroecology: The ecology of sustainable food systems.* CRC Press, Boca Raton, p. 364.

Goers, L., Lawson, J., Garen, E., 2012. Economic Drivers of Tropical Deforestation for Agriculture, in: Ashton, S.M., Tyrrell, L.M., Spalding, D., Gentry, B. (Eds.), *Managing forest carbon in a changing climate.* Springer, Dordrecht, Netherlands, pp. 305–320.

Grunert, K.G., 2006. Future trends and consumer lifestyles with regard to meat consumption. *Meat Science* 74, 149–160.

Hanspach, J., Abson, D.J., Loos, J., Tichit, M., Chappell, M.J., Fischer, J., 2013. Develop, then intensify. *Science* 341, 713.

Henle, K., Alard, D., Clitherow, J., Cobb, P., Firbank, L., Kull, T., McCracken, D., Moritz, R.F.A., Niemelä, J., Rebane, M., Wascher, D., Watt, A., Young, J., 2008. Identifying and managing the conflicts between agriculture and biodiversity conservation in Europe – a review. *Agriculture, Ecosystems and Environment* 124, 60–71.

Herrero, M., Thornton, P.K., Notenbaert, A.M., Wood, S., Msangi, S., Freeman, H.A., Bossio, D., Dixon, J., Peters, M., Steeg, J. van de, Lynam, J., Rao, P.P., Macmillan, S., Gerard, B., McDermott, J., Sere, C., Rosegrant, M., 2010. Smart investments in sustainable food production: Revisiting mixed crop-livestock systems. *Science* 327, 822–825.

Herrero, M., Wirsenius, S., Henderson, B., Rigolot, C., Thornton, P., Havlík, P., Boer, I. de, Gerber, P., 2015. Livestock and the environment: What have we learned in the past decade? *Annual Review of Environment and Resources* 40, 177–202.

Huston, M., 1979. A general hypothesis of species diversity. *The American Naturalist* 113, 81–101.

IAASTD, 2009. *Agriculture at a crossroads.* International Assessment of Agricultural Knowledge, Science and Technology for Development, Washington, DC, p. 95.

Lambin, E.F., Turner, B.L., Geist, H.J., Agbola, S.B., Angelsen, A., Bruce, J.W., Coomes, O.T., Dirzo, R., Fischer, G., Folke, C., George, P.S., Homewood, K., Imbernon, J., Leemans, R., Li, X., Moran, E.F., Mortimore, M., Ramakrishnan, P.S., Richards, J.F., Skånes, H., Steffen, W., Stone, G.D., Svedin, U., Veldkamp, T.A., Vogel, C., Xu, J., 2001. The causes of land-use and land-cover change: Moving beyond the myths. *Global Environmental Change* 11, 261–270.

Lebacq, T., Baret, P.V., Stilmant, D., 2015. Role of input self-sufficiency in the economic and environmental sustainability of specialised dairy farms. *Animal* 9, 544–552.

Mertens, B., Poccard-Chapuis, R., Piketty, M.G., Lacques, A.E., Venturieri, A., 2002. Crossing spatial analyses and livestock economics to understand deforestation processes in the Brazilian Amazon: The case of São Félix do Xingú in South Pará. *Agricultural Economics* 27, 269–294.

Nguyen, T.T.H., Doreau, M., Eugène, M., Corson, M.S., Garcia-Launay, F., Chesneau, G., Van Der Werf, H.M.G., 2013. Effect of farming practices for greenhouse gas mitigation and subsequent alternative land use on environmental impacts of beef cattle production systems. *Animal* 7, 860–869.

Nguyen, T.T.H., Van Der Werf, H.M.G., Doreau, M., 2012. Life cycle assessment of three bull-fattening systems: Effect of impact categories on ranking. *Journal of Agricultural Science* 150, 755–763.

Odum, H.T., 1996. *Environmental accounting: Emergy and environmental decision making.* John Wiley and Sons, New York.

Olea, P.P., Mateo-Tomas, P., 2009. The role of traditional farming practices in ecosystem conservation: The case of transhumance and vultures. *Biological Conservation* 142, 1844–1853.

Oteros-Rozas, E., Martín-López, B., González, J., Plieninger, T., López, C., Montes, C., 2013. Socio-cultural valuation of ecosystem services in a transhumance social-ecological network. *Regional Environmental Change* 1–21.

Oxbrough, A.G., Gittings, T., O'Halloran, J., Giller, P.S., Kelly, T.C., 2006. The initial effects of afforestation on the ground-dwelling spider fauna of Irish peatlands and grasslands. *Forest Ecology and Management* 237, 478–491.

Plieninger, T., Bieling, C., Fagerholm, N., Byg, A., Hartel, T., Hurley, P., López-Santiago, C.A., Nagabhatla, N., Oteros-Rozas, E., Raymond, C.M., Horst, D. van der, Huntsinger, L., 2015. The role of cultural ecosystem services in landscape management and planning. *Current Opinion in Environmental Sustainability* 14, 28–33.

Randall, A., 2002. Valuing the outputs of multifunctional agriculture. *European Review of Agricultural Economics* 29, 289–307.

Renting, H., Rossing, W.A., Groot, J.C., Van der Ploeg, J.D., Laurent, C., Perraud, D., Stobbelaar, D.J., Van Ittersum, M.K., 2009. Exploring multifunctional agriculture: A review of conceptual approaches and prospects for an integrative transitional framework. *Journal of Environmental Management* 90 Suppl 2, S112–123.

Riedel, J.L., Casasús, I., Bernués, A., 2007. Sheep farming intensification and utilization of natural resources in a Mediterranean pastoral agro-ecosystem. *Livestock Science* 111, 153–163.

Ripoll-Bosch, R., Boer, I.J.M. de, Bernues, A., Vellinga, T.V., 2013. Accounting for multi-functionality of sheep farming in the carbon footprint of lamb: A comparison of three contrasting Mediterranean systems. *Agricultural Systems* 116, 60–68.

Ripoll-Bosch, R., Díez-Unquera, B., Ruiz, R., Villalba, D., Molina, E., Joy, M., Olaizola, A., Bernués, A., 2012. An integrated sustainability assessment of Mediterranean sheep farms with different degrees of intensification. *Agricultural Systems* 105, 46–56.

Rodríguez-Ortega, T., Oteros-Rozas, E., Ripoll-Bosch, R., Tichit, M., Martín-López, B., Bernues, A., 2014. Applying the ecosystem services framework to pasture-based livestock farming systems in Europe. *Animal* 8, 1–12.

Schader, C., Muller, A., Scialabba, N.E.-H., Hecht, J., Isensee, A., Erb, K.-H., Smith, P., Makkar, H.P.S., Klocke, P., Leiber, F., Schwegler, P., Stolze, M., Niggli, U., 2015. Impacts of feeding less food-competing feedstuffs to livestock on global food system sustainability. *Journal of The Royal Society Interface* 12, 20150891.

Secretariat of the Convention on Biological Diversity, 2010. Global Biodiversity Outlook 3, Montréal, p. 94.

Soussana, J.F., Tallec, T., Blanfort, V., 2010. Mitigating the greenhouse gas balance of ruminant production systems through carbon sequestration in grasslands. *Animal* 4, 334–350.

Steinfeld, H., Gerber, P., 2010. Livestock production and the global environment: Consume less or produce better? *Proceedings of the National Academy of Sciences* 107, 18237–18238.

Steinfeld, H., Gerber, P., Wassenaar, T., Castel, V., Rosales, M., Haan, C.D., 2006. *Livestock's long shadow: Environmental issues and options.* Food and Agriculture Organization of the United Nations, Rome, p. 390.

Tanentzap, A.J., Lamb, A., Walker, S., Farmer, A., 2015. Resolving conflicts between agriculture and the natural environment. *PLoS Biology* 13, e1002242.

Veysset, P., Lherm, M., Bébin, D., 2011. Productive, environmental and economic performances assessments of organic and conventional suckler cattle farming systems. *Organic Agriculture* 1, 1–16.

Vigne, M., Peyraud, J.-L., Lecomte, P., Corson, M.S., Wilfart, A., 2013. Emergy evaluation of contrasting dairy systems at multiple levels. *Journal of Environmental Management* 129, 44–53.

Vries, M. de, Middelaar, C.E. van, Boer, I.J.M. de, 2015. Comparing environmental impacts of beef production systems: A review of life cycle assessments. *Livestock Science* 178, 279–288.

Weber, K.T., Horst, S., 2011. Desertification and livestock grazing: The roles of sedentarization, mobility and rest. *Pastoralism* 1, 1–11.

Weindl, I., Lotze-Campen, H., Popp, A., Müller, C., Havlík, P., Herrero, M., Schmitz, C., Rolinski, S., 2015. Livestock in a changing climate: Production system transitions as an adaptation strategy for agriculture. *Environmental Research Letters* 10, 094021.

Wezel, A., Bellon, S., Doré, T., Francis, C., Vallod, D., David, C., 2009. Agroecology as a science, a movement and a practice: A review. *Agronomy for Sustainable Development* 29, 503–515.

Wilkinson, J.M., 2011. Re-defining efficiency of feed use by livestock. *Animal* 5, 1014–1022.

Zanten, H.H.E. van, Mollenhorst, H., Klootwijk, C.W., Middelaar, C.E. van, Boer, I.J.M. de, 2015. Global food supply: Land use efficiency of livestock systems. *International Journal of Life Cycle Assessment* 21, 747–758.

Zhang, W., Ricketts, T.H., Kremen, C., Carney, K., Swinton, S.M., 2007. Ecosystem services and dis-services to agriculture. *Ecological Economics* 64, 253–260.

6

THE IMPORTANCE OF GRAZING LIVESTOCK FOR SOIL AND FOOD SYSTEM RESILIENCE

Richard Young

I am a farmer. Inevitably that means I am not an impartial observer. But I hope to demonstrate without bias the extent to which prevailing attitudes and some associated analyses and initiatives intended to make food production and consumption more sustainable fail to take account of several significant issues. Paramount amongst these are the importance of grass and grazing animals for long-term food system security.

During the last decade something close to a consensus has emerged amongst scientists and campaigners, that the best way to reduce greenhouse gas emissions from agriculture, make food production more sustainable and benign, and at the same time address the increasingly serious problem of diet-related disease, is for us all to eat less meat and dairy products.

Critical attention has focused on the problems associated with cattle and sheep, more than on those associated with pigs and poultry. Cattle, sheep and other grazing animals are identified as particularly significant contributors to global warming because they emit the potent greenhouse gas (GHG) methane (CH4), the atmospheric concentration of which now stands at 1.8 ppm – more than 2.5 times pre-industrial levels. While the amount appears small compared with the 400 ppm of carbon dioxide (CO2) in the atmosphere, CH4 is a much more potent GHG than CO2, now calculated to have a global warming potential at least 28 times greater than CO2 over 100 years and 82 times greater over 20 years (IPCC 2014).

Uniquely amongst the three major GHGs, CH4 only persists in the atmosphere for about a decade before most of it is broken down to CO2 and water. Unfortunately, the total amount of CH4 produced most years, from natural and anthropogenic sources, slightly exceeds the capacity of the two major CH4 sinks to break it down – 95 per cent, chemical reactions in the atmosphere, 5 per cent, the energy source of soil methanotrophic bacteria, a sink significantly reduced by the conversion of forests and grasslands to crop production and by ammonium-based nitrogenous fertilisers (Willison et al. 1995, Nazaries et al. 2013). As a result, the atmospheric CH4 level keeps rising.

With methane in mind, Ripple et al. (2014) called for significant reductions in global ruminant numbers, based on the argument that because CH4 has a much shorter life in the atmosphere than the other major GHGs, reducing emissions today would lead to lower atmospheric levels within a decade or two, whereas they argue that much of the CO2 already in the atmosphere will persist for a century or more, unless or until a technological solution is found to remove it. They justify their exclusive focus on ruminants by claiming they are the biggest human-induced source of methane, and explain that a rapid reduction in ruminant numbers globally might just be enough to prevent the planet exceeding fast-approaching climate change tipping points, at least in the short term.

It is worth noting, however, that ruminants only constitute the largest anthropogenic source of methane if one makes an artificial sub-division between methane associated with oil and gas and methane from coal. As their own data show, fossil fuels together are responsible for up to a third more methane than ruminants. Ruminants also only recycle carbon recently photosynthesised from the atmosphere by the plants they eat, whereas fossil fuels inevitably put additional carbon into the atmosphere, as both CO2 and CH4. This becomes particularly significant when one compares the use of forage legumes such as clover with fertiliser nitrogen as sources of nitrogen fertility in agriculture. While the clover needs to be grazed by methane-emitting ruminants to produce food, the production of nitrogen fertiliser is exclusively based on fossil fuel use. In addition, recent research, based on the different combinations of the carbon isotopes C12 and C14 found in methane from different sources, has established that the proportion of CH4 in the atmosphere from fossil fuel extraction, transport and use, and from geological seepage, has been under-estimated by 60–110 per cent, with that from fossil fuels alone under-estimated by 20–60 per cent. The research also finds that the proportion that has come from microbial sources, such as wetlands, ruminants and rice production has been over-estimated by 25 per cent (Schweitzke et al. 2016). Reviewing similar studies, in combination with the latitudinal distribution of CH4, Nisbet et al. (2016) conclude that recent increases in atmospheric CH4 levels, averaging 6 ppb p.a., after a period between 1999 and 2006 when they rose by an average of less than 1 ppb p.a. (NOAA undated), has predominantly been caused by the expansion of wetlands in tropical regions, due to higher than average rainfall.

Livestock trends and meat consumption

For some years, concerns have been raised by the rapid expansion of cattle farming in Brazil, especially on land cleared from former rainforest. Brazil has the second highest cattle population globally (after India) with over 190 million cattle, and beef production increased from 1.4 to 9.6 million tonnes between 1964 and 2014 (FAOSTAT). Most of this has been on land cleared from forest and savanna and is associated with major negative externalities, especially GHG emissions and biodiversity losses. The FAO's influential 2006 report Livestock's Long Shadow calculated that livestock are responsible for 18 per cent of global GHG emissions and almost half (48 per cent) of this figure came from estimation of the GHGs associated with the destruction of rainforest and other virgin land in South America to create new pastures and grow crops to feed farm animals. But while a high proportion of the initial deforestation was associated with cattle, since the mid-1990s, arable farming (much of it on former pastoral land) has been growing much more rapidly than cattle production. Between 1994 and 2014, the arable land area in Brazil increased by 27 million hectares, grazing land by 5 million hectares. Only 13 per cent of Brazil's cattle are raised in feedlots, and of the extra arable cropping, soybeans, in particular, which increased in area from 11.5 to 30.5 million hectares during this period, have been used to increase exports and support a quadrupling of poultry production and a doubling of pork production over the last two decades. By 2013 Brazil was producing 12.5 million tonnes of poultry meat compared with 9.6 million tonnes of beef (FAOSTAT).

In contrast to Brazil, Argentinian beef production has only increased by approximately 5 per cent over the last 30 years, and has slightly declined in recent years. Whereas pork production has more than doubled and chicken production increased six-fold during the same period, on the back of the meteoric increase in soybean production from 12,000 to 19.25 million hectares between 1964 and 2014 (FAOSTAT).

Monogastric animals, such as chickens and (to a lesser extent) pigs, produce little or no methane directly, only small amounts indirectly from manure. They also convert grain, protein feeds and water into meat much faster than cattle and sheep. As a result, estimates of the carbon footprint of chicken and pork are significantly lower than those of ruminants. A range of different figures can be found, but Ripple et al. (2014) put the carbon footprint of a kilo of chicken from intensive systems at about seven times less than that of a kilo of beef from an intensive beef system, 10 times less than beef and 12 times less than lamb from a typical grassland farm, and 17 times less than beef from extensive grazing systems, such as those found in dry rangelands.

Calculations such as these are used to underpin recommendations for general reductions in meat consumption (Popp et al. 2010, Westhoek et al. 2014); taxes on meat (Ripple et al. 2014); differential taxes of 40 per cent on beef and lamb and 9 per cent on chicken and pork (Springmann et al. 2017); and are the scientific basis for an experiment being undertaken by the supermarket Sainsbury's, to find ways to encourage consumers to eat less meat overall and specifically less beef (McKie 2017).

All these issues are given added urgency by the 400 per cent increase in global meat production over the last 40 years. During this period the global population has increased by about 250 per cent, so on average more meat per person is clearly being consumed. But while sheep production increased by only 5 per cent and beef production doubled between 1960 and 2010, both less than the population increase, more pork is eaten than any other meat and global poultry production has increased ten-fold since 1960 (Thornton 2010). Using 2002 data and trends at the time, Thornton (2010) estimated that by 2015 total annual meat consumption in developing countries would be 184 million tonnes, compared with 112 million tonnes in developed countries. However, recent trend data indicates that by 2015, global meat consumption would have reached 320 million tonnes (Poultry Site 2014), 24 million tonnes more than estimated as recently as 2010.

Global production of poultry and pork are similar, at 115 and 120 million tonnes respectively (73 per cent of all meat produced). Beef production is about 67 million tonnes, 20–25 per cent of which comes from cull dairy cows—author's estimate based on dairy cattle numbers in 2014 FAOSTAT and sheep meat production, at about 18 million tonnes, has changed little over several decades. Poultry production is also still growing at a faster rate than all other meats (Poultry Site 2014). In China, where meat consumption is expected to increase further, pork and chicken account for 65 and 15 per cent of all meat consumption, respectively.

Livestock in the drylands

Drylands are characterised by low, and often unreliable, annual rainfall. They cover 40 per cent of the land area, support 30 per cent of the global population, produce 44 per cent of the world's food and include half of all farm animals. Garnett (2010), Neely et al. (2010) and Ripple et al. (2014) are among the authors who recognise the vital importance of livestock, especially grazing animals, in drylands. The inefficiency of ruminants in drylands in terms of methane emissions per kilo of meat or litre of milk is due to the often poor quality of herbage from degraded land and the resulting low productivity, but they are, nevertheless, vital for food security in regions where droughts are frequent and crops can fail completely. Jones and Thornton (2008) suggest that as climate change increases some of the cropland in dryland regions may need to be converted to grassland with grazing animals, to improve food security.

Chatterton and Chatterton (1996) show how the high level of soil degradation in dryland regions is frequently associated with the practice of separating arable and livestock production, which has also characterised so much of global agriculture since 1950. They tell the story of how a group of farmers on degraded soils in northern Australia with declining grain yields, discovered the soil regenerating benefits of ley/arable crop rotations where the grassland phase included self-regenerating legumes, referred to as 'medics' and 'sub-clover'. The farmers had to fight a long battle with technical advisers who initially insisted that increased fertiliser use was the only solution. Eventually the advisers were convinced by the results on the ground and attempts were then made to introduce this system into other dryland regions, particularly in North Africa, where at their time of writing they had been finding only limited success. According to the authors, this was largely because almost all agronomists in the region had also been educated at colleges teaching only the techniques of specialisation and agrochemical use.

Soil degradation

Contrary to common perceptions, continuous crop production is not sustainable. This was the mistake made by a dozen past civilisations which eventually disappeared into the sand, dust and salt-contaminated soils they created (Montgomery 2007, Lal, 2015). You might think we would not be making the same mistakes today, with artificial fertilisers and advanced understanding of soil science. Far from it; we are degrading soils at a faster rate than ever before, and over the last 40 years, 430 million hectares of cropland (about one-third of all current cropland) has had to be abandoned due to soil degradation, much of it in dryland regions (Montgomery 2007).

More than half of all soils globally are now classified as moderately or severely degraded, and every year about 24 billion tonnes of soil (0.7 per cent of the total topsoil) is irrevocably lost into rivers and oceans (Montgomery 2007, UNCCD 2015, HBF and IASS 2015). This comes at an estimated annual cost to the global economy of between $6.3 and $10.6 trillion (ELD 2015). And while the problems are most acute in hot regions with erratic rainfall, they also affect temperate regions such as Europe. Smith (2004) estimated that 300 million tonnes of carbon (1.1 billion tonnes of CO2) is lost annually from European soils as far east as the Urals. Researchers from Cranfield University have estimated that soil degradation in the UK costs the British economy £1.33 billion annually (Graves et al. 2015). Dr Nigel Dunnett and colleagues have calculated that Britain has only enough soil left for 100 more harvests (Case 2014), and Professor John Crawford has calculated that the entire planet only has enough soil left to support the population for another 60 years (World Economic Forum 2012). While those crunch points may be far enough away for politicians to ignore for a little longer, we will be asking more of soils than ever before as climate change and population increase continue, but a high proportion of them are not in a condition to respond well.

Over-grazing by livestock in dry regions is also a significant cause of soil degradation. In some regions the problem is serious, but the factors that give rise to it are often more complex than they appear, as Garnett (2010) and Chatterton and Chatterton (1996) have noted. They can include land grabbing and livestock farmers being forced onto poorer lands so that the better land can be used to grow high-value vegetable and other crops, often irrigated, for export to wealthy developed countries.

The expansion of cattle farming in the Amazon has been responsible for one-eighth of all forest destruction globally in recent times (Greenpeace 2009). But while this destruction is to be bitterly regretted, there were many factors behind it, including illegal logging, the Brazilian government's financial stake in the cattle industry and its determination to increase economic output rapidly (Greenpeace 2009). However, at least the grasslands on which cattle graze are less prone to ongoing soil degradation than the croplands, which have been created in the Amazon and the Cerrado. As a result, while comparative data is lacking, it seems probable that most of the 800 million tonnes of soil lost from Brazilian farmland annually (Merton and Minella 2013) will come from cropland, rather than grassland.

Soil carbon losses risk global food security

While soils have substantial potential to remove carbon from the atmosphere and help to mitigate climate change, losses of carbon from soils under current agricultural methods, plus land use change (LUC) from primary vegetation to croplands constitute the second largest anthropogenic source of atmospheric CO2 after fossil fuels. Conversion of temperate grassland to cropland results in a 40–60 per cent loss of soil organic carbon (SOC) over several decades. Conversion of equatorial forest soil to cropland can result in a 50 per cent loss of SOC within five years (FAO 2015), while conversion to pasture generally results in lower losses (Scharlemann et al. 2014). Globally, soils have lost very large amounts of carbon over time. The FAO (2015) cites a range of estimates: 40, 55, 150, 500 and 537 billion tonnes. Lal (1999) estimated that 66–90 billion tonnes have been lost since 1850. Sousanna et al. (2009) cautiously use a figure of 50 billion tonnes, equivalent to one-fifth of the additional 110 ppm atmospheric CO2 increase since 1850 (not, of course, one-fifth of total carbon lost to the atmosphere in this time – large amounts having been taken up by the oceans with resulting acidification).

Light soils can eventually degrade to desert, while peat-based soils have by far the most carbon to lose, and under continuous arable cropping the soils themselves effectively disappear into the atmosphere in the form of CO2 and nitrous oxide (N2O). Clay soils are significantly more resilient to degradation from carbon losses, and in temperate regions typically plateau at a new level, 40 per cent lower. But losses can still continue where the carbon encapsulated in clay particles is lost through erosion. Clay soils are also vulnerable to compaction and other structural damage from heavy machinery during wet seasons. One only has to watch a few YouTube videos of farmers harvesting crops in wet seasons in European countries to get a feel for how much some heavy soils are being abused.

The decline in soil organic matter and structure can be slowed at a farm scale in several ways, including the use of green manures, but it cannot be halted, let alone reversed in commercial situations where a cash crop is needed every year.

Are no-till systems the solution?

It has frequently been claimed that arable soils under no-till systems can gain carbon. Smith (2004) provides a comprehensive analysis of potential carbon-building approaches, including zero tillage. Much of the evidence for no-till was reviewed by West and Post (2002). They found significant increases averaging 570kg/ha in the top part of the soil profile. This lent support to changes taking place in the major crop growing regions, where farm size was increasing rapidly and the labour force was declining, on the back of simplified methods of crop establishment, based on the direct drilling of crops, with weed control achieved entirely from herbicides, principally glyphosate. While no-till systems are still promoted as a way of building SOC as a result, such interpretation of the evidence has been challenged in recent years. Baker et al. (2007), Angers and Erisen-Hamel (2008) and Luo et al. (2010) all found that increases in the top part of the soil profile were invariably offset by carbon losses lower down. Powlson et al. (2014) reviewed the evidence from 43 sites in temperate regions and found that actual increases were often smaller than reported, occurred only in the top 20cm and were almost always offset by reductions between 20cm and 80cm down.

At the same time, several research groups have found that no-till production results in small decreases in crop yields of 4–9 per cent (Soane et al. 2012, Van den Putte et al, 2010, Pittelkow et al. 2014). This is potentially significant given the need to increase crop yields due to the growing population, though further research is needed to obtain a clearer picture of the impact of no-till in drylands, where its potential to conserve moisture has potential benefits.

Irrigation of crop production

Elsewhere, there continues to be widespread policy support for hydro-electric schemes that flood valleys to store water and then use a proportion of that water for crop irrigation, sometimes turning low-productivity grassland nearby into high-output vegetable or other crop production, often for export. In some instances, as with the Gibe III dam in Ethiopia, long-established pastoralist communities are displaced in the process (Perry 2015).

In a significant proportion of cases, where this takes place in dry regions, and shallow-rooting crops replace deeper-rooting grasses, minerals dissolved in the water build up in the topsoil causing salinisation, due to high evaporation rates. Initially producers change to crops that can better tolerate salt, barley instead of wheat, for example, but eventually levels can become too high for any food production. This is not the only cause of soil salinisation, but on average 2,000 hectares of productive land have been lost to food production from salinisation every day for the last 20 years, at an estimated economic cost of $27.3 billion per year (Qadir et al. 2014).

The vital importance of grass and grassland in producing food, storing carbon and restoring degraded soils

Grassland covers 30 per cent of ice-free land and 70 per cent of agricultural land globally (Neely et al. 2010). It plays a uniquely important role in food system sustainability, in addition to its well-understood roles in relation to nature conservation, water quality catchment management and the culture of some societies. Grass will grow on land that is too steep, too stony, too acidic, too wet and too poor for crop production. As such, grazed grasslands produce food from large areas of land that would otherwise be unproductive (Wilkinson 2011). Soils store four times more carbon than all trees and other life on the planet and three times more than the atmosphere (Lal 2004). Every time grassland is permanently converted to cropland, 40 per cent (Johnston et al. 2009) or more (Lal et al. 2004) of the SOC and much of the reactive nitrogen (Vellinga et al. 2004) is lost to the atmosphere over time, in the form of the CO2 and N2O.

But grass also has another important role, one that has largely been overlooked during the last 60 years. Grass is capable of restoring degraded soils (Smith et al. 2007). Apart from food-bearing trees, grass is arguably the only crop capable of restoring degraded land while also producing food, albeit indirectly. Soil carbon losses can be reduced by the use of cover crops etc., but they cannot be reversed where a cash crop needs to be taken annually and food is to be produced, unless very large amounts of organic material are locally available (something relevant only to a small proportion of cropland). The only solution is for grass and grazing animals to be reintroduced into arable crop rotations and ideally their manures, when housed, mixed with crop residues used for bedding, to be composted and returned to the land.

The importance of grass in restoring degraded land is illustrated by a research project at Rothamsted in the UK which monitored SOC in silty clay loam soil under four different regimes between 1950 and 2000. Land that had been in arable cropping for some time already had a low carbon level and lost little more; grassland that was ploughed and kept in cropping lost 40 per cent of its SOC; grassland that was kept as grassland gained an additional 15 per cent SOC, and cropland that was converted to grass and kept in grass gained the same amount as was lost in the grass to arable trial (Johnston et al. 2009).

A series of experiments starting in 1938 on lighter soils at Woburn in the UK examined the impact of ley-arable rotations on SOC. Where a one-year grazed grass ley was included in a three-year rotation, there was no decline in SOC and after 33 years this increased slightly (1.04 per cent). In a similar trial where a three-year grass ley was alternated with two arable crops, the increase in SOC was 1.26 per cent. In both cases, identical areas to which manure was also applied showed a further 14 per cent increase in SOC. Six similar experiments looking at a wider range of examples, which would be of great value today, were initiated in the 1950s on UK government research farms, but discontinued (Johnston et al. 2009) due, it is assumed, to the belief at the time that all soil fertility could be provided by synthetic fertilisers.

Grass has the potential to increase SOC and therefore build soil organic matter (SOM) under grassland because it produces three to four times as much plant growth below ground as above ground. As roots die off and are replaced by new growth they are broken down to dark stable organic matter. Soil organic matter is critically important because maximum yields cannot be achieved under low SOM conditions (Johnston et al. 2009) though this is more significant on some soil types and for some crops than for others (Hijbeck et al. 2017). Appropriate grazing systems can secure and store carbon in grassland for the long term. In contrast, some carbon additions to arable soils, such as chopped straw, provide only transient increases in SOC and do not increase SOM (Powlson et al. 2008).

Grassland is also not subject to the major soil disturbance and periods of bare fallow, typical of crop production. As a result, photosynthesis takes place over a longer period and hence carbon inputs are greater.

The issue of soil carbon sequestration remains controversial, however, in part because some advocates of mob grazing (approaches which mimic the grazing patterns of wild ruminants) have gone beyond the benefits associated with readily demonstrable levels of sequestration to argue that the widespread uptake of the practice could take atmospheric carbon concentrations down to pre-industrial levels – claims which are not supported by current scientific evidence (Monbiot 2014). Studies also come up with widely varying estimates of how much carbon grasslands can sequester and how long sequestration will continue before a new plateau is reached.

A recent study (Henderson et al. 2015) produces a significantly lower figure than most previous assessments, estimating that even with improved grazing management and the use of legumes, grazing lands globally could sequester only 352 million tonnes of CO2 annually. However, the authors are concerned about the potential N2O emissions from the legumes or nitrogen fertiliser used to increase pasture quality and therefore carbon sequestration, and believe a more realistic figure would be 295 million tonnes CO2 p.a. Follett and Schuman (2005) on the other hand, estimated that 3.5 billion hectares of grassland globally are sequestering 200 million tonnes of carbon (733 million tonnes of CO2) annually, equivalent to offsetting 4 per cent of global GHG emissions. Smith et al. (2008) estimated a global potential for arable and grassland soils to sequester up to 6 billion tonnes of carbon (22 billion tonnes of CO2) annually, but with a realistic maximum potential of about two-thirds this amount, if farmers were paid enough to be carbon stewards.

Such uncertainty and widely varying estimates have existed for a long time. This was the stated reason Dr Pierre Gerber, lead author of the FAO's report (Gerber et al. 2013), Tackling climate change through livestock, and colleagues (and a co-author of the Henderson et al. 2015 paper) did not offset any of the GHG emissions they attributed to cattle, by including beneficial effects of carbon sequestration in grassland in their FAO report. As has been widely reported, Gerber et al. (2013) estimated that, including GHG emissions from rainforest destruction in the Amazon, livestock are responsible for 14.5 per cent of global GHG emissions, with cattle alone accounting for 6 per cent.

However, in a less well-known accompanying report (Opio et al. 2013), Gerber and colleagues effectively acknowledge that by basing their 2013 study on the period 1990–2006, when rainforest destruction was at its peak, the figures they used in 2013 were significant over-estimates. The authors say, 'Given the year of reference (2005), latest trends could not be fully reflected (e.g. reduction of deforestation rates in LUC). A sensitivity analysis was conducted showing that the period of the analysis has an important influence on results' (Opio et al. 2013, p. xv). Gerber et al. (2013) also only included LUC in South America and the Caribbean (see p. 106) not for example LUC in other regions, such as Southeast Asia and Central Africa where the driver is not cattle, but increasing demand for palm oil.

Their assessment is particularly inappropriate for livestock policy considerations in countries like the UK, where 72 per cent of farmland (including common land and rough grazing) is under grass for sound agronomic and environmental reasons. Crop and livestock production together account for 9 per cent of UK GHG emissions (DECC 2016) while LUC is predominantly in the opposite direction to that in the Amazon. At the time that rainforest was being destroyed in Brazil, forests were being planted on UK farmland and the ploughing of grassland took place against a backdrop of falling public and policy support for grazing livestock. Adding together the carbon losses from ploughed land and the current annual gains from grassland and forest comes to 15 million tonnes of CO2 eq. (Miles et al. 2014). Arguably this could all be deducted from the 49 million tonnes produced by UK agriculture as a whole, to give a net figure for all UK agriculture of just 6.2 per cent of UK emissions, based on a similar approach to that used by Gerber et al. (2013). Such figures could be seen as misleading, but the reason for including them is to illustrate the way in which the 14.5 per cent figure and the FAO's 2006 figure of 18 per cent were calculated, since in many respects they are also misleading. The UK figures do not include imported livestock feed or imported fertiliser, but neither of these are needed to any significant extent by grass-based beef or sheep systems.

Assumptions and simplifications necessary to make global estimates of carbon sequestration can overlook other important details at a local level. Data from 486 farms found that where SOC sequestration was included in analyses, it almost halved the carbon footprint of suckler beef farms, but only reduced that of some beef systems by 10–15 per cent (IDELE 2015). Fornara et al. (2016) have shown that grassland to which high applications of dairy cattle slurry are applied is still sequestering substantial amounts of carbon 43 years after the research began. Sousanna et al. (2014) assembled data from carbon sequestration in grassland amounting to 213 site years across Europe and found a mean net sequestration of 760kg of carbon per hectare per year. They argue that grasslands globally have significant potential to sequester and store carbon in the topsoil and at greater depths, if deep-rooting grasses are grown.

One partial explanation for the differences between assessments can be seen from a review of 42 studies (Maillard and Angers 2014). They found that the cumulative effect of carbon from manure applications explained more than half the differences in SOC levels compared with trials using mineral fertilisers or no inputs. Sousanna et al. (2014) also noted the importance of manure application as well as the significance of stocking density in achieving carbon neutrality in grasslands. They found this could be achieved under good conditions at densities of up to 0.85 LU/ha where no manure was applied, at 0.93 LU/ha where 100kg of fertiliser nitrogen was applied, but at up to 1.2 LU/ha where manure was applied. A key reason for the impact of stocking density is that over-grazed grass has less leaf area for photosynthesis.

A further possible explanation relates to the substantial differences in sequestration potential between single species swards and diverse swards, and whether or not legumes are included. Fornara and Tilman (2007) found that including C4 grasses with C3 grasses and legumes increased soil carbon and nitrogen storage by 500 and 600 per cent, respectively, compared with swards growing just a single species; the nitrogen fixed by the legumes stimulated growth in C4 grasses far more than in C3 grasses. C4 grasses cannot be grown successfully in cooler regions, but they are suitable for many parts of the world, and it has been suggested that with climate warming their range is likely to expand (Howden et al. 2008).

Comparative efficiency of ruminants compared with monogastric animals

It is often argued that because about one-third of cropland is used to grow grain for livestock and they are therefore implicated in the major losses of soil carbon that continue to occur, we should reduce livestock numbers globally, especially cattle and sheep, as they convert grain to protein less efficiently than pigs and poultry. In relation, to cattle largely raised on grain this would be prudent. However, as Wilkinson (2011) has shown, when assessed on the basis of human edible food consumption, ruminants can be more efficient than monogastric animals. In large part that is because they make far better use of grass; but in part it is also because even concentrate feed for cattle in the UK, at least, is 50 per cent less dependent on human-edible grain than feed for chickens and pigs – cattle being better suited to the consumption of arable by-products, such as brewers' and distillers' grains, sugar beet pulp and most oilseed by-products, except soybean meal, which is widely used in pig and poultry feed.

It is also the case that many studies compare the efficiency of different livestock systems based only on assessments of protein, even in the case of milk (de Boer 2016), an important source of dietary fats and minerals, or protein and calories, or where the calorific and nutrient value of the fats not intrinsically incorporated within the meat are not included (Shepon et al. 2016). This is most probably because fats like beef tallow and suet are no longer widely consumed. However, even these fats replace vegetable oils in industrial uses.

Agroforestry

Grassland also provides one other substantial form of carbon sequestration potential which is rarely considered when assessing the carbon footprint of milk, different types of meat or food crops. Trees are highly compatible with grazing systems whereas they are generally incompatible with crop production because they get in the way of modern machinery, reduce crop yields and delay ripening. Even large trees, however, take up little ground area when grown at low densities within the grassland itself. Considerable development work has been undertaken on agro-forestry systems worldwide in recent years and their potential to sequester carbon (Mosquera-Losada et al. 2011), but there is a tendency to forget that grass fields with hedgerow field boundaries are a long-established form of agroforestry where the hedges and hedgerow trees play an additional role in providing shelter from cold winds, heavy rain and bright sunshine in hot weather. Hedges and hedgerow trees can store as much carbon underground in root systems as they do above ground in the trunk and branches. The annual leaf loss also provides additional organic matter which in biologically active soils is incorporated into the soil by worms and reduced to dark, stable organic matter by the wide variety of soil-dwelling organisms and micro-organisms that make up 25 per cent of the planet's biodiversity.

Policies encouraging intensification resulted in the removal of approximately 250,000 miles of hedgerows in the UK before the introduction of hedgerow regulations in 1997. While hedges now have some measure of protection, the remaining hedges bordering cropland have no practical value to farmers and constitute an economic burden. As a result, they are cut frequently and hard, and hence have little bulk, thus reducing their biodiversity benefits, carbon sequestration and storage. Some grassland fields have also lost hedgerows, but, since cattle farmers frequently sub-divide larger fields with wire fencing there would be practical, welfare, biodiversity and economic benefits in encouraging the reinstatement of more hedgerows, with specimen trees at appropriate spacing, and also where practical, additional parkland trees within the grassland.

My back of the envelope calculations suggest that, for the typical fields on the small dairy farm where I grew up in the 1950s, up to five hectares in size, adding in hedges and hedgerow trees effectively doubles the carbon sequestration and storage potential of grass fields. The carbon stored in trees and tree roots is also taken out of the atmosphere for many centuries. As such it can also be argued that the relative differences in tree and hedgerow density on grassland and cropland should be taken into consideration when comparing the carbon footprint of beef and lamb with pork and chicken.

Antimicrobials and antimicrobial resistance

Despite countless counter claims from the intensive livestock industry, there is growing recognition that the high dependency of intensive livestock systems on antimicrobials means they are a significant factor in the rise of antimicrobial resistance (AMR) genes in the environment and in the food supply. They contribute to the growing problem of antimicrobial-resistant infections in humans, as well as threatening the long-term viability of the livestock industry due to increasing levels of resistance in livestock pathogens (O'Neill 2015). Despite the incomplete breakdown of use between species in annual data published in the UK by the Veterinary Medicines Directorate (VMD 2016) and some recent reductions in farm antimicrobial use, it can be shown, based on the available data, that between 80 and 96 per cent of farm antimicrobials in the UK are given to pigs and poultry (Nunan 2017), with most of the balance (4–20 per cent, but based on past estimates, probably in the region of 10 per cent) used in milk production, and relatively small amounts used in beef and sheep production. Given that we import 45 per cent of our pork and 25 per cent of our chickens, the global impact on AMR from high chicken and pork consumption in the UK is higher still.

Source of dietary fats

Consideration of the health issues associated with red meat and animal fats is outside the scope of this chapter. However, it is appropriate to point out that on average in the UK we obtain 36 per cent of our energy intake from dietary fats, 1 per cent more than the recommended level (Bates et al. 2014), but down from 41 per cent in the early 1980s (COMA 1984). With the virtual elimination of beef fat from the national diet, dramatic reductions in the consumption of full cream milk over recent decades and greatly reduced availability of lard, due to pressure on pig farmers to produce very lean pork, there has been a major trend away from consuming natural animal fats to consuming vegetable oils, a high proportion of which are also chemically altered. At the beginning of the 20th century almost all dietary fats in the UK came from grassland in the form of dairy products, meat and animal fats or vegetables grown in mixed farming systems. Today, well over half of them come from destroyed equatorial rainforests. The two most widely used vegetable oils globally, palm oil and soybean oil, along with sunflower oil and rapeseed oil are often modified by the industrial processes of interesterification, fractionation and partial hydrogenation, to turn them into solid fats at room temperatures, suitable for inclusion in processed foods, or to create designer fats with special textures and other characteristics for confectionery, margarine, spreads and other products.

Humans evolved over long periods consuming animal fats and the long-term effects of the sudden change to such a high proportion of vegetable oils in the diet, often chemically altered, is unknown. However, leaving aside discussion of whether or not we have been correctly advised on the health issues associated with animal fats and saturated fats in particular (Calder 2016) and the postulated health risks associated with diets high in omega-6 (Dunbar et al. 2014), it is worth pointing out that the escalating use of palm oil, as a result of the rejection of animal fats, increased consumption of processed foods and population growth, is associated with substantial rainforest loss and horrific environmental degradation, GHG emissions, river and air pollution and biodiversity losses, in Southeast Asia, Central Africa and South America. This includes the expected extinction of great apes and threats to the survival of elephants, rhinos, tigers and other endangered species in Southeast Asia (Fitzherbert et al. 2008, WWF 2013, Savilaakso et al. 2014, Woolley 2015, Orangutan Foundation undated). Global palm oil production now stands at 64.5 million tonnes, up a further 9.6 per cent since January 2016 (Global Palm Oil Production 2017). The UK imported 643,400 tonnes of palm and palm kernel oil in 2009 of which 60 per cent was used in processed foods, 8 per cent in frying oils, 23 per cent in intensive livestock feed and the remainder in non-food products (DEFRA 2011). Globally, palm oil now accounts for 56 per cent of all dietary fat consumed (Sime Darby 2014).

Yet half of the fatty acids in palm oil are saturated, approximately the same as beef fat. But while palm oil contains no omega-3 fatty acids to balance its omega-6 fatty acids, something increasingly seen as important to reduce inflammation – a potential initiator of a number of chronic diseases, including dementia (Calder 2006) – beef fat from grazing animals contains modest but valuable amounts of omega-3 fatty acids in an ideal balance of less than 2:1 omega-6 to omega-3, when the animals are predominantly fed on grass and grass products (Enser et al. 1998, Elmore et al. 2004, Daley et al. 2010). And if, for the sake of argument, we ever again come to see animal fats as healthy, or at least recognise that in some situations, such as frying, beef fat could replace palm oil and be no worse for us, this would significantly alter the efficiency calculations about ruminant products.

Conclusions

It is clear from a wide range of sources that the capacities of planetary ecosystems are already being exceeded and that agriculture is one of the major causes of this. As such, it is heartening that increased attention is finally turning to how food systems and consumption patterns can be modified to reduce those pressures. At first sight consuming more chicken and pork and less beef and lamb, or even consuming no livestock products at all, appear to be ways to reduce greenhouse gases, as well as produce more calories, more protein or more fat, depending on the crop under consideration, than from the animals that could be kept on the same area of land.

However, once we recognise that crop production cannot continue indefinitely without degrading soils well past the point of optimum productivity and that all-arable systems are running up against serious agronomic issues, it quickly becomes apparent that a durable and secure food future can only be achieved if we learn to alternate exploitative crops with regenerative ones. Ideally, that means including grass and legumes in arable rotations. As such, we need more sophisticated and open-minded debate about future food systems and what we should eat for a healthy planet than has taken place so far.

There are no simple solutions. In part this is because it is difficult to envisage a limit to population growth on a finite planet without natural disasters and human suffering on an epic scale, at some point in the future. In part, it is because we still lack sufficient data to determine some issues, such as the achievable levels of soil carbon sequestration on a wide range of soils. It is tempting to pick the best examples and hold them up as the way forward. Sousanna et al. (2014) not only find that European grasslands can sequester slightly over three-quarters of a tonne of carbon per hectare annually, they also calculate that at stocking rates of up to 1.2 adult cattle per hectare, under appropriate management, such systems are carbon neutral, even taking CH4 emissions from ruminants and N2O emissions from soil and manure into account. This paints a very different picture to that presented by Henderson et al. (2015). Sousanna and colleagues based their conclusions on actual research, whereas Henderson and colleagues base theirs on modelling which requires broad generalisations. Nevertheless, even if Sousanna's results prove well-founded they relate to optimum climate conditions. In the least optimum conditions they considered, stocking levels needed to fall as low at 0.3 LU/ha to achieve carbon neutrality, and we still do not know how long such rates of sequestration could continue or how widely applicable they might be. We already know that more grassland and less cropland will definitely increase carbon sequestration overall, but more research is clearly needed. Unfortunately, though, it can take many decades to obtain meaningful data from new trials on soil carbon sequestration, and we probably can't afford to wait that long.

There is also no single solution because very different assessments and approaches are needed in different regions, for example in the drylands; in rainforests; in parts of Southern Europe, where grass does not grow particularly well; in regions where it might be possible to double soil carbon sequestration by reintegrating more trees into agriculture without loss of productivity; in countries like the UK and Ireland, where grass is the best and sometimes only suitable crop for much of the land and where the issues associated with LUC are usually now the opposite of those in Brazil – though only because most European forests were felled to make way for agriculture several thousand years ago.

But even if we were to ignore carbon sequestration from both grass and grassland trees and the oversights from the way in which Gerber et al. (2013) calculated that cattle are responsible for 6 per cent of anthropogenic global GHG emissions, does 6 per cent seem so particularly inappropriate, given the importance of ruminants for global food security? Add to this the critically important role grass plays in storing carbon, its potential to regenerate degraded soils, and the fact that technologies exist to reduce the use of fossil fuels and their emissions and we get a broader picture. As such, I find it hard to understand why all cattle systems have been characterised as a problem, when surely the basic distinctions we need to make are not between cattle and chickens, but between animals which depend heavily on grain, and which are therefore in direct competition with humans, and those which eat grass and arable by-products, which we cannot eat.

Continuous crop production is also not sustainable for another reason. Without the genuine break in weed, disease and pest cycles afforded by grass, crop production comes to depend more and more on synthetic chemicals: fertilisers for fertility and pesticides to control weeds, pests and diseases. Quite apart from the finite nature of the resources from which these are manufactured and the established environmental costs associated with their production, transport and use, many of them are no longer working effectively. Just as bacterial pathogens develop resistance to antimicrobials, so weeds develop resistance to herbicides, foliar diseases develop resistance to fungicides and insect pests develop resistance to insecticides. In the UK, for example, more than half (54 per cent) of all cereal crops are now infested with blackgrass, which can reduce yields by 50 per cent in the most severe cases (Farmers Guardian 2017). The weed has become resistant to all in-crop herbicides and some arable farmers are being forced by necessity to convert to organic methods, or to put their most affected fields into grass for several years at a time and graze them, in order to regain some degree of control.

But my major concern about the current approach to these issues is that while the methane emissions from ruminants should not be ignored, they are nothing like as significant as many people have been led to believe. Films such as 'Cowspiracy' claimed that cattle were responsible for 51 per cent of global warming, based on completely highly questionable figures, as explained by vegan carbon specialist Danny Chivers (Chivers 2016).

Whatever the reality in relation to emissions, the carbon put into the atmosphere by ruminants as either CO2 or CH4 is all recycled carbon. This is very different to the fossil fuels used to produce fertilisers for crop production and power our luxury lifestyles. These put new carbon into the atmosphere, carbon which was last removed from it 400 million years ago. Furthermore, while just about everyone has now heard about methane from cattle, how many people, I wonder, realise that apart from being the largest source of CO2, fossil fuels also make up the largest anthropogenic source of methane as well? For me it is vitally important this message is heard because some people I encounter assume it is fine to travel internationally as much as they like because they don't eat red meat.

If viewed from outer space, the mistakes we are making to the soils would be seen to bear an eerie resemblance to those made by the world's first great civilisation, the Sumerians. The only difference – they destroyed a small part of the fertile crescent in the Middle East, while we are destroying most of the fertile soils on the planet.

Since the emergence of modern agriculture, the global population has been relying on the soil organic matter built up under forests and grasslands grazed by herds of wild ruminants over thousands of years, and most people appear to be unaware of just how close we are to the tail end of this natural capital resource, upon which we all depend and why we must husband it more carefully.

There is, though, increasing realisation that converting the last few remaining areas of virgin land to crop production, in significant part to replace the land that is being lost through our own mismanagement and urban growth, comes at an enormous cost in terms of GHG emissions, pollution, biodiversity loss and social upheaval. But in order not to be forced to convert the last remaining natural ecosystems and lose the iconic species that inhabit them – a process already underway – we have to regenerate degraded lands and in most cases that means establishing grass and stocking it appropriately with grazing animals, regardless of their methane emissions. We need to see grass and grazing animals as vital strategic resources that should be deployed where they can best deliver three key objectives: carbon sequestration, food security and social benefits. But this could be balanced by raising significantly fewer ruminants and other livestock species on grain.

If none of this convinces you, all I can say is that instinctively I feel humans will never thrive on meat from animals forced to live bored, short and meaningless lives in total confinement. Whereas we will thrive, as our ancestors did for thousands of years, on the produce of animals that graze diverse grass swards, which we cannot eat, while having reasonably natural and fulfilling lives. There is no science to demonstrate that, only common sense.

References

Angers, D.A. and Eriksen-Hamel, N.S. (2008) 'Full-inversion tillage and organic carbon distribution in soil profiles: a meta-analysis', *Soil Science Society of America* vol 72, pp1370–1374.

Anon (2017) 'Crop nutrition role in blackgrass control', Farmers Guardian, 3 February. p27.

Baker, J.M., Ochsner, T.E., Venterea, R.T. and Griffis, T.J., (2007) 'Tillage and soil carbon sequestration – what do we really know?', *Agriculture, Ecosystems & Environment*, vol 118, pp1–5.

Bates, B., Lennox, A., Prentice, A., Bates, C., Page, P., Nicholson, S. and Swan, G. (2014) *National Diet and Nutrition Survey: Results From Years 1–4 (Combined) of the Rolling Programme (2008/2009–2011/12)*, Public Health England, London.

Calder, P.C. (2006) 'n-3 Polyunsaturated fatty acids, inflammation, and inflammatory diseases', *American Society for Clinical Nutrition*, vol 83, ppS1505–S15195.

Calder, P.C. (2016) 'A hole in the diet-heart hypothesis?', *Nature Reviews Cardiology*, vol 13, pp385–386.

Case, P. (2014) 'Only 100 harvests left in UK farm soils, scientists warn', *Farmers Weekly*, 21 October available at http://www.fwi.co.uk/news/only-100-harvests-left-in-uk-farm-soils-scientists-warn.htm, accessed 16 May 2017.

CGIAR (undated) *The World's Dry Areas*, available at http://drylandsystems.cgiar.org/content/worlds-dry-areas, accessed, 16 January 2017.

Chatterton, L. and Chatterton, B. (1996) *Sustainable Dryland Farming: Combining Farmer Innovation and Medic Pasture in a Mediterranean Climate*, Cambridge University Press, Cambridge, UK.

Chivers, D. (2016) 'Cowspiracy: stampeding in the wrong direction*? New Internationalist*, available at https://newint.org/blog/2016/02/10/cowspiracy-stampeding-in-the-wrong-direction/, accessed 12 January 2017.

COMA (1984) *Diet and Cardiovascular Disease*, Report on Health and Social Subjects, 28, Committee on Medicinal Aspects of Food Policy, HMSO, London.

Daley, C.A., Abbott, A., Doyle, P.S., Nader, G.A. and Larson, S. (2010) 'A review of fatty acid profiles and antioxidant content in grass-fed and grain-fed beef', *Nutrition Journal*, vol 9, pp1–12.

de Boer (2016) 'Minimizing the environmental footprint of livestock production: which measure to use'. Steps to Sustainable Livestock conference, Bristol, available at www.globalfarmplatform.org/wp-content/uploads/2016/04/46-Imke-de-Boer-Steps-to-Sustainalbe-Livestock-Measuring-Efficieny.pdf, accessed, 15 September 2016.

DECC (2016) 2014 UK *Greenhouse Gas Emissions*, available at www.gov.uk/government/uploads/system/uploads/attachment_data/file/496946/2014_Final_Emissions_Statistical_Summary_Infographic.pdf, accessed 23 December 2016.

DEFRA (2011) *Mapping and Understanding the UK Palm Oil Supply Chain*, A Report for the Department of the Environment, Food and Rural Affairs by Proforest, available at http://randd.defra.gov.uk/Document.aspx?Document=EV0459_10154_FRA.pdf

Dunbar, B.S., Bosire, R.V. and Deckelbaum, R.J. (2014) 'Omega-3 and omega-6 fatty acids in human and animal health: An African perspective', *Molecular Cell Endocrinology,* vol 398, pp69–77.

ELD Initiative (2015) The Value of Land: Prosperous Lands and Positive Rewards Through Sustainable Land Management: The Economics of Land Degradation Secretariat, available at www.eld-initiative.org/fileadmin/pdf/ELD-main-report_05_web_72dpi.pdf, accessed 17 January 2017.

Elmore, J.S., Warren, H.E., Mottram, D.S., Scollan, N.D., Enser, M., Richardson, R.I. and Wood, J.D. (2004) 'A comparison of aroma volatile and fatty acid compositions of grilled beef muscle from Aberdeen Angus and Holstein-Friesian steers fed diets based on silage or concentrates', *Meat Science*, vol 68, pp27–33.

Enser, M., Hallett, K.G., Hewett, B., Fursey, G.A.J., Wood, J.D. and Harrington, G. (1998) 'Fatty acid content and composition of UK beef and lamb muscle in relation to production system and implications for human nutrition', *Meat Science*, vol 49, pp329–341.

FAO (2015) *Status of the World's Soil Resources*, FAO, Rome.
FAOSTAT (2013) *Food Balance Sheets*, FAO, available at www.fao.org/faostat/en/#data/FBS, accessed 13 January 2017.
Fitzherbert, E.B., Struebig, M.J., Morel, A., Danielsen, F., Brühl, C.A., Donald, P.F. and Phalan, B. (2008) 'How will oil palm expansion affect biodiversity?', *Trends in Ecology & Evolution*, vol 23, pp538–545.
Follett, R.F. and Schuman, G.E. (2005) 'Grazing land contributions to carbon sequestration.' In 'Grassland: A global resource', Proceedings of the XXth International Grassland Congress, Dublin, Ireland (ed D.A. McGilloway) pp265–277. Wageningen Academic Publishers, Wageningen, The Netherlands.
Fornara, D.A. and Tilman, D. (2007) 'Plank functional composition influences rates of soil carbon and nitrogen accumulation', *Journal of Ecology*, vol 96, pp314–322.
Fornara, D.A., Wasson, E., Christie, P. and Watson, C.J. (2016) 'Long-term nutrient fertilization and the carbon balance of permanent grassland: Any evidence for sustainable intensification?', *Biogeosciences*, vol 13, pp4975–4984.
Garnett, T. (2010) 'Livestock and Climate Change'. In *The Meat Crisis: Developing More Sustainable Production and Consumption*, eds. D'Silva, J. and Webster J. Earthscan, London and Washington DC, pp34–56.
Graves, A.R., Morris, J., Deeks, L.K., Rickson, R.J., Kibblewhite, M.G., Harris, J.A., Farewell, T.S., Truckle, I. (2015). 'The total costs of soil degradation in England and Wales', *Ecological Economics*, vol. 119, pp399–413.
Gerber, P.J., Hristov, A.N., Henderson, B., Makkar, H., Oh, J., Lee, C., Meinen, R., Montes, F., Ott, T., Firkins, J., Rotz, A., Dell, C., Adesogan, A.T., Yang, W.Z., Tricarico, J.M., Kebreab, E., Waghorn, G., Dijkstra, J. and Oosting, S. (2013) 'Technical options for the mitigation of direct methane and nitrous oxide emissions from livestock: A review', *Animal*, vol 7, pp220–234.
Gerber, P.J., Steinfeld, H., Henderson, B., Mottet, A., Opio, C., Dijkman, J., Falcucci, A. and Tempio, G. (2013) *Tackling Climate Change Through Livestock – A Global Assessment of Emissions and Mitigation Opportunities*, Food and Agriculture Organization of the United Nations (FAO), Rome.
Global Palm Oil Production (2017) *Global Palm Oil Production January 2017*, available at www.globalpalmoilproduction.com, accessed 5 February 2017.
Greenpeace (2009), *Slaughtering the Amazon*, available at www.greenpeace.org/international/en/publications/reports/slaughtering-the-amazon/, accessed 4 January 2017.
HBF and IASS (2015) *Soil Atlas: Facts and Figures About Earth, Land and Fields*, Heinrich Böll Foundation and Institute for Advanced Sustainability Studies, Berlin, Germany.
Henderson, B.B., Gerber, P.J., Hilinski, T.E., Falcucci, A., Ojima, D.S., Salvatore, M. and Conan, R.T. (2015) 'Greenhouse gas mitigation potential of the world's grazing lands: Modelling soil carbon, and nitrogen fluxes of mitigation practices', *Agriculture, Ecosystems & Environment*, vol 207, pp91–100.
Hijbeck, R., van Ittersum, M.K., ten Berge, H.F.M., Gort. G., Spiegel, H. and Whitmore, A.P. (2017) 'Do organic inputs matter – a meta-analysis of additional yield effects for arable crops in Europe, *Soil Plant* vol 411, pp293–303.
Howden, S.M., Crimp, S.J. and Stokes, C.J. (2008) 'Climate change and Australian livestock systems: Impacts, research and policy issues', *Australian Journal of Experimental Agriculture*, vol 48, pp780–788.
IDELE (2015) Conference 'L'élevage des ruminants, acteurs des solution climat', 9–10 June 2015, Paris. Summarised in 'Sequestration Fact Sheet (July 2016) SAI Platform, www.saiplatform.org/pressroom/174/46/New-Publication-Sequestration-Fact-Sheet, accessed 20 January 2017.

IPCC (2014) 'Climate Change: Synthesis Report', In *Contribution of Working Groups I, II and III to the Fifth Assessment Report of the Intergovernmental Panel on Climate Change*, eds. Pachauri, R.K. and Meyer, L.A. IPCC, Geneva, Switzerland, p87.

Johnston, A.E., Poulton, P.R. and Coleman, K. (2009) 'Soil organic matter: Its importance in sustainable agriculture and carbon dioxide fluxes', *Advances in Agronomy*, vol 101, pp1–57.

Jones, P. and Thornton, P (2008) 'Cropper to livestock keepers: Livelihood transitions to 2050 in Africa due to climate change', *Environmental Science Policy*, vol 12, pp427–437.

Lal, R. (1999) 'Soil management and restoration for C sequestration to mitigate the accelerated greenhouse gas effect', *Progress in Environmental Science*, vol 1, pp307–326.

Lal, R. (2004) 'Soil carbon sequestration to mitigate climate change', *Geodemera*, vol 123, pp1–22.

Lal, R. (2015) 'Soil carbon sequestration and aggregation by cover cropping', *Journal of Soil and Water Conservation*, vol 70, pp329–339.

Luo, Z., Wang, E. and Sun, O.J. (2010) 'Can no-tillage stimulate carbon sequestration in agricultural soils? A meta-analysis of paired experiments', *Agriculture, Ecosystems & Environment*, vol 139, pp224–231.

Maillard, É. and Angers, D. A. (2014) 'Animal manure application and soil organic carbon stocks: a meta-analysis', *Global Change Biology*, vol 20, pp666–679.

McKie, R. (2017) 'All change in the aisles to entice us to eat more veg', *The Observer*, 22 January, p10.

Merton, G.H. and Minella, J.P.G. (2013) 'The expansion of Brazilian agriculture: Soil erosion scenarios', *International Soil and Water Conservation Research*, vol 1, pp37–48.

Miles, S., Malcolm, H., Buys, G. and Moxley, J. (2014) Emissions and Removals of Greenhouse Gases from Land Use, Land Use Change and Forestry (LULUCF in England, Scotland, Wales and Northern Ireland: 1990–2012, CEH, available at https://uk-air.defra.gov.uk/assets/documents/reports/cat07/1406021226_DA_LULUCF_2012i_pub_version_1.1_300514.pdf, accessed 18 November 2016.

Monbiot, G. (2014) 'Eat more meat and save the world: The latest implausible farming miracle', *The Guardian*, 4 August, available at www.theguardian.com/environment/georgemonbiot/2014/aug/04/eat-more-meat-and-save-the-world-the-latest-implausible-farming-miracle, accessed 22 April 2017.

Montgomery, D. (2007) *Dirt: The Erosion of Civilizations*, University of California Press, Berkeley, CA.

Mosquera-Losada, M.R., Freese, D. and Rigueriro-Rodríguez, A. (2011) 'Carbon sequestration in European agroforestry systems'. In eds. Kumar, B.M. and Nair, P.K.R. *Carbon Sequestration Potential of Agroforestry Systems, Opportunities and Challenges, Advances in Agroforestry*, Vol 8 (ed. Nair, P.K.R.), Springer Dordrecht Heidelberg, London and New York, pp 43–59.

Nazaries, L., Murrell, J.C., Millard, P., Baggs, L. and Singh, B.K. (2013) 'Methane, microbes and models: Fundamental understanding of the soil methane cycle for future predictions', *Environmental Microbiology*, vol 15, pp2395–2417.

Neely, C., Bunning, S. and Wilkes, A. (2010) 'Managing dryland pastoral systems: Implications for mitigation and adaptation to climate change' *Grassland Carbon Sequestration: Management, Policy and Economics* vol 11, pp235–266.

Nisbet, E.G., Dlugokencky, E.J., Manning, M.R., Lowry, D., Fisher, R.E., France, J.L., Michel, S.E., Miller, J.B., White, J.W.C., Vaughn, B., Bousquet, P., Pyle, J.A., Warwick, N.J., Cain, M., Brownlow, R., Zazzeri, G., Lanoisellé, M., Manning, A.C., Gloor, E., Wirthy, D.E.J., Brunke, E.G., Labuschagne, C., Wolff, E.W. and Ganesan, A.L. (2016) 'Rising atmospheric methane: 2007–2014 growth and isotropic shift', *Global Biochemical Cycles*, vol 30, pp1356–1370.

NOAA (undated) National Ocean & Atmosphere Administration website, 'Trends in atmospheric methane', available at www.esrl.noaa.gov/gmd/ccgg/trends_ch4/, accessed 31 January 2017.

Nunan, C. (2017) *Alliance to Save Our Antibiotics Response to the National Pig Association*, available at www.saveourantibiotics.org/media/1770/alliance-to-save-our-antibiotics-response-to-national-pig-association-criticism.pdf, accessed 17 January 2017.

O'Neill, J. (2015) *Antimicrobials in Agriculture and the Environment: Reducing Unnecessary Use and Waste*, Review on Antimicrobial Resistance, London.

Opio, C., Gerber, P., Mottet, A., Falcucci, A., Tempio, G., MacLeod, M., Vellinga, T., Henderson, B. and Steinfeld, H. (2013) *Greenhouse Gas Emissions From Ruminant Supply Chains – A Global Life Cycle Assessment*. Food and Agriculture Organization of the United Nations (FAO), Rome.

Orangutan Foundation (undated) *The Effects of Palm Oil: How Does Palm Oil Harm Orangutans and Other Wildlife?*, available at https://orangutan.org/rainforest/the-effects-of-palm-oil/, accessed 20 January 2017.

Perry, M. (2015) *Dismantling the Omo Valley*, available at http://sustainablefoodtrust.org/articles/land-grabbing-omo-valley/, accessed 28 October 2016.

Pittelkow, C.M., Liang, X., Linquist, B.A., Groenigen, K.J.V., Lee, J., Lundy, M.E., Gestel, N.V., Six, J., Venterea, R.T. and Kessel, C.V. (2014) 'Productivity limits and potentials of the principles of conservation agriculture', *Nature*, vol 517, pp365–368.

Popp, A., Lotze-Campen, H., Bodirsky, B, (2010) 'Food consumption, diet shifts and associated non-CO2 greenhouse gases from agricultural production', *Global Environmental Change* 20, 451–462.

Poultry Site (2014) *Global Poultry Trends 2014: Poultry Set to Become No.1 Meat in Asia*, 2 September, available at www.thepoultrysite.com/articles/3230/global-poultry-trends-2014-poultry-set-to-become-no1-meat-in-asia/, accessed 20 January 2017.

Powlson, D.S., Riche, A.B., Coleman, K., Glendining, M.L. and Whitmore, A.P. (2008) 'Carbon sequestration in European soils through straw incorporation: limitations and alternatives', *Waste Management*, vol 28, pp741–746.

Powlson, D.S., Stirling, C.M., Jat, M.L., Gerard, B.G., Palm, C.A., Sanchez, P.A. and Cassman, K.G. (2014) 'Limited potential of no-till agriculture for climate change mitigation', *Nature Climate Change*, vol 4, pp678–683.

Qadir, M., Quillérou, E., Nangia, V., Murtaza, G., Singh, M., Thomas, R.J., Drechsel, P. and Noble, A.D. (2014) 'Economics of salt-induced land degradation and restoration', *United Nations Sustainable Development Journal*, vol 38, pp282–295.

Ripple, W.J., Smith, P., Haberl, H., Montzka, S.A., McAlpine, C., Boucher, D.H. (2014) 'Ruminants, climate change and climate policy', *Nature Climate Change*, vol 4, pp2–5.

Savilaakso, S., Garcia, C., Garcia-Ulloa, J., Ghazoul, J., Groom, M., Guariguata, M.R., Laumonier, Y., Nasi, R., Petrokofsky, G., Snaddon, J. and Zrust, M. (2014) 'Systematic review of effects on biodiversity from oil palm production', *Environmental Evidence*, vol 3(1), pp1–21.

Scharlemann, J.P.W., Tanner, E.V.J., Hiederer, R. and Kapos, V. (2014) 'Global soil carbon: Understanding and managing the largest terrestrial carbon pool', *Carbon Management*, vol 5(1), pp81–91.

Schweitzke, S., Sherwood, O.A., Bruhwiler, L.M., Miller, J.B., Etiope, G., Dlugokencky, E.J., Michel, S.E., Arling, V.A., Vaughn, B.H., White, J.W. and Tans, P.P. (2016) 'Upward revision of global fossil fuel methane emissions based on isotope database', *Nature*, vol 538, pp88–91.

Shepon, A., Eshel, G., Noor, E. and Milo, R. (2016) 'Energy and protein-to-food conversion efficiencies in the US and potential food security gains from dietary changes', *Environmental Research Letters*, vol 11, p105002.

Sime Darby (2014) *Palm Oil Facts and Figures*, Figure 5, available at www.simedarby.com/upload/Palm_Oil_Facts_and_Figures.pdf, accessed 5 February 2017.

Smith, P.D. (2004) 'Carbon sequestration in croplands: The potential in Europe and the global context', *European Journal of Agronomy*, vol 20, pp229–236.

Smith, P.D., Martino, Z., Cai, D., Gwary, H., Janzen, P., Kumar, B., McCarl, S., Ogle, F., O'Mara, C., Rice, B., Scholes, O. and Sirotenko, O. (2007) 'Agriculture'. In *Climate Change 2007: Mitigation: Contribution of Working Group III to the Fourth Assessment Report of the Intergovernmental Panel on Climate Change*, eds. Metz, B., Davidson, O.R., Bosch, P.R., Dave, R., and Meyer, L.A. Cambridge University Press, Cambridge, United Kingdom and New York, pp499–540.

Smith, P.D., Martino, Z., Cai, D., Gwary, H., Janzen, P., Kumar, B., McCarl, S., Ogle, F., O'Mara, C., Rice, B., Scholes, O., Sirotenko, O., Howden, H., McAllister, T., Pan, G., Romanenkov, V., Schneider, U., Towprayoon, S., Wattenbach, M. and Smith, J. (2008) 'Greenhouse gas mitigation in agriculture', *Philosophical Transactions of the Royal Society B*, vol 363, pp789–813.

Soane, B.D., Ball, B.C., Arvidsson, J., Bash, G., Moreno, F. and Roger-Estrade, J. (2012) 'No-till in northern, western and south-western Europe: A review of problems and opportunities for crop production and the environment', *Soil Tillage Research*, vol 118, pp66–87.

Sousanna, J.-F., Klumpp, K. and Ehrhardt, F. (2014) 'The role of grassland in mitigating climate change, book chapter in EGF at 50 The Future of European Grasslands', Proceedings of the 25th European Grasslands Federation (ed Hopkins, A., Collins, R.P., Fraser, M.D., King, V.R., Lloyd, D.C., Moorby, I.M. and Robson, P.R.H), Aberystwyth, Wales, 7–11 September, 2014.

Sousanna, J.-F., Tallec, T. and Blanfort, V. (2009) 'Mitigating the greenhouse gas balance of ruminant production systems through carbon sequestration in grasslands', *Animal*, vol 4, pp334–350.

Springmann, M., Mason-D'croz, D., Robinson, S., Wiebe, K., Godfray, H.C.J., Rayner, M. and Scarborough, P. (2017) 'Mitigation potential and global health impacts from emissions pricing of food commodities', *Nature Climate Change*, vol 7, pp69–74.

Steinfeld, H., Gerber, P.J., Wassenaar, T. and De Haan, C. (2006) *Livestock's Long Shadow: Environmental Issues and Options*, United Nations Food and Agriculture Organization, Rome.

Thornton, P.K. (2010) 'Livestock production: Recent trends, future prospects', *Philosophical Transactions of the Royal Society B*, vol 365, pp2853–2867.

UNCCD (2015) Desertification, Land Degradation & Drought (DLDD): Some Global Facts and Figures, United Nations Conventions to Combat Desertification.

Van den Putte, A., Govers, G., Diels, J., Gillijns, K. and Demuzere, M. (2010) 'Assessing the effect of soil tillage on crop growth: A meta-regression analysis on European crop yields under conservation agriculture', *European Journal of Agronomy*, vol 33, pp231–241.

Vellinga, Th.V, Polo-van Dasselaar, A.van den and Kuikman, P.J. (2004) 'The impacts of grassland ploughing on CO2 and N2O emissions in the Netherlands', *Nutrient Cycling in Agroecosystems*, vol 70, pp33–45. Kluwer Academic Publishers.

VMD (2016) UK-VARSS UK *Veterinary Antibiotic Resistance Sales and Surveillance*, Report, available at www.gov.uk/government/uploads/system/uploads/attachment_data/file/582341/1051728-v53-UK-VARSS_2015.pdf

West, T.O. and Post, W.M. (2002) 'Soil organic carbon sequestration by tillage and crop rotation: A global analysis', *Soil Science Society of America Journal*, vol 66, pp1930–1946.

Westhoek, H., Lesschen, J.P., Rood, J., Wagner, S., De Marco, A., Murphy-Bokern, D., Leip, A., Grinsven, H. van, Sutton, M.A. and Oenema, O. (2014) 'Food choices, health and environment: Effects of cutting Europe's meat and dairy intake', *Global Environmental Change*, vol 26, pp196–205.
Wilkinson, J.M. (2011) 'Re-defining efficiency of feed use by livestock', *Animal*, vol 5, pp1014–1022.
Willison, T., Goulding, K., Powlson, D. and Webster, C. (1995) 'Farming, Fertilizers and the Greenhouse Effect', *Outlook on Agriculture*, vol 24, pp241–247.
Woolley, J. (2015) *How Palm Oil Companies Have Made Indonesia's Forest Fires Worse*, Greenpeace, available at http://energydesk.greenpeace.org/2015/11/20/how-palm-oil-companies-have-made-indonesias-forest-fires-worse/, accessed 20 January 2017.
World Economic Forum (2012) 'What if the world's soil runs out?', *Time*, 14 December, available at http://world.time.com/2012/12/14/what-if-the-worlds-soil-runs-out/, accessed 20 January 2017.
WWF (2013) *Palming Off and National Park, World Wide Fund for Nature*, Riau, Sumatra, Indonesia.

PART II

Farming practices and animal welfare

7

BEEF AND DAIRY

The cattle story

John Webster

Introduction: the cattle story in time and space

There is abundant evidence that the nature and extent of current practices for the production and consumption of food from animals (in this case, cattle) are unhealthy, unsustainable and, in many respects, unethical. However, the aim of this chapter and this book is not simply to add to the chorus of those who cry havoc but to review the evidence, from this draw attention to the major problems but also seek solutions through strategies based on the principles of good husbandry. These may be categorised as efficiency in the use of resources, compassion for the animals and farmers involved in livestock production and sympathetic stewardship of the living environment. Caring passionately *about* animals and their welfare is easy. Caring *for* them properly requires a great deal of knowledge and understanding.

It is important that we do not base our evaluation of cattle husbandry and welfare solely on current production practices, especially the intensive practices that have come to dominate production in the developed world. We must view a far wider perspective in time and space. In traditional cultures the rearing of ruminants and similar grazing species (cattle, sheep, goats, buffalo, yak, llamas and other camelids) provided not just food but clothing, work, fuel and fertiliser for present needs but also a vital reserve of capital wealth. These cultures evolved in nomadic and pastoral communities where the land was free, but the produce of the land, principally grasses, was not directly available for human consumption. The indigenous people of North America coexisted entirely sustainably with the American bison until colonists destroyed the ecosystem by killing off the animals and taking away the land. Even today grasslands, shrub and parklands (grass and trees) make up approximately 70% of land potentially available for agriculture. Grasses are supremely efficient, robust and sustainable in their ability to harvest energy from the sun. Since we are unable to reap this harvest directly for ourselves due to our inability to digest cellulose, it makes sound environmental sense to avail ourselves of this resource at second hand as meat, and especially milk from grazing animals. Pastoral systems, and especially silvo-pastoral systems, can also play a significant role in carbon sequestration. I shall return to this later.

Nomadic cultures relied on the ruminants that walked with them to provide most of their needs. Within many settled village communities, the most valuable of non-human animals was (and still is) the milk cow. She is a daily provider of food in the form of milk to be consumed at once or conserved as butter, cheese, ghee or yoghurt. Farmers and their families invest time and labour to grow, cut, carry and conserve food for the house cow, and the cow repays this investment through the production of milk for home consumption and for sale. Throughout history and worldwide, dairy production has offered those who work the land a currency that could lift them from subsistence agriculture towards some freedom of choice in the marketplace. At best therefore, a family could thrive on the wealth provided by their milch cow. She was their greatest asset and valued accordingly. Jack's mother was quite right to be appalled on hearing that her son had exchanged the house cow for a bag of beans.

The first threat to traditional livestock farming came from the enclosures, whereby common land was taken from the people and passed into private ownership. This severely restricted the ability of families to acquire their food and wealth from animals that supported themselves by grazing food that humans couldn't eat from land that they didn't own. In the UK the practice and legalisation of enclosures took place in the 18th century. In the third world, the annexation of forests and other common land for urbanisation and industrial agriculture continues to present a massive and current global threat to the sustainability of the land and the communities that draw their living directly from the land.

The second agricultural revolution, that of the 20th century, included the industrialisation and extreme intensification of most forms of livestock production. This has been extremely successful in its primary aim; provision of more food, cheaper food and more choice throughout the seasons to a far greater number of people living in towns and cities out of touch with the realities of farming. However, it has generated a new set of problems concerning human health, animal welfare and environmental degradation.

In the developed world of industrialised agriculture, dairy herds of more than 100 animals are the norm and massive dairy factories in which cows are permanently confined in herds of over 1,000 animals are becoming increasingly common. In the last 30 years annual lactation yields of the most productive herds of dairy cattle have increased from less than 5,000 to over 10,000 litres per cow. These total yields correspond to peak daily yields of approximately 25 and 50 litres/day. This has been achieved by parallel processes of genetic selection for increased yield and changes in diet and feeding practice designed to increase nutrient supply.

The most conspicuous illustration of the industrialisation of beef production has been the development of massive feedlots for 'finishing' animals typically on diets consisting mainly of corn (maize) and soya. In the US (1998) beef-cattle sales were

26.8 million head, 85% of which were produced in larger commercial feedlots with capacities of more than 1,000 animals. It is important, however, to point out that the great majority of these animals spent only about 150 days on feedlot having been born to and raised naturally by beef cows living on open range and subsisting primarily on pasture. In Europe at least 50% of beef comes from calves born to dairy cows. They are taken from their mothers at birth, artificially reared and the majority of these calves spend most of their lives in sheds. The consequences of these two systems for the welfare of the animals and the environment will be considered later.

Cattle welfare

Animal welfare is a big subject that has been worked over many times by many people. Much of the debate relates to animal welfare as a human concern. However, here (and elsewhere Webster 1994, 2005) I am more interested in how they feel than how we do. I shall consider animal welfare as perceived by the animals themselves and how best we may seek to promote it. In this regard I have for 25 years operated on the basis of the 'Five Freedoms' (FAWC 1993). A more recent pan-European study by the Welfare Quality® group (Botreau et al. 2007) proposed a set of four principles and eleven criteria (Table 7.1). The two approaches are essentially the same. Both are based on a comprehensive list of outcome measures of physical and emotional welfare, namely proper nutrition; a satisfactory physical environment; absence of pain, injury and disease; freedom from fear and stress; and opportunities to exercise natural, socially acceptable behaviour. The last may perhaps be better expressed as 'freedom of choice'. I have always stressed that these criteria should not be viewed as unachievable criteria of excellence but as a practical template for the investigation and resolution of welfare problems on an individual farm or within a production system (e.g. production of white veal (Webster 2005). The approach has been widely adopted for use in risk management and quality control procedures at the level of the system or individual farm. (Main 2009; Welfare Quality 2009).

TABLE 7.1 Three approaches to categorizing the elements of farm animal welfare

Five Freedoms (FAWC 1993)	*Welfare Principles (Botreau et al. 2007)*	*Five Domains (Mellor and Beausoleil 2015)*
Hunger & thirst	Good feeding	Food and water
Discomfort	Good housing	Environmental challenge
Pain, injury & disease	Good health	Disease & injury
Fear and stress	Appropriate behaviour	Behavioural restriction
Natural behaviour		
		Mental state

TABLE 7.2 Comparison of the magnitude of welfare risks *incurred as a direct consequence of management practices* to lactating dairy cows, beef cattle on feedlots and beef cattle (cows and calves) at pasture or on range. (n.s. = not significant). Some of the welfare problems associated with traditional methods of rearing calves for white veal have been reduced through legislation and public demand – see text.

	Dairy cows	*Beef on feedlot*	*Beef at pasture*	*'White veal' (traditional)*
Nutrition problems	+++	+++	+/–	+++
Physical discomfort	++	+	+/–	+++
Pain and injury	++	+	n.s.	+++
Infectious disease	+	++	n.s	+++
Fear and stress	n.s.	+	n.s.	+++
Restricted behaviour	+	++	n.s.	+++
Exhaustion	++	n.s.	n.s.	n.s.

An alternative approach to the evaluation of animal welfare, the 'Five Domains' has been proposed by Mellor and Beausoleil (2015). This identifies physical and psychological challenges within four domains, then integrates them within a fifth domain, 'Mental State'. This approach may well get closer to an analysis of how we think they feel. However, that is not the prime purpose of the Five Freedoms, which are intended for use as a comprehensive protocol for examining the different elements of animal welfare and what we should do about each of them in turn.

No system of animal production can guarantee absolute freedom from suffering and ill health. However, many risks to health and welfare arise *as a direct consequence of the management system.* Table 7.2 uses the principles of the Five Freedoms to briefly summarise these risks for dairy cattle, beef cattle and calves reared by traditional methods for the production of white veal. Where the letters n.s. appear in Table 7.2 this does not mean that the problem will never arise but that it is unlikely to present as a significant anthropogenic risk for that population.

The three major problems of health and welfare for dairy cattle, namely infertility, mastitis and lameness are typically described as 'production diseases', which acknowledges that they are a direct consequence of the production system imposed on the animals. These potential sources of poor health and welfare can be interdependent and additive. For example, the high genetic merit dairy cow, housed in cubicles and fed a diet based on wet grass silage and concentrate in parlour, may suffer both from hunger and chronic discomfort, partly because the quality of feed has been inadequate to meet her nutrient requirements for lactation and she has lost condition, partly because the wet silage has contributed to poor hygiene and predisposed her to foot lameness and partly because genetic selection has created a cow too big for the cubicles.

The main health risks for beef cattle on feedlots are associated first with the stresses of transport from ranch to feedlot, then with the switch to high-energy rations based on starchy cereals. The primary problems are severe respiratory disease, typically *pasteurella* pneumonia, commonly described as 'shipping fever' and chronic digestive disorders, especially ruminal acidosis. Moreover this can precipitate laminitis, a severely painful condition, probably affecting all four feet.

Beef cows and calves given access to pasture may have few welfare problems provided that the pasture is reasonably sufficient and they have access to shelter (freedom of choice) from the worst stresses of heat and cold. Because cattle living outdoors are extremely well adapted to climatic stresses, most heat stress can be avoided by providing shelter from direct sunlight, cold stress by shelter from wind and precipitation. It is natural for ruminants, wild and domestic, to experience seasonal food shortages (winter in the temperate zones, the dry season in the tropics).

Column 5 in Table 7.2 considers the traditional method for rearing calves for the production of white veal on all-liquid diets and rates it as +++ bad according to all of the Five Freedoms. The extreme restriction on behaviour that enraged Ruth Harrison (1964) and led to the publication of the Brambell Report (1965) was sufficient evidence to rate the system as unacceptable. This, however, was but one of their problems. The diet was deficient in iron with the deliberate intention of inducing anaemia. The lack of dietary fibre also predisposed them to chronic digestive disorders, including severely painful abomasal ulcers. Diet and environment (high stocking density) contributed to major respiratory problems, and the calves were only kept alive through routine daily administration of antibiotics. It was my sense of outrage over white veal production that led me to propose the Five Freedoms in their current form. I have presented the argument in full elsewhere (Webster 1994).

The Five Freedoms have proved to be an exceptionally valuable tool for assessing the welfare state of an animal, or a herd of animals, at a moment in time. However, for many farm animals, and for dairy cows in particular, some of the most severe welfare problems arise from the long-term consequences of trying, and ultimately failing, to cope with the exacting physiological and behavioural demands of everyday life. Exhaustion, the final welfare concern listed in Table 7.2, is not identified within the Five Freedoms, but for dairy cows it is probably the biggest welfare problem of all. It describes the cow broken down in body, and probably in spirit, through a succession of stresses arising from improper nutrition, housing, hygiene and management exacerbated in many cases by inappropriate breeding due to selection for production traits at the expense of fitness.

Dairy cows at the limit

No farm animal is worked harder than the dairy cow. The proof of this contention is provided by Table 7.3, which compares the daily food energy requirements and energy expenditure (i.e. work, expressed as heat production) of a range of humans and farm animals. To simplify the comparison, values for energy intake and heat production are expressed in relation to that of an adult sedentary human (e.g. a typical office worker or university student).[1] Relative to an adult sedentary male, a lactating mother will eat 38% more food energy and work 13% harder; 25% of the

TABLE 7.3 'How hard do animals work?' This table compares the daily food energy requirements (expressed as metabolisable energy, ME), energy expenditure as work (heat production), 'food' energy outputs, expressed as weight gain in meat animals, eggs or milk. The sedentary adult human (e.g. office worker) is taken as the basis for comparison (ME intake and work output as heat = 1.0). Energy exchanges of all other classes are expressed as multiples of this standard sedentary human. (For further explanation of scaling terms see Webster 2005, p. 103.)

Species	*Activity*	*Energy exchange*		
		ME intake	*Work/heat*	*"Food"*
Human	Sedentary	1.00	1.00	
	Working miner	1.25	1.25	
	Lactating woman	1.53	1.28	0.25
	Endurance cyclist	2.60	2.90	–0.30
Pig	Grower	2.10	1.30	0.80
	Lactating sow	3.20	1.73	1.47
Birds	Broiler chicken	2.10	1.18	0.92
	Laying hen	1.73	1.30	0.43
	Passerine feeding chicks	3.03	3.03	
Cow	Suckler with one calf	2.22	1.32	0.91
	Dairy cow, 50l/day	5.68	2.14	3.53

food energy she consumes will be carried into her milk. Miners digging coal by hand worked about 25% harder than sedentary individuals, but slightly less than the mothers of their children. Only those engaged in extreme sports such as the Tour de France work to their absolute limits, and then not on a full-time basis. Growth in farm animals is not a particularly energy-demanding process. Even in the rapidly growing broiler, heat production is less than 20% above maintenance. The laying hen, producing one egg per day, is faced by considerable metabolic demands, e.g. in relation to calcium metabolism. However, the energy cost of egg-laying is not particularly severe (heat production 30% above maintenance). All these costs pale into insignificance when set against the cost to a dairy cow of sustaining a milk yield of 50 litres/day. She has to consume an amount of feed nearly six times that of maintenance and her work load (heat production) exceeds twice that of maintenance. Synthesis of so much milk not only presents the dairy cow with an enormous metabolic load, the need to consume enough feed to meet this metabolic demand (five to six times that required for maintenance) drives the digestive system to its limits and can seriously compromise their need to rest and sleep. The demands of lactation for a sow feeding ten piglets (or a bitch feeding eight puppies) are also high. However, they do not approach that of the high-yielding dairy cow. Moreover they are unlikely to persist longer than about eight weeks by which time the sow, or bitch, will almost certainly have lost a lot of condition. The dairy cow has the added problem of sustaining the metabolic demands of lactation for most of her working life. The only animal species that I have discovered to work harder than dairy cows are birds while feeding their young in nests. This too is a process that doesn't last too long. It is little wonder that dairy cows break down with signs of exhaustion.

Another potential welfare problem for the high-yielding Holstein cow is the fact that her energy demands greatly exceed her maximum possible energy intake from pasture. If a cow is to sustain a yield of 50 litres/day or more she must have near continuous access to a highly nutritious diet (a Total Mixed Ration, TMR) containing a high proportion of mechanically harvested cereals and protein supplements such as soya. This leads to the practice of zero-grazing, whereby cows are confined through most or all of lactation and may be allowed out to pasture (if at all) during a period of about two months at the end of lactation and before the birth of their next calf. Having accepted a management system that keeps dairy cows off the land and feeds them entirely on mechanically harvested feed, there is in theory no limit to herd size. It is now common for herd size in intensive dairy units to exceed 1,000 milking cows. These animals are obviously denied natural behaviours at pasture, including freedom of choice. However, in terms of the other four freedoms, I do not believe that one can condemn large, zero-grazing dairy systems simply for being large and zero-grazing. Each element of welfare (nutrition, comfort, health, behaviour) has to be assessed within each individual enterprise. I am generally sympathetic to systems that support lower-yielding, more robust cows that derive much of their nutrition (and satisfaction) from pasture, mainly on grounds of sustainability, measured both in relation to the ecosystem and the survival of rural communities. However, I have to concede that in many such traditional farms both cows and farmers are currently suffering from overwork and under-investment, both of which states are unsustainable.

However well formulated the diet for high yielding dairy cows, metabolisable energy (ME) demand in early lactation exceeds that which can be achieved by the cow within the constraints of appetite and the cow loses condition. She 'milks off her back'. The physiological demand for nutrients to support lactation creates a condition of 'metabolic hunger' and the intensity of this hunger increases as body condition falls. The loss in body condition and increase in hunger is more extreme when cows are injected with bovine growth hormone (BST) to stimulate increased milk yield (Chalupa and Gallingan 1989).

It is salutary to consider these stresses on the physiology of digestion and metabolism in terms of how it feels for the high-yielding cow. She is motivated to eat by metabolic hunger (a function of both milk yield and body condition). She is motivated to *stop* eating by sensations (conscious or unconscious) associated with gut overload and the conflicting desire to do something other than eat, such as rest. At pasture, the first constraint on food intake is the rate at which the cow can physically consume the grass. Here the motivation for the cow to stop eating is most likely to arise from the desire to rest than from the sensation of gut fill. Very high-yielding cows confined within a zero-grazing system are presented with the conflicting problems of metabolic hunger, gut overload and the need to rest in a more extreme form and face a more difficult compromise as they seek to minimise the discomfort involved in reconciling these three stresses.

This summary of the conflicts between metabolic need, digestive capacity and the need for rest provokes a number of difficult practical questions concerning dairy cow welfare.

- Is it more stressful to a dairy cow to produce 55 l milk/day than 25 l/day?
- Is it stressful to restrict a cow with the genetic potential to produce 55 l/day to a diet that can only sustain 25 l/day?
- Is it stressful to restrict a cow to a zero-grazing system for most or all of her adult life?

There are no easy answers to these questions. The use of high genetic merit Holsteins (60 l/day potential) has presented welfare problems manifested most obviously by infertility and early forced culling (Pryce et al. 1998). This is particularly evident on pastoral systems (e.g. in New Zealand) where ME intake cannot keep pace with metabolic demand (Harris and Winkelman 2000). Many dairy farmers operating this system are now working towards a better balance between supply and demand both by improving the quality of the pasture and by selection within the Holstein breed, or through cross-breeding to produce a more robust cow with a lower potential yield but an improved lifetime performance.

Currently less than half the "high genetic merit" dairy cows in the developed world manage to sustain a working life of more than three years (three lactations). The three main causes of enforced culling (removal of unproductive cows from the herd) are infertility, mastitis and lameness (Esslemont and Kossaibati 1996). As stated earlier, these may all be considered as 'production diseases' for which the major risks arise from hazards intrinsic to the system and management. A major hazard for infertility is loss of body condition associated with inadequate nutrition in early lactation. Mastitis is caused by infections with bacteria arising from the environment or sequestered within the udder of carrier cows and transmitted at the time of milking. The costs to the farmer of mastitis are obvious and immediate: discarded milk, costs of treatment and loss of production in the longer term. Consequently most farmers operate a strict mastitis control policy through attention to good hygiene and the elimination of infected carrier cows with high somatic cell counts (SCC). In many countries this strategy is rewarded through an economic policy of carrot and stick: increased milk price for low SCC, financial penalties when SCC in the bulk tank is high.

Lameness is the most severe welfare problem for the dairy cow by virtue of the pain involved and its prevalence. On random inspection of the milking cows on a modern commercial dairy farm over 25%, on average, are likely to show visible signs of lameness (Cook 2003, Whay et al. 2003). This is a complex problem involving a multiplicity of hazards associated with housing, hygiene, nutrition, breeding and management. There is less incentive to control lameness than mastitis because the economic costs are less apparent and usually there is no financial incentive to take remedial action. Many farmers have assumed fatalistically that some degree of lameness is an inevitable consequence of a system that involves concrete floors and lots of slurry. However, recent research has consistently revealed that the most important risk factors for lameness are associated with failures of foot care; improper or non-existent foot trimming and failure to treat new cases at the first sign of abnormal locomotion (Bell et al. 2009, Smith et al. 2007). One can sympathise with farmers and stockpeople who work long hours and can find little time to attend to cows' feet. However, they should be aware that the best approach to the problem simply requires them to spend more time with their cows. There is no need to rebuild the farm.

While these three great production diseases can be attributed mainly to failures of nutrition, housing and management, there is no denying that things have been made worse for both farmers and their cows through a breeding policy that selected cows overwhelmingly on the basis of increased productivity (milk yield in first lactation) without sufficient attention to fitness traits such as fertility, resistance to mastitis, sound locomotion, etc., that would reduce their susceptibility to the major production diseases and enable them to sustain a longer working life, while feeling better in the process.

Table 7.4 (from Pryce et al. 1998) describes the phenotypic and genotypic correlations between selection for increasing milk yield, calving interval (a measure of infertility), mastitis and lameness in UK Holstein/Friesian cows. The phenotypic correlation describes the association as it appears on farm. The genotypic correlation describes that which is attributable to breeding rather than management and this is positive and highly significant in all cases. The negligible phenotypic effects on mastitis and lameness reveal that farmers are just managing to keep things under control through improvements to husbandry designed to compensate for the genetic deterioration in fitness. In the case of infertility, the battle is being lost.

Fortunately for all, dairy farmers and breeders are becoming increasingly aware of the need to modify selection indices to produce a more robust cow. Whereas ten years ago over 75% of selection pressure would typically be directed towards production *per se* (yields of milk protein and fat), modern selection indices give increasing emphasis to traits linked to robustness and leading to improved lifetime performance. Indeed within Holstein UK, fitness traits now contribute just over

TABLE 7.4 Phenotypic and genotypic correlations between milk yield and three indices of fitness in the dairy cow (from Pryce et al. 1998)

	Phenotype	*Genotype*
Calving interval	+0.20	+0.39
Mastitis	–0.01	+0.26
Lameness	+0.04	+0.17

50% to the selection index. This is undoubtedly a step in the right direction though it is still too soon to assess the results.

Beef cows and their calves

It is my belief that beef cows who spend most of the year on well-managed pastures in temperate climates, give birth to one calf per year and feed it for about six months may experience a better quality of life than any other class of animal reared under commercial conditions. (I exclude the "pets" reared for the pleasure of hobby farmers.) Indeed I have argued that if the calves in the slaughter generation are also finished at grass, it may be more humane to eat beef than cheese. As illustrated in Table 7.2, these animals are able to experience most of the Five Freedoms, most of the time. Admittedly most of the beef cows of the world are unlikely to experience the comforts of the county of Hereford. Beef cattle can thrive wherever grass can grow, from the extreme heat of Texas and Queensland to the severe cold of the northern prairies and the steppes of central Asia. The physical stresses imposed on these animals – heat, cold, malnutrition – may be intense and prolonged and in poorly managed enterprises; these stresses may be exacerbated through overgrazing, failure to provide adequate shelter or control parasites. There is not space here to review in detail welfare issues for beef cattle on range, but see EFSA 2012. In brief, it can be said that beef cattle have a very wide zone of thermal comfort and the upper and lower limits shift up and down during acclimatisation to summer and winter conditions (Webster 1976). Cattle, in common with all ruminants, are also extremely well adapted to the experience of seasonal undernutrition during winter in the higher latitudes, or the dry season in the tropics. They should, of course, not be left to starve (although some times and in some places this is unavoidable). However, it is normal at this time for the diet to be restricted in quantity and poor in quality. Ruminants have an elegant physiological mechanism for coping with limited quantities of high-fibre, low-protein forages. When all mammals lose weight, body protein is broken down to urea. In ruminants this urea is not lost to the system, but recycled into the rumen and used to maintain the population of microbial protein to sustain digestion of fibrous feeds. Moreover the urea, which would be a waste product in simple-stomached animals is recycled, via microbial protein, back to the animal in the form of amino acids to replace lost body proteins (Webster 2009). The successful overwintering of beef cows illustrates the difference between stress and suffering. The former is a natural phenomenon. Suffering occurs when an animal is unable to cope (or has great difficulty in coping) with stress. Beef cows on well-managed pastures all over the world are well able to cope with natural stresses most of the time. This reflects not only the extent of their physiological powers of adaptation. They are also able to enjoy perhaps the most important of the freedoms: freedom of choice.

Significant, anthropogenic welfare problems for beef cattle born and raised on range begin when calves are removed and transported to feedlots to be fed intensively to slaughter weight on high-energy rations, typically based on corn (maize) and soya. The first and greatest risk is 'shipping fever'. This condition typically manifests as severe pneumonia and pleurisy. The incidence of this form of bovine respiratory disease in groups of cattle in feedlots in US has been reported to range from 4–44%, with a median value of about 15% (Snowder et al. 2006). Although mortality rates in treated animals are generally low (< 1%) the performance and welfare of these cattle are likely to be compromised throughout the finishing period. The aetiology is complex. Several viruses are involved in the pathogenesis but most damage is done by the bacteria *pasteurella multocida*. The traditional name 'shipping fever' implied that transport *per se* is the major precipitating stress. Later research shows that treatment after arrival on feedlot is the major risk, especially an abrupt change of diet from grass to corn. These days it is customary for feedlot operators to increase access to corn feeding more gradually to reduce the risk of respiratory disease. Nevertheless high-starch, low-fibre diets are inconsistent with healthy rumen digestion. Some degree of ruminal acidosis is almost inevitable. In many cases this leads to chronic damage to the rumen wall (parakeratosis) and predisposes the animals to liver abscesses and painful lameness associated with laminitis (EFSA 2012). In the US (especially) millions of dollars are spent on feed additives that claim to 'enhance performance' but in fact attempt, with more or less success, to offset the harmful effects of a fundamentally unhealthy diet.

Beef, veal and "bobby calves" from the dairy herd

The majority of beef produced in Europe and UK comes from calves born to dairy cows, separated from their mothers shortly after birth, reared at first on milk replacer, then weaned onto a mixed ration of forage and concentrates. The exact system of feeding and housing will be governed in part by local conditions of climate and feed availability. However, the main factor determining the rearing system will be the phenotype (body shape) of the calf. The traditional Friesian dairy cow was, in fact, a dual-purpose animal. Male calves born to Friesian calves mated with Friesian bulls are sufficiently well muscled to make good-quality beef, although, unlike classic beef breeds such as Hereford and Aberdeen Angus, they are typically fattened in yards on a mixture of concentrates and conserved silage because it is unprofitable to finish them at grass.

Over the last 40 years, the pressure on the dairy industry to produce more and more milk per cow has produced the modern Holstein, a conspicuous collection of bones supporting a large udder. Male Holstein calves (and those from other extreme dairy breeds such as Jerseys) that do not have the conformation to make them worth rearing for beef have little value. In many parts of the world their fate has been to become 'bobby calves': transported off farm and to slaughter within the first two weeks of life. Because they are of such low value, they receive little or no care and their welfare is dreadful. In the second half of the 20th century, the combination of surplus male Holstein calves and surplus milk products led to a massive expansion in the white veal industry, especially in Holland and Italy. This may have been a bonus for dairy farmers because it increased the value of their surplus calves. For the calves, however, it only prolonged their suffering. The development of alternative systems for the production of pink veal from calves reared in groups on a mixture of liquid feed and forage can undoubtedly improve calf welfare (Webster 1994). However, the uptake of these systems has been small, largely because it is difficult to make a profit.

The constant endeavour of good farmers throughout history has been to care for the land: to manage it in such a way as to be profitable, efficient and sustainable. On a mixed farm, this has traditionally involved the growing of crops, the management of pastures and the husbandry of animals: milk from dairy cows as a major enterprise but with beef as an excellent extra source of income. The traditional, robust Friesian cow was ideal for this purpose. With a typical working life of six lactations, and only needing one Friesian heifer calf to replace her in the herd, she could give birth to four calves sired by beef bulls (e.g. Hereford or Charolais), with the conformation required to produce high-quality beef largely from pasture on the home farm.

The modern, large specialist dairy production unit, with populations of 1,000 or more Holstein cows yielding 8,000–10,000 litres of milk per lactation, housed continuously in sheds and consuming total mixed rations brought to them by feeder wagons, may be efficient within its own terms of reference, but it can no longer be said to be farming the land. Moreover it is unlikely that these units will include facilities for rearing male calves. The problem for the calves is compounded by the fact that the working life of the modern Holstein is likely to be three lactations or less. Thus she is unlikely to be mated more than once (if at all) with semen from a beef bull to produce a calf that can be reared for beef in a manner that is consistent with satisfactory welfare.

These problems were addressed within a Calf Forum involving a balanced mix of producers, professionals and welfarists (CIWF/RSPCA 2008). Their report describes how it is quite possible to remove the problem of surplus male calves destined for veal production or condemned to become bobby calves or killed on farm prior to registration. First, breed a more robust cow, able to sustain six lactations or more. Inseminate her as a heifer either by natural mating or by artificial insemination (AI) from a relatively small beef breed (e.g. Hereford) to reduce the risk of obstetric problems at first calving. Inseminate her for the second time with sexed semen from a dairy bull to produce a heifer replacement for her in the herd and use semen from beef bulls thereafter. Henceforth (if not quite at a stroke) no more bobby calves.

Resources: demand and sustainability

Many of the chapters in this book rightly draw attention to the urgent threats both to human health and the living environment arising from the ever-increasing demand for meat and milk. The sheer size of the industry has led to the destruction of forests and permanent pastures to create vast tracts of maize and soya bean grown for livestock feed. Moreover, the size of the international dairy industry will continue to increase as increasingly affluent consumers, especially in Asia, come to discover the pleasures of milk and milk products. Meat and dairy production from ruminants draw particular criticism on two grounds. Cattle appear to convert animal feed to human food less efficiently than pigs and poultry. They also produce large amounts of methane as a natural consequence of fermentation of carbohydrates in the rumen, and the global warming effect of methane is 21 times that of carbon dioxide. I suggest, however, that it is not sufficient simply to add up the environmental demands of livestock production and define them (e.g.) in terms of a Global Footprint (e.g. *Livestock's Long Shadow*, FAO 2006). The sustainability of demand can only be properly assessed in relation to the capacity of the land, the water and the sun to supply that demand. Before one dismisses dairy and beef production as especially flagrant examples of man's inhumanity to other animals and to the sustainable environment, it is necessary to examine three big questions (at the very least).

1. To what extent can we feed animals on feeds that are complementary to, rather than competitive with, food grown for human consumption?
2. What are the other major environmental demands for livestock production (especially fossil fuels)?
3. What is the balance between demand for resources (e.g. energy, nitrogen, water) and the production of pollutants (e.g. greenhouse gases) and the capacity of the land sustainably to accommodate these demands?

There is not space to review these issues in any detail. They are addressed elsewhere in this book and I have expressed my own thoughts at greater length in *Animal Husbandry Regained: The Place of Farm Animals in Sustainable Agriculture* (Webster 2013). I present here brief examples to illustrate these three big issues.

Competitive and complementary feeds

Table 7.5 compares efficiencies of production (output/input) for four major foods of animal origin: eggs, pork, milk and beef. Output is measured in terms of food energy and protein for man. Input is measured in terms of total feed energy and protein and 'competitive' energy and protein, i.e. that which could have been consumed directly by humans. Production of milk and eggs is inherently more efficient than meat production as a source of protein for humans because it doesn't involve killing the animals. Milk production is by far the most efficient when measured in terms of food energy and protein supply to humans, relative to consumption of food directly available to man. This is because a typical well-balanced ration for dairy cows can be formulated (and, in the UK, typically is formulated) on the basis that over 75% comes from feed that is complementary to, rather than in

TABLE 7.5 Efficiency of energy and protein conversion in meat, milk and egg production (from Webster 2013). For each system, efficiency is described by the ratio of output to input, where output is defined by energy and protein in food for humans; inputs are described in terms of total and 'competitive' intake of ME and protein, where 'competitive' describes energy and protein from feed sources that could be fed directly to humans.

	Eggs	*Pork*	*Milk*	*Beef*
Production unit	1 hen	22 pigs	1 cow	1 calf
Support unit	0.05 hens	1 sow	0.33 heifers	1 cow
Output/year (kg food)	15	1300	8000	200
MJ food energy	130	13000	28000	2500
kg protein	1.65	208	264	32
Input/year (MJ ME in total)	389	67038	67089	29850
MJ 'competitive' ME	351	53630	20127	10268
Input/year (kg protein in total)	5.2	818	946	361
kg 'competitive' protein	5.0	736	236	108
Efficiency				
Food energy/total feed ME	0.33	0.19	0.42	0.08
Food energy/'competitive' feed ME	0.35	0.24	1.39	0.24
Food protein/total feed protein	0.32	0.25	0.28	0.09
Food protein/'competitive' feed protein	0.33	0.28	1.12	0.30

competition with, the needs of people. In the example provided by Table 7.5, milk energy and protein yields are 1.39 and 1.12 energy and protein inputs from 'food for humans'. By this criterion, the dairy cow becomes the most sustainable of farm animals, more so than the hen. Even beef production becomes no more inefficient than pork when expressed in the relation to consumption of competitive energy. I acknowledge at once that this argument (like all the others) is incomplete, but it is more comprehensive than some.

Life cycle analysis

It is, of course, necessary to review the efficiency and sustainability of cattle production in terms of all demands on resources (e.g. energy and water) and potential threats to sustainability (e.g. greenhouses gases, GHG). These themes appear throughout this book. The demands and threats (if not the capacity to sustain these demands and threats) are described in detail in *Livestock's Long Shadow* (FAO 2006). This topic is massive in scope. Here I shall present only a brief example of the principle of Life Cycle Analysis as developed by Pelletier (2008; Pelletier et al. 2010a, b) to analyse the environmental costs of the major inputs and emissions involved in animal production systems. The most

TABLE 7.6 Life cycle assessment of inputs and emissions required to produce 1 tonne of meat in broiler, pig and beef production systems (from Pelletier 2008, Pelletier et al. 2010a,b)

Output (1 tonne meat)	*Energy use (GJ)*			*GHG*
	ME total	*ME competitive*	*Fuel energy*	*CO_2 equiv*
Broiler chickens	36	32	14.9	1.39
Pork, commercial	52	41	9.7	2.47
Pork, niche	68	49	11.4	2.52
Beef, feedlot finished	149	51	84.2	32.7
Beef, pasture finished	194	20	114.2	45.3

important inputs are energy, protein and water. It is, however, necessary to distinguish between (relatively) sustainable and unsustainable sources of these three resources. Energy inputs are classified as total feed energy, 'competitive' feed energy and fossil fuel energy. The sources of feed energy itself may be subdivided into 'free energy' (solar energy converted into plant matter by photosynthesis) and 'fuel energy' used in the production, fertilisation, harvesting and processing of plant material for animal feed.

Table 7.6 presents some examples of the application of LCA to examine total energy use in livestock production systems. It has been adapted (and greatly simplified) from Pelletier (2008; Pelletier et al. 2010a,b). The examples include three intensive ('commercial') systems – broiler chicken, pork and feedlot beef – and two more 'traditional' alternatives – 'niche' pork (equivalent to organic or free range) and pasture-finished beef production. The output of the system in every case is one tonne of meat. The data have been drawn from units operating in the central belt of the US. This is important because much of the demand for fuel energy derives from the production of feed crops (corn and soya) from fertilised, irrigated pastures. Clearly the demand for fuel energy in particular will vary enormously according to the extent to which animals can harvest feed for themselves, relative to that which depends on machines.

In these examples, broiler poultry production is the most efficient in terms of meat production relative to energy intake, whether measured in terms of total or competitive ME. However, it is slightly less efficient in terms of fuel energy use, attributable mainly to increased energy use in feed production and environmental control. Intensive beef production (feedlot finished) is extremely inefficient in relative terms, measured in terms of total ME and fuel energy use. In these examples the two 'traditional' or 'alternative' systems, niche pork production and pasture-finished beef, were significantly less efficient than their intensive comparison, when assessed both in terms of feed energy and fuel energy. This shows that one cannot necessarily make a case for less intensive livestock farming on the basis of energy cost when fossil fuels are taken into account. However, I repeat:

every evaluation is likely to be case specific. My intention here is merely to highlight the questions we need to ask.

Methane production and carbon sequestration

One of the major environmental concerns arising from livestock production relates to the production of methane (CH_4), which is approximately 18 times as potent a greenhouse gas (GHG) as carbon dioxide (CO_2). The major "culprits" in the matter of methane production are the ruminants (Table 7.4), or to be more specific, the microorganisms responsible for the anaerobic fermentation of plant material in the rumen. It is an inescapable fact that ruminant animals are significant contributors to GHG production and the more extensive the system, the greater the production of GHG relative to production of meat and milk. There is considerable capacity to manipulate the production of methane by rumen microorganisms through manipulation of diet or the use of licensed pharmaceuticals. However dietary manipulation can create health problems for the animals resulting from unstable rumen fermentation; pharmacological manipulation can also create real health problems for some animals, and present concerns (real or apparent) to consumers and legislators anxious to ensure the production of safe, 'natural' food from animals.

The fashionable assault on ruminants as major contributors to global warming is perhaps the most extreme example of my especial bête noire, namely argument from inadequate premises. For a start, it is nothing new, not even in degree. The cattle population of the US in 2007 was approximately 100 million, of which 42 million were adult cows. In the 17th century the population of American Bison was ca. 60 million. Given that feedlot animals finished on high starch rations produce relatively less methane than animals at pasture one can estimate, with considerable uncertainty, that methane production from ruminants in the US is probably no more than 20% greater than it was 300 years ago.

More critically, and more scientifically, it is meaningless to consider methane production in isolation. Well-managed grasslands constitute a significant carbon sink, the extent of carbon sequestration depending on factors such as the intensity of grazing and the balance between grasses and legumes (clovers and alfalfa). Several recent studies of C and GHG balance (production and sequestration) in a wide range of grassland systems throughout Europe have indicated that dairy production, dependent in part on permanent pastures, can be approximately GHG neutral (e.g. Soussana et al. 2010). Beef production on range with good pasture management can achieve net sequestration of GHG equivalents. However, a far more effective way to combine cattle production with carbon sequestration is through the development of silvo-pastoral systems such as those currently operating in South America where cattle graze grass and browse shrubs within the shelter of larger trees (Kumar and Nair 2011). So far as cattle welfare is concerned these systems can be extremely attractive, providing balanced nutrition, thermal and physical comfort, good social contact and, above all, freedom of choice.

Living off the land: 'emergy' analysis

It is easy to criticise much analysis of ecology and sustainability on the grounds that it is based on limited metrics. The limited metric that I have applied in this chapter is energy. This has the merit that the same units can be used to quantify the inputs of sunlight, animal feed and fossil fuels and to measure the efficiency of their conversion to food for humans. It is also salutary to remind the reader that despite the constant endeavour of popular journalists, pedlars of food supplements and others with a relaxed attitude to the truth, over 80% of the digestible food that we eat is used for fuel energy and consumed to support the fire of life. However, the analysis so far has not taken into account other vital resources such as water, minerals, etc. There is, however, a new approach to analysis of ecosystems based on the concept of embodied energy or 'emergy'. This concept seeks to express all the work processes and resources (sunlight, water, fossil fuels, minerals, etc.) used in the generation of a product in terms of a common unit of measurement (Zhao et al. 2005). The approach does involve a lot of assumptions that inevitably carry a deal of uncertainty. However, I believe it to be a most elegant way of assessing the efficiency and sustainability of farming the land for food.

In this case resources are defined as follows:

- Renewable emergy (R) = emergy equivalents 'off the land' from sustainable sources e.g. sunlight, free water, etc.
- Unrenewable emergy (UR) = loss of emergy from land degradation (etc.).
- Purchased goods and services (F) = bought in feed, fuel, labour, etc.
- Yield (Y) = food for human consumption.

Table 7.7 uses the concept of emergy transformations to compare yield and sustainability of different agricultural processes, corn production in US, conventional and organic pig production in Sweden (Pereira and Ortega 2012), intensive and

TABLE 7.7 Yield and sustainability within agricultural systems assessed in units of embedded energy ('Emergy') from Pereira et al. 2012[a], Rotolo et al. 2007[b], Vigne et al.[c] 2013). EYR = emergy yield ratio, ELR = environmental load ratio, ESI = environmental sustainable index. These ratios are dimensionless. For further explanation see text.

	EYR	*ELR*	*ESI*
Corn[a] (US)	1.07	18.8	0.06
Conventional pig[a] (Sweden)	1.04	22.3	0.05
Organic pig[a] (Sweden)	1.13	7.80	0.15
Intensive dairy[c] (Brittany)	1.35	3.25	0.42
Extensive dairy[c] (Mali)	1.89	1.25	1.57
Grazing cattle[b] (Argentina)	3.73	0.55	6.80

extensive dairy production in Brittany (France) and South Mali respectively (Vigne et al. 2013) and beef cattle grazing in Argentina (Rotolo et al. 2007). Three dimensionless ratios are used to compare the contribution of local resources to yield and sustainability:

- EYR (emergy yield ratio) = (R + NR + F)/F: contribution of local resources ('land') to product.
- ELR (environmental load ratio) = (NR + F)/F: ratio of non-renewables to renewables in product.
- ESI (emergy sustainable index) = EYR:ELR: (yield:environmental compatibility).

The ratios in column 1 (EYR) in Table 7.7 show that the relative contribution of local renewable resources to yield did not differ greatly between corn, conventional and organic pig production. The contribution of local resources was greater for dairy production, especially low-intensity dairy production in South Mali. This should not be a surprise given what has been written earlier (e.g. Table 7.5). The grazing of beef cattle was by far the most efficient in terms of the contribution of renewable resources. The most striking differences between systems are revealed in ESI, the measure of yield relative to environmental compatibility. By this measure extensive, small-scale dairy production is more sustainable than intensive production even in the relatively pasture-based systems that operate in Brittany. However, beef from permanent pasture far outstripped all other systems by these measures of sustainability. This may come as a surprise to the urbanites of today but would seem like a complicated proof of the obvious to the traditional gauchos of the Pampas or the indigenous races of North America living in perfect symbiosis with the bison.

Coda: husbandry regained

Whatever some may wish, milk and beef production are not going to go away. It follows therefore that our responsibility is to do these things better. This does not imply, as some may claim, simply going back to traditional farming nor, as others will assert, continuing to develop down the same intensive route.

Intensive dairy production: I offer the following steps towards improved husbandry for cows, farmers and the land:

1. Improvements to the provision and formulation of diets through better use of food sources that are complementary to, rather than competing with, the food needs of humans.
2. Improvements to building design to give cows more comfort when lying down and softer, less abrasive walking surfaces to reduce the risk of foot injuries.
3. Better attention to hygiene and management, especially foot care and early treatment of lame cows.

4 Reduction of pollution and energy costs, e.g. through the use of anaerobic digesters to ferment manure and other wastes and capture methane as an energy source.
5 Improved lifetime performance and welfare through increased emphasis on selection for robustness relative to milk yield.
6 Reduced production of male calves of extreme dairy type that are unfit for beef production.

Pastoral systems: Dairy systems in New Zealand show that it is still possible, on the right land and in the right climate, to produce milk from grass. It is, however, important to point out that this system can be less idyllic than it may appear. Herds in excess of 500 animals are being kept on monocultures of grasses and walked very long distances to and from the milking parlour. These large herds are creating new problems for the cows, especially increased prevalence of lameness, and for the environment, through destruction of mixed, sustainable ecosystems.

An environmental audit of dairy farming systems designed solely to produce income from the sale of milk and milk products will show that pasture-based systems operating at maximum output pose a greater potential threat to the environment (per unit of milk produced) than intensive, zero-grazing systems through such things as increased nitrogen pollution, increased production of methane and increased fossil fuel consumption for the production of artificial fertilisers. If dairy cows are to be let out into fields, rather than confined in milk factories, then the best way to realise the principles of good husbandry is to accommodate dairy production within all the other elements that contribute to sustaining the quality of the living countryside. There is a real place for extensive, lower-output, dairy production within the context of a mixed farm and a broader definition of sustainable agriculture, where income from food production makes a significant but not dominant contribution to the cost of sustaining the living environment.

The commercial production of beef, involving extensive use of fertilisers, irrigation and the feeding of large quantities of cereals and soya to fatten stock is, by most measures, the most profligate of all major systems of livestock production. However, it is also the case (Table 7.7) that grazing cattle on well-managed ranges can be a highly sustainable process. Silvo-pastoral systems in which cattle graze and browse within the comfort of a parkland environment are even more environment-friendly because they can make significant contributions both to carbon sequestration and water management. However, their output, measured simply in terms of food sales, is likely to be too low to meet the need of the farmers to sustain a reasonable standard of living. This is a main reason why so many pastoral systems in so many parts of the world have suffered from overgrazing and desertification.

I think most would concede that cattle at pasture, whether beef or dairy, have made an invaluable contribution to the sensitive, sustainable and downright beautiful stewardship of the countryside. Where I live, the cows are moved through small fields with high hedges, which are a Mecca for wildlife and the lanes between the fields explode with wildflowers. When the cows come in for milking, they bring in the muck but the muck attracts the insects and the insects attract the swallows and martins, who nest in the eaves and the swifts who soar, and sleep, in the sky. If this is what the people not actively engaged in food production wish to preserve for our own peace of mind, we must be prepared to acknowledge that these things are worth more than the price we pay for milk and beef. One way to reward farmers for greater attention to animal welfare and more 'natural' husbandry systems is, of course, through higher prices for food that is recognised as higher value by virtue of organic status, high welfare or local provenance. This quality assurance must, of course, be supported by robust independent procedures for quality control (Webster 2012). This approach permits the individual consumer to reward the producer for holding to standards that he or she holds dear. It does not impose on all the cost necessary to meet the standards of those who can afford them. One may argue that this approach cannot guarantee improved welfare for all the farm animals. However, as we have seen with free-range eggs, consumer pressure has been far more effective than legislation in bringing about change in the interests of the animals.

It is not, however, realistic to expect the individual consumer to pay the costs of sustaining the long-term quality of the living environment, not least because it brings no immediate reward. It is a generally accepted maxim of governments when facing environmental issues that 'the polluter should pay'. By the same logic society should be prepared to reward the 'anti-polluters': those who are actively engaged in the conservation of wildlife, management of water and sequestration of carbon since they offset the anthropogenic insults of the rest of us. This can be best achieved via taxation through redirection of agricultural subsidies. The strategists whose job is to underpin the Common Agriculture Policy of the European Union have recognised this in principle (European Commission 2012). In practice, however, the amount of money allocated in support of policies directed towards improved animal welfare and environmental quality is derisory and largely directed towards actions designed to make the countryside look prettier. Most subsidy is dished out mindlessly in proportion to farm size. The big issues of sustainability of land, water and energy are as yet untouched. If we are to sustain the quality of the life of the land we, as a society, have no option but to make it possible for those who work the land to be good stewards of the land.

Note

1 For a more complete explanation of this comparison based on the concept of metabolic body size (weight, $kg^{0.75}$) see Webster (2005), p. 133.

References

Bell, N.J., Bell, M.J., Knowles, T.G., Whay, H.R., Main, D.J. and Webster, A.J.F. (2009) The development, implementation and testing of a lameness-control programme based on HACCP principles and designed for heifers on dairy farms. *The Veterinary Journal* 180, 178–188.

Botreau, R., Veissier, I., Butterworth, A., Bracke, M.B.M. and Keeling, L. (2007) Definition of criteria for overall assessment of animal welfare. *Animal Welfare* 16, 225–228.

Brambell, F.W.R. (1965) *Report of technical committee to enquire into the welfare of animals kept under intensive husbandry systems.* (Cmnd. 2836) London: H.M. Stationery Office.

Chalupa, W. and Gallingan, D.T. (1989) Nutritional implications of somatotropin for lactating cows. *Journal of Dairy Science* 72, 2510–2524.

Compassion in World Farming and Royal Society for the Prevention of Cruelty to Animals (2008) *Beyond Calf Exports Stakeholders Forum.* Report on Conclusions and Recommendations.

Cook, N. (2003) Prevalence of lameness among dairy herds in Wisconsin as a function of housing type and stall surface. *Journal of the American Veterinary Association* 223, 1324–1328.

Esslemont, R.J. and Kossaibati, M.A. (1996) Incidence of production diseases and other health problems in a group of dairy herds in England. *Veterinary Record* 139, 484–490.

European Commission (2012) *The Common Agriculture Policy after 2013.* http://ec.europa.eu/agriculture/cap-post-1913/index_htm

European Food Safety Authority (2012) Scientific opinion on the welfare of cattle kept for beef production and the welfare of calves in intensive farming systems. *EFSA Journal* 10(5), 2669, (166pp).

Farm Animal Welfare Council (FAWC) (1993) *Second report on priorities for research and development in farm animal welfare.* London: DEFRA.

Food and Agriculture Organisation (FAO) (2006) *Livestock's long shadow: Environmental issues and options.* Rome: FAO.

Harris, B.L. and Winkelman, A.M. (2000) Influence of North American Holstein genetics on dairy cattle performance in New Zealand. *Proceedings New Zealand Large Herd Conference* 6, 122–136.

Harrison, R. (1964) *Animal machines.* London: Stuart.

Kumar, B.M. and Nair, P.K.R. (eds.) (2011) *Carbon sequestration potentials of agroforestry systems: Opportunities and challenges.* Advances in Agroforestry 8. New York: Springer.

Main, D. (2009) Application of welfare assessment to commercial livestock production. *Journal of Applied Animal Welfare Science* 12, 97–104.

Mellor, D.J. and Beausoleil, N.J. (2015) Extending the 'Five Domains" model for animal welfare to incorporate positive welfare states. *Animal Welfare* 24, 239–251.

Pelletier, N. (2008) Environmental performance in the US broiler poultry sector: Life cycle energy use and greenhouse gas, ozone depleting, acidifying and eutrophying emissions. *Agricultural Systems* 98, 67–73.

Pelletier, N., Lammers, P., Stender, D. and Pirog, R. (2010a) Life cycle assessment of high and low-profitability commodity and deep-bedded nache swine production systems in the Upper Midwestern United States. *Agricultural Systems* 103, 599–608.

Pelletier, N., Pirog, R. and Rasmussen, R. (2010b) Comparative life cycle environmental impact of three beef production strategies in the upper Midwestern United States. *Agricultural Systems* 103, 380–389.

Pereira, L. and Ortega, E. (2012) A modified footprint method: The case study of Brazil. *Ecological Indicators* 16, 113–127.

Pryce, J.E., Veerkamp, R.F. and Simm, G. (1998) Expected correlated responses in health and fertility traits to selection on production in dairy cattle. *Proceedings on the 6th World Congress on Genetics applied to Animal Production* 23, 383–386.

Rotolo, G.C., Rydberg, T. and Lieblein, G. (2007) Emergy evaluation of grazing cattle in Argentina's Pampas. *Agriculture, Ecosystems and Environment* 119, 383–395.

Smith, B.L., Kristula, M.A. and Martin, D. (2007) Effects of frequent functional foot trimming on the incidence of lameness in lactating dairy cattle. *The Bovine Practitioner* 41, 137–145.

Snowder, G.D., Van Vleck, L.D., Cundiff, L.V. and Bennett, G.L. (2006) Bovine respiratory disease in feedlot cattle: Environmental, genetic and economic factors. *Journal of Animal Science*, 84, 1999–2008.

Soussana, J.F., Allec, T. and Blanfort, V. (2010) Mitigating the greenhouse gas balance of ruminant production systems through carbon sequestration in grassland. *Animal* 4(3), 334–340.

Vigne, M., Peyraud, J.-L., Lecomte, P., Corson, M.S. and Wilfart, A. (2013) Emergy evaluation of contrasting dairy systems at multiple levels. *Journal of Environmental Management* 129, 44–53.

Webster, A.J.F. (1976) The influence of the climatic environment on metabolism in cattle. pp103–120 in *Principles of cattle production.* Eds. H. Swan and W.H. Broster. Butterworths, London.

Webster, J. (1994) *Animal welfare: A cool eye towards Eden.* Blackwell Science, Oxford.

Webster, J. (2005) *Animal welfare: Limping towards Eden.* Wiley Blackwell, Oxford.

Webster, J. (2009) Animal welfare and nutrition. pp113–132 in *Welfare of production animals: Assessment and management of risks.* Eds. F.J.M. Smulders and B. Algers. Wageningen, the Netherlands: Wageningen Academic Publishers.

Webster, J. (2013) *Animal husbandry regained: The place of farm animals in sustainable agriculture.* UK: Earthscan from Routledge, London and New York, p243.

Webster, J. (2016) *Livestock production systems: Animal welfare and environmental quality.* Ch 7, pp137–152 in *The Routledge handbook of food and nutrition security.* Eds. B. Pritchard, R. Ortiz and M. Shekar. Routledge, London and New York.

Welfare Quality (2009) *Assessment protocols for cattle, pigs and poultry.* Lelystad, The Netherlands: Welfare Quality Consortium.

Whay, H.R., Main, D.C.J., Green, L.E. and Webster, A.J.F. (2003) Assessment of the welfare of dairy cattle using animal-based measurements. *Veterinary Record* 153, 197–202.

Zhao, S., Li, Z. and Li, W. (2005) A modified method of ecological footprint calculation and its application. *Ecological Modelling* 185, 65–75.

8

HOW CAN WE SUSTAIN THE DEMAND FOR EGGS?

Claire A. Weeks and Ian J. H. Duncan

Introduction

Traditionally, hens have lived alongside human families literally scratching a living from the scraps available. Harvest time provided a bonanza of spilt grain to be gleaned from the fields where it was sustainably gathered using low-tech human energy. Threshing and milling on a small scale allowed further opportunities for the canny hen to fill her crop. She supplemented her diet with worms, grubs and insects thereby controlling many of the insects competing for crops destined for the human table. Importantly, the hens still laid their eggs in batches and were occasionally allowed to hatch a brood of chicks thereby providing cockerels for the table and replacement hens for the flock. In time, often several years old, the hens would be dispatched for the pot to provide yet more nutrient-rich meals of chicken stew and broth. This ecologically sound and sustainable method of production continues in so-called backyard flocks. In the west these tend not to be sustainable, as their affluent owners purchase commercial chicken feed and frequently lose their birds to predation. In less developed parts of the world hens continue to provide highly nutritious food at next to no cost to the humans alongside whom they subsist. These hens are breeds that have evolved to be fit and robust whilst still producing more eggs than their jungle fowl ancestors. The chicks are able to follow their mother high into trees shortly after hatching to escape predators. Production may also be scaled up to no more than a couple of hundred hens whereby the eggs are hatched in wood-fired brooders and the hens are kept in simple, naturally ventilated houses. It remains a part-time business using family labour and can make a substantial contribution not only to the family income but to the local economy and diet. The scaling-up of family-run hen populations has been greatly facilitated in Africa by a policy of dispensing Newcastle Disease vaccines managed by the village ladies. Often the most effective route to increased sustainable efficiency is through disease control rather than intensification *per se*.

Egg production has evolved to supply the demands of an increasingly industrialised, urban and expanding human population. For example, in 1950 when global human population was 2.5 billion, egg production remained small scale and largely free range. In several countries, including the UK, small mobile houses were the norm, with manual egg collection and frequent pasture rotation on mixed farms alongside other livestock and crop enterprises. With the growth of industry, not surprisingly, many agricultural workers chose to swap working in dark, wet and muddy conditions for the relative comfort of the factory environment. The way of keeping hens followed suit with the development of cage production systems in which the birds were kept warm and dry, producing clean eggs to meet an ever-rising demand. The housing change resulted also from the various problems encountered with free-range production that included 'fowl sick' land, *Salmonella pullorum*, red and scaly leg mite, coccidiosis, worms, comb frostbite, crop binding and losses to predators (Elson, 1988), which caused high mortality (Robinson, 1961) and reduced margins. The health benefits of cage housing accrued by keeping hens away from their faeces and from these parasites and diseases picked up from contaminated ground, not to mention protection from predators. Automated feed and water delivery and egg collection further reduced labour costs. Moreover the value of supplementary lighting and lighting regimes became recognised (e.g. Morris and Fox, 1958) enabling reliable, year-round production. Genetic selection stepped up a gear with the emphases on breeding out batch-laying characteristics, increasing egg output and reducing the feed required to produce each egg (i.e. the feed conversion efficiency). For any animal, a principal way to reduce its feed requirement is to reduce its body size and keep it in thermally comfortable conditions thereby reducing the amount of food needed to maintain body temperature and key body functions. Hens were inevitably selected for reduced body size and more were put in each cage to keep each other warm. Unfortunately the selection for controlled environment production now leaves current genotypes at a disadvantage when exposed to cold, wet weather in free-range environments. Environmental control became possible in insulated houses with fan ventilation. The drive to reduce fixed costs and capital requirements pushed as many birds into each cage as was physically possible. High-rise hen production in batteries of cages, often more than seven tiers high, mirrored the demise of the back-to-back housing for humans in cities and their replacement with tower apartments.

This all happened astonishingly rapidly and largely away from the public eye, yet supported and encouraged by the governments of the day. In the early 1960s a small lady living in London somehow became aware of the industrialisation of agriculture and questioned the morality of pursuing a predominantly economic model. This lady was Ruth Harrison and her book *Animal Machines* (Harrison, 1964) criticised intensive systems of production, such as the battery cage, in which animals were kept crowded together in a very unnatural environment, were denied access to fresh air and sunlight and often had no space to move. In the UK, the publication of these facts led to such public outrage that the British Government formed a committee to investigate the whole topic of intensive animal production systems. They published their findings in a report that is generally known as *The Brambell Report* (Command Paper 2836, 1965). This report was also very critical of battery cages. For example, the report stated:

> Much of the ingrained behaviour is frustrated by caging. The normal reproductive pattern of mating, hatching and rearing young is prevented and the only reproductive urge permitted is laying. They cannot fly, scratch, perch or walk freely. Preening is difficult and dust-bathing impossible. . . . The caged bird which is permitted only to fulfil the instinctive urges to eat and drink, to sleep, to lay and to communicate vocally with its fellows, would appear to be exposed to considerable frustration.
>
> *(Command Paper 2836, 1965, pp. 18–19)*

However, the Brambell Committee's conclusions, although descriptive of the hens' situation, were not based on much hard evidence, as little was available at the time. In the subsequent 50 years, scientists and industry have been working to find an economically viable method of production that meets both the health and behavioural aspects of hen welfare. This has proved to be a real challenge with no one system ticking all the boxes. Both the Laywel project (www.laywel.eu) and Lay et al. (2011) have considered many aspects of egg production systems and noted that while some non-cage systems offer greater potential for meeting behavioural needs, in practice the wide variation in performance and of welfare outcomes offsets this. In this chapter we shall consider some aspects of the husbandry of hens, in particular examining the pros and cons of various housing systems including their sustainability. The industry tends to concentrate on the economic dimension of sustainability and adopt a relatively short-term view based on the financial viability and resilience of current methods of egg production (Burton et al., 2016). We favour a more long-term view with an emphasis on the environmental dimension, whereby ecological balance is supported by avoiding the depletion of natural resources and pollution. However, the social aspects of sustainability (Figure 8.1) need also to be considered,

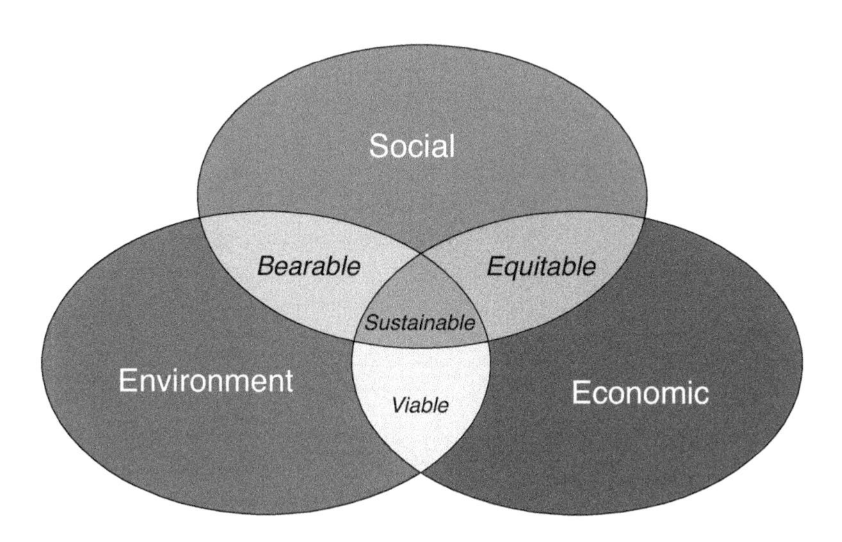

FIGURE 8.1 Sustainable development

Source: Johann Dréo https://commons.wikimedia.org/w/index.php?curid=1587372

particularly given the demands of an expanding human population of over 7.5 billion – three times greater than in 1950 – and consuming more than 75 million tonnes of commercially produced eggs per annum.

Housing systems

The welfare advantages and disadvantages of housing systems will now be discussed briefly and have recently been reviewed by Lay et al. (2011) and Elson (2015). One issue that prevails across housing systems is that of injurious pecking and the prevalent means of controlling its impact, which is beak trimming. We use the term *injurious pecking* to include feather pecking, cannibalism and vent pecking but not aggressive pecking, which is thought to have a different underlying motivation. The most widely accepted theory is that injurious pecking is redirected foraging or ground-pecking behaviour (Blokhuis, 1989; Dixon et al., 2008), but it has also been proposed that feather pecking is a normal behaviour that plays a role in social exploration (McAdie and Keeling, 2002). Certainly there is a genetic component to the expression of the behaviour and it has been possible to select low- and high-feather pecking lines within a few generations (Kjaer et al., 2001), but although production is in general reduced in low-feather pecking lines, modern genetic techniques such as quantitative trait location (QTL) may lead to specific selection against a high propensity either to inflict or receive injurious pecking. In the meantime the predominant method of controlling the damage inflicted by injurious pecking behaviour is to remove the tip of the beak: in particular the sharp, curved upper mandible. Infrared treatment at one day old has been shown to be less painful and have fewer long-term consequences for bird welfare, but hot-blade trimming of a larger proportion of the beak is also practised and leads to neuromas and chronic pain (Hughes and Gentle, 1995). In some parts of the world such as the EU, the societal view is that animals should not be mutilated and this has led to legislation banning beak trimming. However, it is also recognised that the consequences of not beak-trimming might outweigh its practice so a derogation is currently allowed on a country basis. After many decades of research, scientists are beginning to understand the underlying mechanisms associated with feather pecking (reviewed by Rodenburg et al., 2013) and importantly to identify risk factors and ways of managing hens to reduce the incidence of injurious pecking (Nicol et al., 2013) so that it may soon become possible to manage productive flocks of intact beak birds.

Conventional (battery) cages

We have already outlined the advantages of cages in terms of hygiene and, thereby in general, of health. Keeping animals in large numbers and in close proximity enables virulent pathogens to spread rapidly, so good biosecurity is paramount to reduce the risk of disease outbreaks affecting the flock. Productivity is greatest in cage systems for several reasons including good feed conversion efficiency, a thermally comfortable environment, better levels of health and, on average, reduced mortality and no mislaid eggs. With so much automation, the system makes fewer demands of those caring for and managing the birds, leaving less room for error. Further, hens with pecking tendencies have fewer potential 'victims' with no more than six birds per cage. The number of hens kept in both conventional and furnished (colony) cages is much closer to the basic social unit of 10–20 birds seen in jungle fowl (Collias et al., 1966) and feral domestic fowl (McBride et al., 1969), than that occurring in loose housing systems, which commonly have thousands of hens in the one group (Blokhuis and Metz, 1992). Of course, domestic fowl may be able to adapt to life in large groups and so their welfare may not be adversely affected by extensive husbandry systems on that basis.

What do the birds themselves prefer? Early preference tests showed that hens prefer smaller rather than larger groups and familiar hens over strangers (Hughes, 1977; Dawkins, 1982). However, these tests used only very small groups (up to six birds for the large groups). Other preference tests have shown that, when available space is properly controlled, most hens prefer a group size of 70 birds to one of four birds (Lindberg and Nicol, 1993, 1996). Of course this group size is still very much smaller than the large groups of several thousand hens typical in non-cage systems. It is unclear whether or not hens are stressed by large group sizes *per se* as there inevitably are confounding factors that make investigating the matter complex, not least recognising and tracking individual birds.

However, these potential advantages of cages are offset by the extreme restriction of space, the barrenness of the environment and the lack of opportunities to express important behavioural needs such as nesting, foraging, perching and dust-bathing (Weeks and Nicol, 2006). Further, having only a wire floor to stand on is physically uncomfortable and can lead to foot and claw abnormalities only partially reduced by providing abrasive materials adjacent to the feed trough. The extreme lack of space prevents hens from exercising, leading to weakened bones (so-called disuse osteoporosis), which is only partially resolved by dietary interventions and genetic selection (Whitehead, 2004). Further, the low height of battery cages prevents hens from adopting the 'standing alert' posture that is very common in their repertoire (Dawkins, 1985). In other experiments in which cage height and cage area were manipulated independently, some other less obvious effects were revealed. When height was reduced to that of battery cages, the incidence of head stretching, head scratching and body shaking were reduced, and, surprisingly, the length of time that hens spent sitting was also reduced. When cage area was reduced to that of battery cages, head scratching, body shaking and feather raising were performed at a lower rate and cage pecking at a higher rate (Nicol, 1987a). In other trials, it was found that behaviour patterns that had been shown at a low incidence when space was restricted showed a 'rebound' effect when the hens were given more space, suggesting that the spatial restriction had resulted in a build-up of motivation to perform these patterns (Nicol, 1987b). All of these results suggest that the dimensions of normal battery cages may compromise welfare by restricting the behavioural repertoire of the birds.

Another approach to investigating the effects on welfare of the restrictive space available in battery cages has been to 'ask' hens how much space they prefer. Both Hughes (1975) and Dawkins (1981) have shown that hens prefer more space than that available in conventional battery cages. The fact that the argument can be made 'the hen herself prefers more room' is even more powerful evidence that battery cages provide insufficient space.

The shortcomings of conventional (battery) cages have been discussed by several authors including Baxter (1994), and Duncan (2010) in the first edition of this book. Indeed, recognition of these has led to considerable research by scientists into alternative systems that might better meet the needs of hens, whilst also being commercially viable. In a ground-breaking change of attitude, the research into what hens need, prioritise and value led to pioneering methodology beginning with simple preference tests (Dawkins, 1977) but later using a variety of methods to test hens' motivation to access resources such as more space, nestboxes, perches and dustbaths, using consumer demand theory as one of the underpinning rationales for the approaches. This research, reviewed by Weeks and Nicol (2006), led to the development of the furnished cage system (Appleby et al., 2002) and has influenced the design of other alternative systems such as aviaries.

Furnished cages

This housing system has evolved as a pragmatic compromise that retains the relative ease of management, low labour input and health benefits of cages whilst to some extent meeting the most pressing behavioural needs of the birds. Scientific trials have indicated that hens particularly value and need more space plus opportunities to express nesting, perching, foraging and dust-bathing behaviour. Thus, over time, cages larger in all dimensions and containing a discrete nesting area and perches have evolved. Providing foraging and dust-bathing opportunities has proven more challenging and most often is given as a token scattering of feed on an artificial turf pad. From the hens' perspective this is most likely better than nothing, but not as good as substrate to peck and scratch in and properly dust-bathe. Early designs of furnished cages provided trays containing sand (Abrahamsson and Tauson, 1997) but a small proportion of birds laid eggs in them and the sand proved damaging to egg- and manure-belt drives when scaled up to commercial production. Providing litter or dust-bathing substrates may also lead to faecal contamination, dirty eggs and a dusty aerial environment which are all downsides to the generally more hygienic and healthier environment provided by the cage system.

Current designs of commercial furnished cages accommodate 40 to 80 birds per cage and are often referred to as colonies, possibly in a bid to escape the 'cage' nomenclature which is anathema to welfarists (CIWF, 2010). Recent research has indicated that there can be competition for nest sites in these large furnished cages, which might result in frustration (Hunniford et al., 2014). However, as well as satisfying their desire to roost, perches improve the bone strength of hens housed in furnished cages (Abrahamsson and Tauson, 1993). Others have also reported that hens kept in furnished cages and non-cage systems have stronger bones than hens in battery cages (Michel and Huonnic, 2003; Rodenburg et al., 2008; Sherwin et al., 2010; Lay et al., 2011; Freire and Cowling, 2013).

Non-cage housing systems for laying hens

There are several options, with variations in design and layout, but basically these consist of keeping the birds indoors with access to one or more tiers with variants that also provide a veranda or access outdoors. These have been gradually increasing in popularity as the general public becomes aware of the extreme behavioural restrictions associated with conventional cages. Legislation and standards are increasingly prohibiting the use of these systems, as has happened in the European Union since January 2012 (European Commission, 1999), whereby all hens must have a nest, perching space, litter to allow pecking and scratching and unrestricted access to a feed trough. In alternative (i.e. non-cage) systems in the EU, the stocking density may not exceed nine laying hens per m^2 usable area, with at least one nest for every seven hens and adequate perches. It is interesting that there remains considerable research to be done in order to determine what constitutes suitable perch design and provision; however, a panel of experts concluded that 'an adequate perch is elevated, accessible and functional (providing sufficient overview)' (EFSA, 2015). Some organic systems operate small flocks (typically 500–2,000 birds) in mobile, free-range houses reverting to the tradition whereby the enterprise can be integrated with crops in rotation.

The proportion of laying hens housed in non-cage systems in the EU increased from 8.7 per cent in 1995 (Agra CEAS, 2006) to 44.3 per cent in 2014 (EEPA, 2016). Figure 8.2 illustrates the percentage of hens kept in the principal housing systems in the EU in 2014. Moreover major retailers and restaurants in the US have recently pledged to increasingly source cage-free eggs, aiming to achieve this within ten years. Egg Farmers of Canada (EFC) announced in early 2016 on behalf of the more than 1,000 Canadian egg farms that a coordinated, systematic, market-oriented transition from conventional egg production toward other methods of production for supplying eggs will begin. They anticipate the current proportion of 10 per cent cage-free will shift to about 50 per cent within eight years and become totally cage-free by 2036 depending on market demands. Cage-free housing is increasing Australia (30 per cent in 2012), with other countries set to follow suit.

Most of the loose-housing systems are based on the traditional 'deep litter' barn with a single-tier raised slatted area. Increasingly, the economic advantages of keeping more hens per unit area and using the warmth from the metabolic heat of the birds are being realised in multi-tiered indoor housing, including those with access to a range. The winters in northern Europe and much of North America prevent free range from being used throughout the year, so often a 'Wintergarten' or veranda attached to the house provides more space and fresh air for the hens during the winter and they may be given access to free range during the summer.

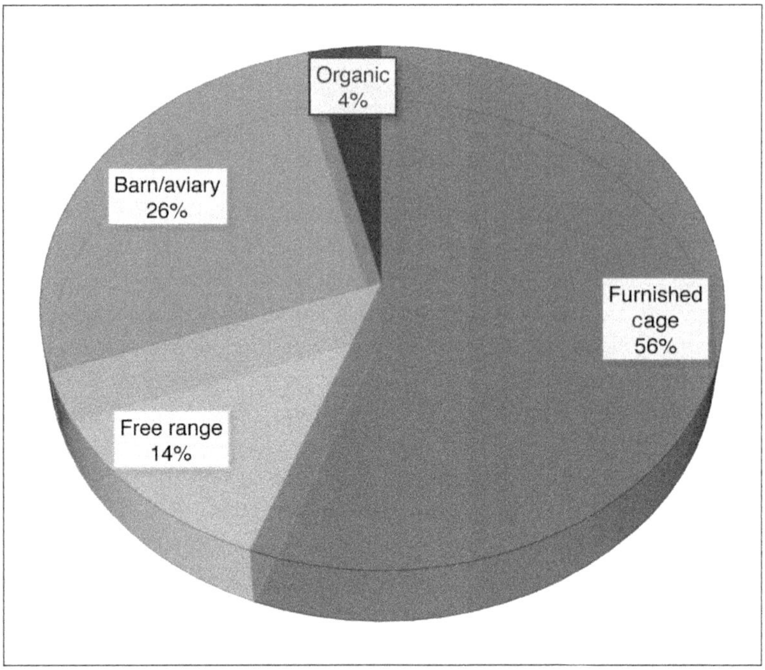

FIGURE 8.2 Number of laying hens in 2014 by way of keeping (Based on data from 26 member states of the EU)

Source: European Egg Processors Association (www.eepa.info/Statistics.aspx)

A description of prevalent housing systems was given by the Laywel project that compared these in the EU (www.laywel.eu).

Free range

This system offers the greatest potential for good welfare if the range is of high quality offering shelter from both predators and extreme weather, and providing a diversity of plant and insect foraging opportunities. The provision of natural shelter, in particular trees, has been shown to increase ranging and improve welfare. For example Bright et al. (2011, 2016) have found improved plumage in flocks with at least 5 per cent of the range area planted with trees providing a good canopy. This has been linked with improved egg quality and production (Bright and Joret, 2012). Trees often improve pasture drainage and absorb dust and ammonia emissions, thereby improving the environmental conditions. Hens are more likely to be able to express full nesting and dust-bathing behaviour and to perch high in a well-designed free-range system. Moreover, the hens can usually space themselves according to the activity they are engaging in, and can often escape from bullies and choose a microclimate.

The welfare disadvantages are that the hens may be exposed to weather extremes and also to predation. There is a relatively high risk of infection by internal parasites particularly *Coccidia* spp. and of infestation by external parasites especially Red Mite (*Dermanyssus gallinae*) (Rodenburg et al., 2008; Fossum et al., 2009). The risk of feather pecking and cannibalism is also greater in all non-cage systems. This is probably because this behavioural abnormality can be culturally transmitted. Therefore, if there are a few primary peckers in a population of hens, their feather pecking behaviour can spread widely if they are in a very large group, but it is greatly restricted when they are divided up a few hens to a cage. Moreover they have many more potential 'victims'.

Loose-housing (indoor) systems

Some of the behavioural advantages of free range are also present for the various barn systems. Hens can choose nesting sites and show nesting behaviour. They have more room than in battery cages, but high stocking densities may restrict spatial freedom. The majority offer some foraging potential in littered areas provided these are kept clean and friable. Usually foraging opportunities will be available to hens in barn systems but not always. In an attempt to improve hygiene and air quality some barn systems are completely slatted with no loose substrate for foraging. Considering that hens spend 60–70 per cent of their active time foraging (Savory et al., 1978), an all-slatted system deprives the birds from satisfactory foraging and also prevents the hens from dust-bathing. There is considerable evidence that a lack of suitable foraging opportunities leads to injurious pecking (see Lambton et al., 2013; Nicol et al., 2013).

The majority of barn systems make use of the height dimension and may have raised perches or slats so that birds can show roosting behaviour. At the end of a laying year, bones of hens from barn systems are much stronger than those of hens from battery cages (Knowles and Broom, 1990; Nørgaard-Nielsen, 1990) meaning that they are at much lower risk of suffering bone breakage during catching and transportation. However, this should be balanced against the fact that hens in these systems have been shown to suffer from a higher incidence of broken bones during the laying year (Nicol et al., 2006; Petrik et al., 2015). Nicol et al. (2006) found that 60 per cent of hens in aviaries had old fractures (mainly of the sternum) at the end of the laying year, presumably sustained when they collided with objects in the barn. Barn systems also protect hens from extreme weather and from predators. It seems particularly important to offer ramps (ideally full-width) for hens to access each tier and to avoid aerial perches, which have the highest rate and severity of keel fractures (Wilkins et al., 2011).

The welfare disadvantages of barn systems are that the presence of a loose substrate, essential for foraging and dust-bathing, can lead to high levels of ammonia and dust (Appleby et al., 1988), which may lead to respiratory problems in both hens and humans. The group size in barn systems is often several thousands of hens. This is much larger than the group size of 50–100 hens for which there is some indication of preference (Lindberg and Nicol, 1993, 1996). However, there is also evidence that hens in very large groups (3,000–16,000) can be very calm and non-aggressive (Whay et al., 2007). Average levels of feather pecking and cannibalism and of mortality are higher than in cages. There is also a small risk of infection with internal parasites, but this is lower than in birds on free range. A considerable problem is the risk of Red Mite (*Dermanyssus gallinae*) infestation. Not only does this parasite pose a welfare risk through the direct effect of blood loss, but it is also being implicated as a vector of other diseases (De Luna et al., 2008). Currently there is an international effort to seek a solution to this problem (Mul et al., 2009).

Comparisons of housing systems

The basis of comparisons has varied between studies. A review by European scientists focussed on welfare, noting, 'The problem of how different indicators should be weighed against each other to come to a final conclusion as to whether or not the housing system promotes good bird health and satisfies the behavioural priorities of the bird is difficult, since there is still no generally accepted methodology for such integration of indicators' (EFSA, 2005, p8). Their evaluation highlighted the serious problem of injurious pecking in many systems which is especially difficult to control in large-group furnished cages and in non-cage systems. They noted a higher level of bone fractures sustained during lay in non-cage systems and greater bacterial contamination on the eggshells from alternative systems. The latter was confirmed in a study of three strains of bird in three housing systems which found differing levels of microbial contamination between breeds and housing systems but the lowest levels in conventional cages (Jones and Anderson, 2013).

Another pan-European study, Laywel (www.laywel.eu) attempted to measure productivity as well as physiology, health and behaviour when comparing systems, noting great variability in most measures for non-cage systems, which influenced the risk for poor welfare occurring in a given system. This study concluded that: 'with the exception of conventional cages, all systems have the potential to provide satisfactory welfare for laying hens. However this potential is not always realised in practice. Among the numerous explanations are management, climate, design, different responses by different genotypes and interacting effects' (Blokhuis et al., 2007, p110).

Sherwin et al. (2010) also employed several measures to evaluate welfare in four housing systems, finding that the lowest prevalence of welfare problems was found in furnished cage housing and the highest in single-tier barn systems. They too found positive and negative aspects to each system and suggested that the welfare of modern genotypes was poor based on a high prevalence of emaciation, loss of plumage, fractures and evidence of stress across all housing systems.

As the North American market begins to move away from caged egg production systems, some recent studies have evaluated alternatives, including the review by Lay et al. (2011). Using outcome measures of welfare, developed by the European

Welfare Quality® project, Blatchford et al. (2016) compared two strains of hens in colony cages, conventional cages and aviaries. Their findings were that birds in aviaries had overall better feather cover but were dirtier, birds in conventional cages had more foot but fewer keel abnormalities. Important key indicators, such as mortality were not considered in this study, but Weeks et al. (2012) found significant differences in liveability between housing systems and wide variation within systems when looking at UK records for a whole year. On average the levels of mortality in free range (9.52 per cent), organic (8.68 per cent) and barn (8.55 per cent) flocks were significantly greater than in cage systems (5.39 per cent). This led Claire Weeks to consider the sustainability of loose-housed systems and to gather a large database from 3,851 flocks to model. This confirmed other reports, again finding that producer-recorded cumulative mortality at 60–80 weeks of age was highest in free-range flocks (mean 10 per cent range 0–69 per cent) and lowest in flocks housed in conventional cages (Weeks et al., 2016). These authors also found that mortality was higher in flocks with intact beaks and variation between breeds, although both these risk factors were confounded by their unequal representation across housing systems. However, others have noted strain effects (e.g. Aerni et al. (2005) when comparing aviaries and conventional cages. Weeks et al. (2016) restricted the life cycle analysis to free-range flocks, as this system appeared to have the greatest potential for improvement, and their models indicated that if all producers could reduce mortality to the levels currently achieved by the first quartile (mean = 5 per cent), flock greenhouse gas emissions could be reduced by as much as 25 per cent. Clearly this would also enhance hen welfare and better meet the expectations of egg consumers, for whom animal welfare is a concern (e.g. Eurobarometer, 2016). There is scope for a more rigorous examination of the environmental impacts of different housing systems, as was concluded by Xin et al. (2011) who examined environmental impacts of egg production systems in the US, finding that non-cage systems were less efficient in their use of resources such as feed, energy and land.

The future

The demand for eggs is unlikely to reduce in the foreseeable future. Eggs provide humans with versatile, convenient and affordable nutrients, including protein of high biological value. Moreover, with a high food conversion ratio, hens compete less with humans for resources than other animals, particularly beef cattle, when grains are used as the main part of their diet. Yet in many countries humans are dictating cage-free systems without being prepared to pay any more for their eggs. Several studies have indicated that egg production from alternative systems costs more, with a recent estimate by Matthews and Sumner (2015) finding total costs in aviaries to be 36 per cent and for furnished cages 13 per cent higher than for conventional cages, but operating costs of furnished cages were only about 4 per cent higher than conventional cages. In the UK the margins for free-range eggs have reduced in recent years owing to retailer competition. The response of industry has been to move towards houses accommodating more birds – 32,000 is now common whereas a few years ago 8,000 was typical. Concurrently there seems to be a reduction in the contact time of those caring for the birds. Yet we have evidence that the skill, commitment and attention to detail of both managers and stockmen/women is crucial to the success of any flock both financially and in terms of bird welfare. For example a high uptake of measures such as provision of additional foraging materials reduces the incidence of injurious pecking and of mortality (Lambton et al., 2013).

To produce eggs sustainably and with good welfare for the birds several approaches are likely to be needed. Strains of hens should be developed which are better suited to alternative systems – i.e. robust and less prone to feather pecking, laying floor eggs and smothering. Scandinavian experience suggests white genotypes may be more suitable, in which case consumers will need educating that white eggs have equal nutritional value to those with brown shells. In an ideal world consumers would also learn to value and pay for high-quality food. We and others (e.g. Elson, 2015) feel there is scope to refine and develop existing housing systems to meet the behavioural needs of the hens and provide plenty of space with access to fresh air and sunshine whilst better protecting them from predation and diseases such as avian influenza, which is predominantly transmitted by wild birds. The Rondeel system (www.rondeel.org) shows promise in this respect and manages relatively small flocks of hens with intact beaks. The round system comprises five sectors each with an aviary and a transparent, covered veranda offering natural daylight to a flock of typically 1,500 birds. In good weather hens may also forage and dust-bathe in a small outside area of sandy soil planted with a few trees. Importantly the birds are fully protected from potential predators by netting. The Roundel system markets its eggs as locally as possible and has a number of sustainable underlying constructs but remains a niche market in the Netherlands. To be more widely adopted further development would be needed so that it could scale up and be cheaper to construct and easier to manage.

Finally there is a need for improved knowledge transfer, for stimulating change, innovation and uptake of ideas and for motivating managers and poultry carers to adopt a proactive approach to flock husbandry so that they achieve the good results that a proportion of the industry has already demonstrated is both realisable and sustainable. This is likely to require training those who care for hens to not only acquire the relevant skills and knowledge but also to develop a professional attitude and behaviour (Hemsworth and Coleman, 2011). These authors also note that society should value their skill and contribution to animal well-being and food safety and afford stockmen the status and salary commensurate with this.

References

Abrahamsson, P. and Tauson, R. (1993) Effect of perches at different positions in conventional cages for laying hens of two different strains. *Acta Agriculturæ Scandinavica, Section A, Animal Science*, 43, 228–235.

Abrahamsson, P. and Tauson, R. (1997) Effects of group size on performance health and birds' use of facilities in furnished cages for laying hens. *Acta Agriculturæ Scandinavica, Section A, Animal Science*, 47, 254–260. DOI: 10.1080/09064709709362394

Aerni, V., Brinkhof, M.W.G., Wechsler, B., Oestler, H. and Frohlich, E. (2005) Productivity and mortality of laying hens in aviaries: A systematic review. *World's Poultry Science Journal*, 61, 131–143. DOI: 10.1079/WPS200450

Agra CEAS Consulting (2006) Trends in laying hen numbers and the production and consumption of eggs from caged and non-caged production systems. Final Report for Eurogroup for Animal Welfare, Agra CEAS Consulting, Wye, UK.

Appleby, M.C., Hogarth, G.S., Anderson, J.A., Hughes, B.O. and Whittemore, C.T. (1988) Performance of a deep litter system for egg production. *British Poultry Science*, 29, 735–751.

Appleby, M.C., Walker, A.W., Nicol, C.J., Lindberg, A.C., Freire, R., Hughes, B.O. and Elson, H.A. (2002) The development of furnished cages for laying hens. *British Poultry Science*, 43, 489–500.

Baxter, M.R. (1994) The welfare problems of laying hens in battery cages. *Veterinary Record*, 134(24), 614–619.

Blatchford, R.A., Fulton, R.M. and Mench, J.A. (2016) The utilization of the Welfare Quality® assessment for determining laying hen condition across three housing systems. *Poultry Science*, 95, 54–163.

Blokhuis, H.J. (1989) *The development and causation of feather pecking in the domestic fowl*. Ph.D. Thesis, Wageningen Agricultural University, Wageningen, The Netherlands.

Blokhuis, H.J., van Niekerk, T.F., Bessei, W., Elson, A., Guémené, D., Kjaer, J.B., Levrino, G.A.M., Nicol, C.J., Tauson, R., Weeks, C.A. and de Weerd, H.A.V. (2007) The Laywel project: welfare implications of changes in production systems for laying hens. *World's Poultry Science Journal*, 63, 101–114.

Blokhuis, H.J. and Metz, J.H.M. (1992) Integration of animal welfare into housing systems for laying hens. *Netherlands Journal of Agricultural Science*, 40, 327–337.

Bright, A., Brass, D., Clachan, J., Drake, K. and Joret, A. (2011) Canopy cover is correlated with reduced injurious feather pecking in commercial flocks of free range laying hens. *Animal Welfare*, 20, 329–338.

Bright, A., Gill, R. and Willings, T.H. (2016) Tree cover and injurious feather-pecking in commercial flocks of free-range laying hens: A follow up. *Animal Welfare*, 25, 1–5.

Bright, A. and Joret, A.D. (2012) Laying hens go undercover to improve production. *Veterinary Record*, 170, 228. DOI: 10.1136/vr.100503

Burton, E., Gatcliffe, J., O'Neill, H.M. and Scholey, D. (eds) (2016) *Sustainable Poultry Production in Europe*, CAB International, Oxford, UK. ISBN-13: 9781780645308.

CIWF (2010) Joint statement against modified or 'enriched' cages. www.ciwf.org.uk/news/2010/08/enriched-cages-condemned/

Collias, N.E., Collias, E.C., Hunsaker, D. and Minning, L. (1966) Locality fixation, mobility and social organization within an unconfined population of red jungle fowl. *Animal Behaviour*, 14, 550–559.

Command Paper 2836 (1965) Report of the Technical Committee to Enquire Into the Welfare of Animals Kept Under Intensive Livestock Husbandry Systems, Her Majesty's Stationery Office, London.

Dawkins, M.S. (1977) Do hens suffer in battery cages? Environmental preferences and welfare. *Animal Behaviour*, 25, 1034–1046. http://dx.doi.org/10.1016/0003-3472(77)90054-9

Dawkins, M.S. (1981) Priorities in the cage size and flooring preferences of domestic hens. *British Poultry Science*, 22, 255–263.

Dawkins, M.S. (1982) Elusive concept of preferred group size in domestic hens. *Applied Animal Ethology*, 8, 365–375.

Dawkins, M.S. (1985) Cage height preference and use in battery-kept hens. *Veterinary Record*, 116, 345–347.

De Luna, C.J., Arkle, S., Harrington, D., George, D.R., Guy, J.H. and Sparagano, O.A.E. (2008) The poultry Red Mite *Dermanyssus gallinae* as a potential carrier of vector-borne diseases. *Annals of the New York Academy of Sciences*, 1149, 255–258.

Dixon, L.M., Duncan, I.J.H. and Mason, G. (2008) What's in a peck? Using fixed action pattern morphology to identify the motivational basis of abnormal feather-pecking behaviour. *Animal Behaviour*, 76, 1035–1042.

Duncan, I.J.H. (2010) Cracking the egg. In D'Silva, J. and Webster, J. (eds) *The Meat Crisis: Developing More Sustainable Production and Consumption*, Earthscan, London and Washington, 117–132.

EEPA (2016) www.eepa.info/Statistics.aspx (accessed May 2016).

EFC (2016) www.eggfarmers.ca/wp-content/uploads/2016/02/EN-FINAL-Egg-Farmers-of-Canada-Housing-announcement.pdf (accessed May 2016).

EFSA European Food Safety Authority – AHAW (2005) The welfare aspects of various systems of keeping laying hens. *Annex to the EFSA Journal*, 197, 1–23.

EFSA European Food Safety Authority – AHAW (2015) Scientific opinion on welfare aspects of the use of perches for laying hens. *EFSA Journal*, 13(6), 4131 [71 pp.]. DOI: 10.2903/j.efsa.2015.4131

Elson, H.A. (1988). Poultry management systems – looking to the future. *World's Poultry Science Journal*, 44, 103–111.

Elson, H.A. (2015) Poultry welfare in intensive and extensive systems. *World's Poultry Science Journal*, 71, 449–459. DOI: 10.1017/S0043933915002172

Eurobarometer (2016) Attitudes of Europeans towards animal welfare. Ref: 442. http://ec.europa.eu/COMMFrontOffice/PublicOpinion/index.cfm/Survey/getSurveyDetail/yearFrom/1973/yearTo/2015/search/animal%20welfare%20/surveyKy/2096 (accessed May 2016).

European Commission (1999) Council Directive 1999/74/EC laying down minimum standards for the protection of laying hens. *Official Journal of the European Communities*, L203, 53–57, 3.8.1999, http://eur-lex.europa.eu/LexUriServ/LexUriServ.do?uri=OJ:L:1999:203:0053:0057:EN:PDF

Fossum, O., Jansson, D.S., Etterlin, P.E. and Vagsholm, I. (2009) Causes of mortality in laying hens on different housing systems in 2001 to 2004. *Acta Veterinaria Scandinavica*, 51, 3–11.

Freire, R. and Cowling, A. (2013) The welfare of laying hens in conventional cages and alternative systems: First steps towards a quantitative comparison. *Animal Welfare*, 22, 57–65.

Harrison, R. (1964) *Animal Machines*, Vincent Stuart, London.

Hemsworth, P. and Coleman, G. (2011) *Human Livestock Interactions*, CAB International, Oxon, UK. ISBN-13: 9781845936730.

Hughes, B.O. (1975) Spatial preference in the domestic hen. *British Veterinary Journal*, 131, 560–564.

Hughes, B.O. (1977) Selection of group size by individual laying hens. *British Poultry Science*, 18, 9–18.

Hughes, B.O. and Gentle, M.J. (1995) Beak trimming of poultry: Its implications for welfare. *World's Poultry Science Journal*, 51, 51–61.

Hunniford, M.E., Torrey, S., Bedecarrats, G., Duncan, I.J.H. and Widowski, T.M. (2014) Evidence for competition for nest sites by laying hens in large furnished cages. *Applied Animal Behaviour Science*, 161, 95–104.

Jones, D.R. and Anderson, K.E. (2013) Housing system and laying hen strain impacts on egg microbiology. *Poultry Science*, 92, 2221–2225.

Kjaer, J.B., Sørensen, P. and Su, G. (2001) Divergent selection on feather pecking behaviour in laying hens (Gallus gallus domesticus). *Applied Animal Behaviour Science*, 71, 229–239.

Knowles, T.G. and Broom, D.M. (1990) Limb bone strength and movement in laying hens from different housing systems. *Veterinary Record*, 126, 354–356.

Lambton, S.L., Nicol, C.J., Friel, M., Main, D.C.J., McKinstry, J.L., Sherwin, C.M., Walton, J. and Weeks, C.A. (2013) A bespoke management package can reduce levels of injurious pecking in loose-housed laying hen flocks. *Veterinary Record*, 17, 423. http://dx.doi.org/10.1136/vr.101067

Lay, D.C., Fulton, R.M., Hester, P.Y., Karcher, D.M., Kjaer, J.B., Mench, J.A., Mullens, B.A., Newberry, R.C., Nicol, C.J., O'Sullivan, N.P. and Porter, R.E. (2011) Hen welfare in different housing systems. *Poultry Science*, 90, 278–294.

Lindberg, A.C. and Nicol, C.J. (1993) Group size preferences in laying hens. In Savory, C.J. and Hughes, B.O. (eds) *Proceedings of the Fourth European Symposium on Poultry Welfare*, Universities' Federation for Animal Welfare, Potters Bar, 249–250.

Lindberg, A.C. and Nicol, C.J. (1996) Space and density effects on group size preferences in laying hens. *British Poultry Science*, 37, 709–721.

McAdie, T.M. and Keeling, L.J. (2002) The social transmission of feather pecking in laying hens: Effects of environment and age. *Applied Animal Behaviour Science*, 75, 147–159.

McBride, G., Parer, I.P. and Foenander, F. (1969) The social organization and behaviour of the feral domestic fowl. *Animal Behaviour Monographs*, 2, 125–181.

Matthews, W.A. and Sumner, D.A. (2015) Effects of housing system on the costs of commercial egg production. *Poultry Science*, 94, 552–557. DOI: 10.3382/ps/peu011

Michel, V. and Huonnic, D. (2003) A comparison of welfare, health and production performance of laying hens reared in cages or aviaries. *British Poultry Science*, 23, 775–776.

Morris, T.R. and Fox, S. (1958). Artificial light and sexual maturity in the fowl. *Nature* 181, 1522–1523.

Mul, M., Van Niekerk, T., Chirico, J., Maurer, V., Kilpinen, O., Sparagano, O., Thind, B., Zoons, J., Moore, D., Bell, B., Gjevre, A.-G. and Chauve, C. (2009) Control methods for *Dermanyssus gallinae* in systems for laying hens: Results of an international seminar. *World's Poultry Science Journal*, 65, 589–599.

Nicol, C.J. (1987a) Effect of cage height and area on the behaviour of hens housed in battery cages. *British Poultry Science*, 28, 327–335.

Nicol, C.J. (1987b) Behavioural responses of laying hens following a period of spatial restriction. *Animal Behaviour*, 35, 1709–1719.

Nicol, C.J., Bestman, M., Gilani, A.-M., Haas, E.N. de, Jong, I.C. de, Lambton, S.L., Wagenaar, J.P., Weeks, C.A. and Rodenburg, T.B. (2013) The prevention and control of feather pecking: Application to commercial systems. *World's Poultry Science Journal*, 69, 775–787.

Nicol, C.J., Brown, S.N., Glen, E., Pope, S.J., Short, F.J., Warriss, P.D., Zimmerman, P.H. and Wilkins, L.J. (2006) Effects of stocking density, flock size and management on the welfare of laying hens in single-tier aviaries. *British Poultry Science*, 47, 135–146.

Nørgaard-Nielsen, G. (1990) Bone strength of laying hens kept in an alternative housing system compared with hens in cages and on deep litter. *British Poultry Science*, 31, 81–89.

Petrik, M.T., Guerin, M.T. and Widowski, T.M. (2015) On-farm comparison of keel fracture prevalence and other welfare indicators in conventional cages and floor-housed laying hens in Ontario, Canada. *Poultry Science*, 94, 579–585.

Robinson, L. (1961) *Modern Poultry Husbandry*, Crosby Lockwood, London.

Rodenburg, T.B., Tuyttens, F.A.M., Reu, K.D., Herman, L., Zoons, J. and Sonck, B. (2008) Welfare assessment of laying hens in furnished cages and non-cage systems: An on-farm comparison. *Animal Welfare*, 17, 363–373.

Rodenburg, T.B., Van Krimpen, M.M., De Jong, I.C., De Haas, E.N., Kops, M.S., Riedstra, B.J., Nordquist, R.E., Wagenaar, J.P., Bestman, M. and Nicol, C.J. (2013) The prevention and control of feather pecking in laying hens: Identifying the underlying principles. *World's Poultry Science Journal*, 69, 361–374.

Savory, C.J., Wood-Gush, D.G.M. and Duncan, I.J.H. (1978) Feeding behaviour in a population of domestic fowls in the wild. *Applied Animal Ethology*, 4, 13–27.

Sherwin, C.M., Richards, G.H. and Nicol, C.J. (2010) Comparison of the welfare of layer hens in 4 housing systems in the UK. *British Poultry Science*, 51, 488–499.

Weeks, C.A., Brown, S.N., Richards, G.J., Wilkins, L.J. and Knowles, T.G. (2012) Levels of mortality in hens by end of lay on farm and in transit to slaughter in Great Britain. *Veterinary Record*, 170, 647. http://dx.doi.org/10.1136/vr.100728

Weeks, C.A., Lambton, S.L. and Williams, A.G. (2016) Implications for welfare, productivity and sustainability of the variation in reported levels of mortality for laying hen flocks kept in different housing systems: A meta-analysis of ten studies. *PLoS One*, 11(1), E0146394. http://dx.doi.org/10.1371/journal.pone.0146394

Weeks, C.A. and Nicol, C.J. (2006) Behavioural needs, priorities and preferences of laying hens. *World's Poultry Science Journal*, 62, 296–307.

Whay, H.R., Main, D.C.J., Green, L.E., Heaven, G., Howell, H., Morgan, M., Pearson, A. and Webster, A.J.F. (2007) Assessment of the behaviour and welfare of laying hens on free-range units. *Veterinary Record*, 161, 119–128.

Whitehead, C.C. (2004) Skeletal disorders in laying hens: The problems of osteoporosis and fractures. In Perry, G. (eds) *Welfare of the Laying Hen*, Poultry Science Symposium Series, Volume 27, 259–278, CABI Publishing, Wallingford, Oxford, UK.

Wilkins, L.J., McKinstry, J.L., Avery, N.C., Knowles, T.G., Brown, S.N., Tarlton, J. and Nicol, C.J. (2011). Influence of housing system and design on bone strength and keel bone fractures in laying hens. *Veterinary Record*, 169, 414.

Xin, H., Gates, R.S., Green, A.R., Mitloehner, F.M., Moore, P.A. and Wathes, C.M. (2011) Environmental impacts and sustainability of egg production systems. *Poultry Science*, 90, 263–277. DOI: 10.3382/ps.2010–00877

9

CHEAP AS CHICKEN

Andy Butterworth

Chickens are the most common farmed animal on solid earth. In 2016, around 50 billion chickens were reared for meat. This means that in the year 2016, more chickens were reared for meat than some people estimate the number of humans who have ever lived on the planet – ever. How has it come to be that chicken has taken such a global hold, consuming vast amounts of cereal and protein, and, in turn, being consumed in vast numbers? In this chapter I discuss chickens reared exclusively for meat. Chicken has become a barometer for least cost production and can be purchased in many supermarkets for less money by weight than some fruits and vegetables. With this quite astounding mass of animals in the 'care' of mankind, is it inevitable that the global chicken business will keep as its central philosophy – 'cheap as chicken'?

Chicken history

The history of chicken intensification builds on the importance of two key ingredients – the move of rural people to towns and cities and electricity – enabling increased poultry house size and use of fossil fuel to enable the harvesting and transport of feed from previously unachievable distance. But first, the conventional history. In Asia today you will see backyard birds that are identical in nature to the first domesticated chicken, the red jungle fowl – light, agile birds, still able to fly for short distances and to fly up into trees, rear young and produce eggs and (a little) meat.

The Ancient Egyptians appear to have reared poultry in large groups and to have developed technology for incubating large numbers of eggs. But the first birds with a lineage to the current birds reared on a commercial scale were imported from Asia to the US and Europe and can still be traced through existing lines such as the Java chicken. However, most chickens were reared in backyards and small flocks until the 1930s where expanding city populations in the US created a demand for fresh poultry meat, and around cities like New York and Chicago, farms started to rear increasingly large numbers of birds in large outdoor flocks and housed in small group coops.

In the 1930s most farms did not consider the use of electricity for provision of services to animal houses and so the use of automated systems for ventilation were rare. Farmers at this time were aware of the effects of poor air and house environment on their birds, and by the late 1930s farmers were beginning to experiment with keeping birds in more 'controlled environments'. By 1940 many birds were still given access to the outdoors, but the 'range houses' that they used at night were becoming increasingly large and complex, with feeding systems, lighting and ventilation systems starting to develop as electricity became more widely used. A quantum change in philosophy became apparent in the 1950s with the development of the first widely used fully housed poultry systems – and chicken rearing started to move entirely into houses. To enable this, systems to provide food automatically, to control ventilation and to regulate house temperature were developed, and by 1960, the house design used throughout the world was established and would be quite recognizable to many poultry farmers today. As the birds moved indoors, people began to forget poultry as regular 'farmyard' animals and started to see poultry as a low-cost food available in the food market, rather than at the farmer's gate.

Today, globally over 75 per cent of poultry meat now comes from birds reared entirely indoors. Of the 25 per cent not reared under controlled conditions, the majority are farmed at family or local farm or subsistence level (particularly in Africa and Asia) – however, a small percentage of birds are beginning to 'return to the paddock' as consumers in the developed world choose to purchase free-range or organic poultry. Poultry plays an important role in the livelihood of rural communities in developing countries and rural, small-scale poultry accounts for about 80 per cent of the world's poultry stocks in some developing countries, and can contribute by providing income, satisfying religious requirements, using family labour and providing for the family and local nutritional needs. Africa's poultry meat consumption has grown rapidly, with more than 2 million metric tons of poultry products valued at nearly US $3 billion being supplied to meet domestic demand in 2012.

Chicken houses

If so many thousands of millions animals are kept indoors, are these houses good places for them to live out their lives? Although there are variations on what constitutes a modern chicken house there are some generally recognizable features. Birds are most commonly kept on a floor covered in a layer of litter, but in some countries where it is permitted, broilers are increasingly being reared on wood slats, or plastic or wire mesh floors with no litter. Litter can be wood shavings, rice hulls (the husk of the rice grain), chopped straw, peat or chopped newspaper. Around the world, wood shavings and rice hulls are the dominant material. The floor under the litter is concrete in many countries, but in some places the floor is earth. The birds are kept under a low roof. The roof might be supported by solid walls, or by mesh or netting walls in tropical countries. In some countries, particularly in Asia, some broiler houses are now 'double' or even 'triple deckers' with two or three floor levels under one roof. Some houses are made from very modern materials – steel and concrete, with steel or aluminium sheet clad walls and roof, whilst others, even some very large houses, particularly in South America and Asia, are made from local timber, with clay tiles on the roof.

Light is usually provided by electric lights, and in fully enclosed houses, light levels are generally quite low – at around 20–40 lux, with a minimum light level of 20 lux (over 80 per cent of the useable floor area) now required in Europe (European Union, Council Directive, 2007/43/EC) – just a bit more than the minimum you would need to read this book. In houses with mesh sides, or with pop holes to the outdoors, light levels can be very high. One reason commonly given for keeping birds at low light levels has been that this keeps them 'calmer' and so less likely to become excitable and to 'pile up' and suffocate. The vast differences in light levels seen in different poultry houses around the world make this argument a bit hard to follow, and in some European countries retailers are requiring poultry producers to put windows into their houses to provide some element of natural light.

In most large poultry houses artificial ventilation is required. Ventilation brings in fresh air and removes ammonia and dust – and in countries with high temperatures, ventilation is combined with cooling in the form of evaporative cooling and tunnel ventilation to reduce house temperatures. Almost all current ventilation systems rely on electricity, and in some countries electrical energy is one of the highest unit costs for poultry production. Without electricity, the houses used to produce most of the world's chicken could not function.

At the beginning of life for many chicks, particularly in cooler northern or southern countries, the poultry house is heated using gas, oil, biomass or electrical heaters to provide the warmth for the young chicks. As the chicks grow they produce heat (the litter also produces heat as it breaks down) and so quite quickly the 'heating' can usually be turned off and needs to be replaced by ventilation – even in cold countries.

To feed the birds, two main types of feeders are used, one of which is pan feeders, which look like bowls and are supplied with feed by screw augers that carry the feed from silos outside the house. In the other (less common now) system, a metal U-shaped track contains a chain and as the chain is pulled around the track it carries food from a silo outside the house. In the smaller poultry houses seen in some countries, or in free-range mobile houses, the feed can be provided for the birds in 'hopper feeders' – small hoppers of feed that may need to be filled from sacks by hand.

Water is provided to the birds via pipes with 'nipples' or 'nipples and cups' or (less commonly) via 'bell drinkers' – all of these systems allow a centralized supply of water and drinking points throughout the house. The water system is also used to supply vaccinations and sometimes soluble antibiotics, to the birds via the water.

The control systems for the temperature, ventilation, light, feed and water are usually centralized and controlled by electronic sensors that measure the humidity and temperature in the house. Sample groups of birds are weighed so that the farmer can see how they are growing in comparison with 'expected performance' and sometimes feeding patterns or lighting patterns are adjusted to alter the rate of growth. Today the birds in many houses can be found at a density of up to 20 birds for every metre square (birds m^2), with the maximum number of birds per square meter often being achieved before the very final 'harvest', and some of the birds in the house being removed at an earlier stage of the production cycle in a process known as 'thinning' – which allows maximization of the use of the floor area. In broiler production language, the stocking rate of the birds is usually converted to 'kg per metre squared' (kg/m^2), and in the EU, broiler birds may be kept at up to 42 kg/m^2 (European Union, Council Directive, 2007/43/EC). Some EU countries choose to stock at rates at or below this level based on local national decisions, for example in the UK, birds are predominately stocked at up to 38 kg/m^2 on the basis of industry standards. The use of stocking density may be seen as a removal of the reference to the animal as an individual, and turning the discussion into one about how much 'biological mass in kg' a certain space can carry. Some studies have shown that not only is the space available a factor, but that the way in which the farmer cares for the animals is critically important (Jones et al., 2005; Dawkins et al., 2004).

The whole chicken farm is often part of a vertically integrated business where the chicks and the feed are supplied by the company and the grown birds are taken to the company slaughterhouse. Around the world, variations on this 'recipe' for intensive poultry production exist – some birds are kept in mixed-sex groups (as they were hatched) whilst some are kept in single-sex groups after having been sexed at the hatchery. If birds have been separated into single-sex groups, then they will usually be fed under different 'programmes' to match the different rates of growth of males and females.

Chicken litter

Chickens in most intensive systems live their lives on a bed of litter. In well-managed litter, birds can rest without becoming dirty and they can care for their feathers by preening. If the litter is dry and deep, birds can, and will, dust-bathe, and can forage and scratch – although there is nothing for them to eat in litter. Poorly managed litter can make the birds cold, wet and dirty; can prevent them from cleaning themselves and preening; make dust-bathing impossible; and contact with the litter can produce skin lesions on the feet, hocks and breast. Litter can become wet and sticky, or caked with a hard surface and even oily or greasy. Conversely, litter can also become very dusty – making the house atmosphere damaging to the birds' lungs and respiratory system. Litter 'quality' is at the heart of a chicken's life experience – and, unfortunately, litter quality is also often poor.

Poultry farmers are fully aware of the importance of litter to their birds – but they must juggle the temperature and ventilation in the house, the supply of water via the drinkers, the gut health of the birds and the labour required to manually manage litter. If the farmer drops any of these multiple juggling balls, then litter quality can change very fast – and the life of the birds can become uncomfortable, wet, sticky, dirty and, if skin lesions become established, pain-filled.

Chicken – a 'low margin per head' business

As the intensive poultry house has developed, two major trends have emerged. The first trend is towards large farms, managed by only a handful of people. The second trend is towards a 'low margin per bird' but 'lots of birds' philosophy.

Some farms in northern Europe and the US may have 400,000 birds and be managed by two people, and the largest farms in the world can have up to 2 million birds on the farm at one time. In fact, the man-to-bird ratio can fall to almost unbelievable levels – the grass is cut by contractors, the birds are taken from the house for slaughter by visiting catching teams, the houses are cleaned by a cleaning gang at the end of the growing 'cycle' and the houses and machinery are repaired by outside technicians when required. The farmer walks the houses looking for sick birds, keeps an eye on the monitoring system and plans the feed deliveries and the schedule for slaughter and restocking the houses. The farmer in fact becomes a skilled technician with vast numbers of animals under his or her technical care. Does this matter? If the automated machinery can ventilate and feed the birds, then is there an issue? When a person can farm so many animals, can it be realistic to expect that sick or disadvantaged animals will receive a sensible degree of 'care'? I call this dilemma the 'margin for care problem'.

Some animals, for example some pigs and cows, are kept with care and compassion and even with affection, and then killed and eaten – but some animals are kept with routinely only the smallest 'margin for care' – they are considered as economic 'particles', whose needs are met within the constraints of economic capacity. I suggest that a fundamental concept of animal care in farming systems could, and should, be the concept of 'margin for care'.

What is the margin for care in chicken farming?

1 Making care a virtue: if society only portrays farmers as efficient and shrewd businessmen and technicians, but fails to portray them as people who are 'permitted' or expected and 'enabled to care' for farmed animals, then farm-

ers may lose sight of the fact that at the heart of their business is the care of animals – creation of places and systems where animals find a place of care to live out their time on Earth. Can farmers be given permission by society and by the farming community to recognize the need for care? If so, how can we (society) reward farmers who show a real ability to 'care' for animals rather than an ability to make systems work and to make (small) profit margins from each animal?

2 An economic margin for care: farming is a business and some farming businesses operate on the tightest of economic margins – if a lone farmer can be given authority to care, with technical assistance, for 250,000 animals, should it be required that the business can show sufficient economic margin to provide the basics of an animal's life – light, space, thermal and physical comfort and low levels of fearfulness or disease? If there is almost no economic or conceptual margin, then the care capacity may be pared back to a skeleton. If there is no margin, then there is little or no capacity to invest in improvements in animals' lives, or to create environments that do more than provide the absolute basics. If a business that looks after so many sentient animals cannot show that it can provide acceptable, or even high, levels of these requirements, then is the farm, and the farming system, showing contempt for the concept of 'margin for care' – in other words, is it operating on a basis and a platform based on unsustainably low levels of animal concern?

The idea that 'care' is at the very core of farming seems alien to some people – some may say that farming is a serious business. Farmers might say, 'We don't have time for these cosy concepts, the farming world is a hard cold place, these are farm animals not pets, and we need to provide only what is necessary to achieve production goals'. But is that right? It may be that this philosophy (farming as a tough economic activity) erodes a very simple basic principle – that if we permit animal-derived food to become a commodity alone, we shift the concept of margin to its economic meaning only and we fail to ask or even to expect that farming provides sufficient 'margin for care'. Without a concept of chickens (or other farmed animals) as worthy of investment of care, countless animals across the world will live their lives (and quality of life is important to each animal) with only the thinnest separation from the bottom of the care barrel.

Animals farmed in a minimal margin system may 'produce' – they may weigh sufficient at the time of slaughter, they may grow as expected – but that may be all we can say. We probably aren't able to say that we (as society) showed high levels of care – we provided only as much care as the low levels of margin permitted.

Chicken business

The chicken business is now global. Although many companies rear chickens in their own country, the birds are all part of a global bird family linked by a small number of broiler chicken genotypes – the selected lines of chicken genetics which provide the great-grandparent, grandparent, breeder birds and finally the eggs that will hatch out to be the birds that are reared for meat.

From the 1930s to the 1950s, cross-breeding of different lines of poultry derived from Cornish and White Plymouth Rock birds resulted in dramatic changes in the characteristics of the bird. In the 1950s almost all chicken was sold as 'whole birds', for roasting or 'broiling', and the whole production system was named after this – the broiler industry. Today, in 2017, and in contrast to the 1950s, whole bird sales now form only a small percentage (between 10 and 30 per cent depending on country) of the poultry meat market. The majority of chicken meat is now sold as fillets, breast portions and cuts, or as a part of processed dishes. Some restaurant chains like KFC and Nandos have built their brand on chicken as an easy, and sometimes fast, food. Well, chickens are fast – fast-growing. In the 1950s broilers birds took about 70 days to reach a body weight of about 1.5 kg. In 2017, a broiler bird takes about 34 days to reach about 2.2 kg and can put on up to 100 g of weight a day towards the end of the production period. This is a phenomenal rate of growth – most birds on the supermarket shelf are less than 40 days old!

It is not even that simple – because there is a part of the chicken that has actually developed its growth rate faster than the rest of the bird. The breast muscle is the most valuable part of the bird, and the yield of breast meat has increased much beyond that expected by overall bird growth. The yield (a measure based on percentage of the bird's weight) of the pectoralis major, the breast muscle, has doubled in the last 30 years from 8.3 per cent (1977) to 15.4 per cent (2005), whilst the yield of meat in the leg has not changed much since 1957 (7.5 per cent) compared to 8.2 per cent in 2005 (Canadian Poultry, 2009).

Chicken production races

Feed is the single most expensive input into poultry production, and so, not surprisingly, the rate at which feed can be converted into fowl has its own vocabulary in poultry production language. The 'performance' of a chicken producer can be assessed using a production efficiency factor (PEF), and feed conversion efficiency (FCE) or feed conversion ratio (FCR) are measures used to describe (and to compare) how efficiently chicken can turn feed into flesh. The EPEF (European Production Efficiency Factor) uses daily weight gain, mortality and feed conversion to provide a figure that can indicate a flock's overall performance. In the UK a "400 Club" exists which recognizes high-performing broiler producers – a quote from a poultry trade journal "To achieve a score of 400 is exceptional. It needs everything going your way, and is ultimately down to the management of the farm" (Farmers Weekly, 2013).

Relatively high feed conversion is sometimes used as an argument for chicken as an efficient world feeder – converting cereal and plant-based protein and energy into concentrated animal protein at a ratio of 1 kg chicken for about 2 kg feed – but what does this actually mean?

If you give chickens 2 kg of feed containing about 20 per cent protein, you will get about 1 kg of chicken meat. Only fish have a higher 'feed conversion rate', as ruminants usually require about 7 or 8 kg of feed for each kg of beef or lamb produced. However, although the chicken 'conversion deal' sounds OK, there are a number of catches.

- Catch 1: dry feed is turned into 'wet' chicken, in other words the chicken growing from the feed is made up largely from water (as all living animals are) but the feed fed is dry, so the actual 'conversion ratio' of feed to chicken meat is much higher than first apparent.
- Catch 2: chicken feed is the final product of a long chain; as the cereals, soya, vegetable proteins, fats and fish meal are harvested, collected and processed, there are losses at every stage, so the true 'conversion ratio' – the amount of carbohydrate and protein in total required to rear a chicken – is much greater than that at first made apparent in feed conversion ratios.
- Catch 3: the broiler is not made up entirely of high-value 'breast meat' but also legs, bones, intestines and all the parts which make up a whole animal. Because breast meat provides the highest economic returns, there is profound pressure to increase breast muscle 'yield' in disproportion to the other parts of the bird, but there are also parts of the birds that are not well used as food. This means that the actual final 'true' conversion rate for the edible parts of the bird can be much lower, at around 1 kg for 4.5 kg of feed.

The practical impact of Catch 3 is that the broiler breeders strive to create high breast muscle mass, potentially to the detriment of other characteristics. The balancing act that the poultry geneticists engage in is now very complex. They juggle fertility characteristics (hatchability, liveability of chicks) with skeletal shape, growth rate, muscle conformation of the different parts of the animal (yield), nutritional 'needs', disease-resistance characteristics and overall survival to production age. What has been created over numerous generations is a highly mouldable farm creature, the characteristics of which can be altered within only a few generations to suit changes in the market.

One, rarely considered, outcome of this selection is the loss of flight. The most common farmed animal is a bird – which can't effectively fly! A race of non-flying birds with hyper-developed flight musculature but nowhere to fly to and no capacity to fly anyway! Of course, chickens are not alone in being functionally flightless – but broiler chickens (and farmed turkeys) have been very selectively created this way, thus tethering them to the farm.

In a 2010 report on broilers, the European Food Safety Authority confirmed some of the major welfare problems of broilers and the impact of breeding and feeding practices, saying: 'the major welfare concerns for broilers are leg problems, contact dermatitis, especially footpad dermatitis, ascites and sudden death syndrome. These concerns have been exacerbated by genetic selection for fast growth and increased food conversions' (EFSA, 2010, p50) (EFSA, 2012).

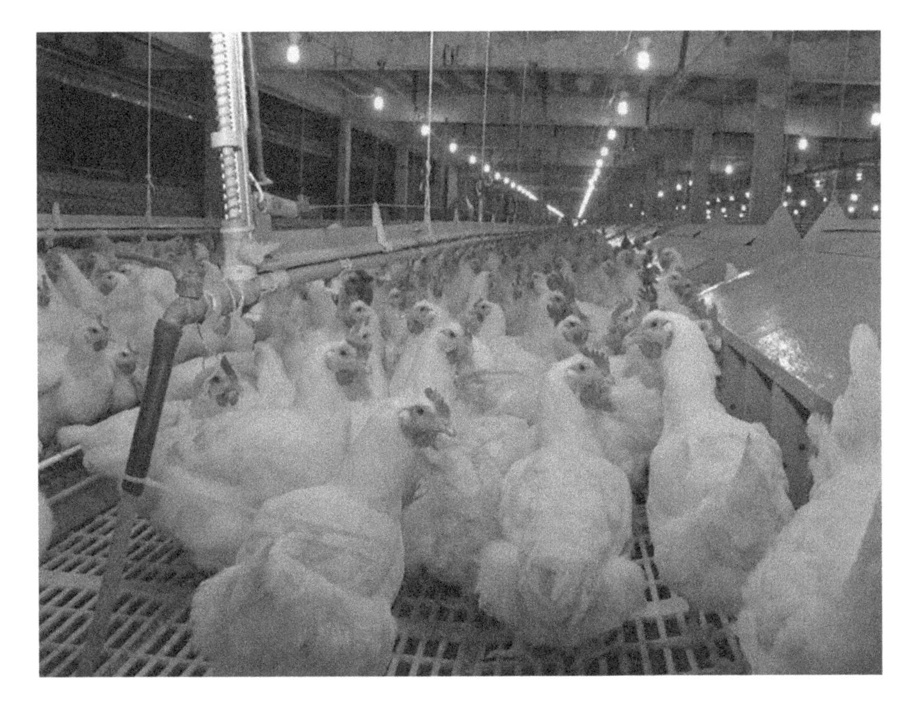

FIGURE 9.1 Broiler breeder birds: mixed males and females in a house with nest boxes

Breeder birds

An important part of the meat chicken system is the parent stock – the birds that produce the eggs that will then hatch and be placed on the production farms. These birds are kept on farms that look more like laying hen farms, with both male and female birds (in a ratio of about 1:10) and with nest boxes for collecting the fertilized eggs. These birds are kept at high levels of biosecurity, but in general must be kept at variable levels of feed restriction so that the males do not become too big, heavy or lame, and so that fertility levels are kept 'high'. The degree of feed restriction can be quite severe. In some countries 'skip a day' feeding is permitted, where the male birds are only fed every other day, or on a rotation of feeding days. The levels of frustration and hunger induced by restricted feeding are difficult to 'measure', but when feed is provided, it is clear from the behaviour of the birds that they are highly motivated to feed!

In a court case brought by Compassion in World Farming in 2003, the judge agreed that such birds were in a state of 'chronic hunger' – while dismissing the case (*R (Compassion in World Farming Limited) v Secretary of State for Environment, Food and Rural Affairs*).

Chicken journeys

The global poultry business has some strange aspects. The chickens themselves are closely related – originating in the elite stock of the breeder companies in countries including Scotland, the US and Australia – and the relatives of these birds are spread by truck and aeroplane across the whole globe. They find themselves finally, after another generation, in broiler breeder sites where they grow (but more slowly than their productive offspring) and mate to produce the fertile eggs that hatch to make the broiler chickens that will be eaten in huge numbers.

The eggs produced by the breeder birds are handled on a grand scale in hatcheries. For every chicken eaten (50 billion a year) more than one egg is required because a percentage do not make it to the farm. The chicks pip their way into the world fuelled only on yolk and their inbuilt genetic knowledge. Everything they do is self-learned – no teenage chicken siblings to transfer knowledge, no adult birds passing on feeding, nesting and living tips. The chicks are a single age group. This results in their own (perhaps instinctive) decisions and reactions arising without any input from previous generations. You may think that this is, well, obvious – but I think this needs some reconsideration. Amongst farmed animals, only fish abandon their young (and not all of them do this) – pigs, cattle, sheep, goats – and chickens if given the option – nurture and *teach* their young. But in the automated, grand-scale production of chickens, this natural and quite fundamental generation step is completely sidestepped. Broiler chickens receive all of their 'being a broiler' education from their peers, and from the inherent behaviours and physiological skills that they carry in their DNA.

Perhaps it should not be forgotten that one aspect of the centralized intensive farming of chickens is the complete severing of this transmission of 'learned knowledge' from animal generation to generation. Who knows what the long-term effects of this may be? Perhaps these animals will slowly lose the 'inherent DNA knowledge' on which we rely at present to give them the 'out of the shell' skills to feed, sleep and grow for human gain. Perhaps by severing this link we eventually create animals so dependent on human support that they can no longer be self-supporting. Perhaps we have already. Some people would say that some strains of broiler chicken are so hyper-adapted that they cannot in fact survive in outdoor systems, or to maturity, without support, shelter, feed control and restriction. This might be a warning alarm.

Another surprising aspect of global chicken production is the fact that cargo ships are criss-crossing the world's oceans carrying (a) feedstuffs for chickens and (b) chicken meat. This sounds quite expected, but it is not. In Asia, leg meat is widely eaten and valued, whilst in the developed world, the price differential between leg meat and white breast meat is very large. So the developed world produces leg meat and exports it to other parts of the world, whilst the countries that will import leg meat export breast meat to the developed world. As well as this 'crossing' of trade, the feed required by chickens also makes some surprising journeys: soya from Brazil, Argentina and India crosses with ships carrying cereals from Russia, Canada, the US and Australia. These cross with boats carrying poultry products to Asia from Europe, from Europe to Asia and from South America to Australia, Europe and Eurasia.

The criss-crossing of feed and chicken product creates complex spider web patterns across the globe and the carbon cost, food miles and economic implications of this meshwork become almost impossible to unravel. Global decisions based on cost and availability determine whether cereals, soya and fish protein are sold to people or to feed animals. The routes that the big boats carrying these foods steer dictate fat or famine for many people across the globe. The chicken in your pre-prepared dish is a relative of a great-grandparent bird grown in Australia from Scottish ancestors. The chicken may have eaten soya from Brazil, cereal from the Ukraine and been transported to you around the Pacific, and then by road from a factory in Holland where it was packaged.

Compare that travelogue with the story of your chicken in 1928 – you went to the butcher and bought a whole, but quite expensive bird, grown by a farmer 20 km away using local corn. How can it be sensible to do all this cross transporting? It can, and clearly does, make 'economic sense' whilst:

- fuel is cheap;
- chicken is a commodity that can be 'grown' in almost any country;
- feed mills search for least cost and maximized efficiency feed formulations;
- the carbon consumptive and globally unsustainable networks of poultry trade are considered 'the norm'.

If any of these things change, the spider web of the poultry trade will get thinner until it cannot hold up and the links between consumer and chicken will probably become more direct again.

Chicken ills

Chickens can suffer disease, like any other animal. The difference is that, if disease enters a poultry house containing 25,000 birds, then it is *not* possible to hospitalize or to examine and treat individuals, so chickens are always considered as a mass, rather than as individuals. Chickens are routinely protected from some diseases, for example Infectious Bursal Disease Virus, by vaccination at the hatchery, or via vaccination in the drinking water on the farm. They may also be protected from some parasitic diseases by vaccination and until recently (and still the case in some countries) by using anti-parasiticidal drugs acting against the gut parasite, coccidia.

Broilers can also suffer a range of 'production' diseases, including lameness (sometimes called leg weakness), skin lesions on the feet (pododermatitis) and on the back of the scaly part of the leg (hock burn), skin damage due to poor litter (breast blister and cellulites) and also respiratory and heart disease affected by diet, genetic susceptibility and by house air and litter quality. Of these, lameness is probably the most widely seen disorder (Broom and Reefmann, 2005; EFSA, 2010 EFSA, 2012). The prevalence in broilers from moderate to severe lameness (scores of three to five in a lameness scoring scale) close to the time of slaughter has been reported

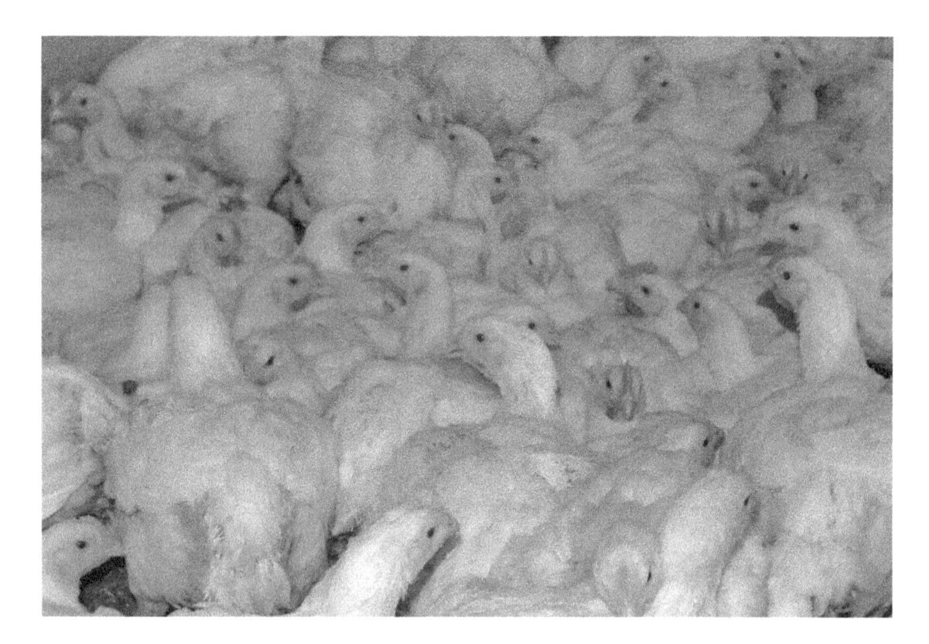

FIGURE 9.2 Broiler (meat) chickens

to range up to 27.3 per cent (Knowles et al., 2008). In other words over a quarter of chickens experience discomfort, compromised ability to walk and/or pain for several days before slaughter.

In general, the philosophy in intensive indoor-reared chicken is to protect by vaccination and to make farms into fortresses that block access to most visitors – and so hopefully to block uninvited pathogens and disease. This fortress farm philosophy may protect the animals from disease, but it makes the poultry business almost invisible. Houses containing 25,000 animals (Fig. 9.2) may have no windows and be indistinguishable from commercial storage sheds. This, in my opinion, raises a simple philosophical dilemma; as the poultry business has disappeared inside, the mental and 'actual' contact between chickens and consumers has disappeared. There is no longer a clear view of what a 'chicken farm' is or even of how a farmed chicken looks and behaves. This invisibility is in direct contrast to the actual dominance of chicken in the food market. This is clearly not an intentioned hiding away, but it may finally have disturbing implications, with so many animals and such a dominant arm of farming effectively 'hidden'.

Chicken needs

Linked to the issue of invisibility is another question that concerns some people, but which does not occur to many. Is it right and just that the most common farmed animals on the planet very often *never*, in their entire lives, see the sun that warms the houses where they live, and powers the plants that produce the cereal and protein that they eat? Some people may consider this a fundamental aspect of a real life – to be illuminated by the sun, whilst others would consider this an irrelevant or even subversive question – bringing a widely used farming system into question. Many scientists would question whether sunlight *per se* is of any importance at all. If an animal can see, if enough artificial light is provided, then why is there an issue? Some studies have shown that birds can see with different spectral sensitivity to mammals and that sunlight may be more essential to them than previously thought (Bennett, 2007).

Most farmers would say that they provide all that is required for the bird's life, including adequate light. I still think that keeping the most numerous farmed animal on the planet mostly hidden from the sun is an almost 'spiritual' issue that should be considered in the debate on what we, as mankind, do to the animals we use for our purposes.

In the same vein, it is clear that chickens are provided with the anatomy and physiology required for a life outdoors. They have feathers that can provide waterproofing, thermal cover and the ability to fly (a little), they can forage and dust-bathe and nest and fight. Some birds are asked to use all of their physiological adaptations and we see that free-range and backyard birds shrug off rain, they bathe in dust and puddles, react to wind and calm and sun and cold by choosing where they lie, sit, perch, roost, fight and sleep. For the majority of the enormous population of chickens farmed, these adaptations are only just skimmed and the birds are provided with a highly moderated environment and protected from these real challenges, but also never asked to use the physiological adaptations and systems that they brought with them from the egg.

A practical farmer might say, 'Yes, isn't it great, we have made their lives so much easier, they don't need to worry about birds of prey or foxes, they are protected from disease, food is only a step or two away, and the day is pretty much free from any unexpected challenges. The birds can mostly eat and *grow*'.

An ethologist may say, 'Here's a list of things I know that chickens can (and do) do when given a chance – scratching, foraging, dust-bathing, clambering, perching, taking shade, seeking heat, avoiding wet, etc., and I've just been watching the birds in the poultry house, and mostly they seem to do little but kick back and *grow*, whilst those outdoors are exercising their physiological capabilities'.

A third person may come along and ask, 'All I want to know is – how many survive, and how much do they weigh, how do they *grow*?' – and for both systems (indoor reared and free range) figures can be provided. Another enquirer might say, 'Well, it's clear, these indoor birds really can *grow*, and fewer die because we can slaughter them earlier because they have grown so well!'

And a fourth person may say, 'Well, this growing thing is OK, but what about the *life* of these birds – if we give them a choice by opening the doors of the house out into paddocks, what do the chickens choose? We find that some chickens choose to spend a lot of their time outside and some don't, and that on warm dry days many do, and on cold wet days, many don't'.

So we have some complex decisions – do we (as a society of chicken eaters) think that growth rate and 'cheap chicken' are so overwhelmingly important that we forget choice, body conformation and the ability to express physiological capacities?

What do chickens actually need? Nobody can truly say, but we can probably hazard some pretty good guesses. Chickens are sentient, capable of feeling pain and avoiding sources of stress, discomfort and distress when they are given a choice. Free-range and backyard birds show a large range of adaptive behaviours that are not 'engaged' in intensive indoor conditions. Society asks a lot of the chicken and it expects that there will be affordability, availability and practical invisibility. The chicken is expected to perform at phenomenal levels – from egg to plate in 40 days – and to return something to the farmer in the way of 'margin' but to be at the level of 'readily affordable' for most consumers.

These are the 'average human' expectations of the chicken. What the chicken actually needs is probably quite different, and applying human expectations is of course likely to attract criticisms of 'anthropomorphism', but it is probably fair to consider that a chicken, like almost any animal, will seek safety, some degree of comfort, both physical and thermal, and avoidance of fear, bullying, pain and disease (when possible – disease is a part of many animals' lives, including humans), space to exercise the physiological capabilities that it has been provided with and company. Food, water, light, air that is not damaging to breathe and a surface to live on that does not cause skin lesions and that enables some behaviours that chickens commonly perform: dust-bathing, scratching, pecking and foraging. If the systems that we create for the lives of this enormous number of animals do not meet these quite uncomplicated criteria, then it is possible that we are permitting, in fact promoting, a quite extraordinary failure – the chickens are providing what we expect, and we are not returning a large part of their 'needs'.

If we as consumers wish to make a difference through our purchases, we can. We can identify chicken reared to specific standards (free range, RSCPA Assured, Organic Food, *Label Rouge*, Devonshire Red, etc.) or which come from systems of production that we perceive as being likely to offer better living conditions for the birds. We might choose to purchase only 'fresh meat' if we are concerned about transportation of poultry meat, as fresh poultry is unlikely to have been transported over long distances. We can also make choices on the content of processed food containing chicken – where does it come from and what was the system of production? Moves are starting to be made in assurance systems and labelling to provide information not only on the type of farm where the animal was kept, but also information on the welfare status of the animal from these farms (animal outcome-based assessment), the method of slaughter, the carbon cost of production, and although this type of information is not yet common on poultry products, in the future this may allow the discriminating consumer to make more informed ethical purchasing choices for chicken. Finally, we could avoid chicken that is 'cheap as chicken'. As long as consumers search for poultry meat at the very lowest cost, then production systems that create low margins per bird and low individual 'animal value' will remain dominant.

Summary

- Meat chickens come from a family of closely related 'genotypes'.
- The global chicken business relies on a network of feed supplies – with complex interlinked effects of transport and local effects in the places where the feeds are grown.
- In some countries, notably in Africa, the 'non-intensive' production of meat chickens is growing significantly as local small- and medium-scale producers step up their production methods and number of birds to supply local 'wet markets' with live birds.
- There is a huge amount of cross-country and cross-continent transport of feed and of refrigerated poultry product.
- The need for high levels of biosecurity, and the types of closed housing systems used, has led to 'fortress farming', and so poultry production has now become almost 'invisible' despite its massive scale.
- Birds live in an environment completely controlled by man, reliant on electrical ventilation, and the quality of their lives can be hugely impacted by litter, air and feed and water quality and the technical influence of the farmer.
- Systems of production, although similar in many parts of the world, do make big differences to the life experience of the birds, and it is possible to provide consumers with information not only on the system of production – but also the welfare status of the birds from different farms.
- Using system and welfare information, we can make ethical purchasing decisions that influence a shift away from 'cheap as chicken'.
- In 2015, around 50 billion chickens were reared for meat. If the systems that we create for the lives of this enormous number of animals do not meet quite uncomplicated criteria for animal 'comfort, care and welfare', then it is possible that we are permitting, in fact promoting, a quite extraordinary failure – the chickens are providing what we expect, but we are not returning a large part of their 'needs'.

References

Bennett, A. T. D. (2007) Avian color vision and coloration: Multidisciplinary evolutionary biology. *The American Naturalist*, vol 169, Supplement 1. S1–S6

Broom, D. M. and Reefmann, N. (2005) Chicken welfare as indicated by lesions on carcasses in supermarkets. *British Poultry Science*, vol 46, issue 4, pp407–414.

Canadian Poultry (2009) www.canadianpoultrymag.com/content/view/953/38/, last accessed 23 March 2009.

Case Note, Reported in The Times August 9, 2004, available at https://www.google.co.uk/?gws_rd=ssl#q=Compassion+in+World+Farming+Limited+v.+Secretary+of+State+for+Environment,+Food+and+Rural+Affairs+(2004)+EWCA+Civ+1009, last accessed 21 April 2017.Compassion in World Farming Limited v. Secretary of State for Environment, Food and Rural Affairs (2004) EWCA Civ 1009.

Dawkins, M. S., Donnelly, C. A. and Jones, T. A. (2004) Chicken welfare is influenced more by housing conditions than by stocking density. *Nature*, vol 427, pp342–344.

EFSA (European Food Safety Authority) (2010) 'Scientific opinion on the influence of genetic parameters on the welfare and the resistance to stress of commercial broilers', EFSA, Parma, adopted 24 June 2010.

European Union, Council Directive 2007/43/EC of 28 June 2007 laying down minimum rules for the protection of chickens kept for meat production. Official Journal of the European Union L 182/19.

Farmers Weekly (2013) 'First farm to record EPEF over 400 for two successive crops', available at http://www.fwi.co.uk/poultry/first-farm-to-record-epef-over-400-for-two-successive-crops.htm, last accessed 20 April 2017. Jones, T. A., Donnelly, C. A. and Dawkins, M. S. (2005) Environmental and management factors affecting the welfare of chickens on commercial farms in the UK and Denmark stocked at five densities. *Poultry Science*, vol 84, pp1155–1165.

Jong, de I. C., Berg, C., Butterworth, A., Estevéz, I. and Bokkers, E. A. M. (2012) *Scientific report updating the EFSA opinions on the welfare of broilers and broiler breeders. Supporting Publications. EFSA Journal*, vol 9, issue 6. DOI:10.2903/sp.efsa.2012.EN-295

Knowles, T. G., Kestin, S. C., Haslam, S. M., Brown, S. N., Green, L. E., Butterworth, A., Pope, S. J., Pfeiffer, D. and Nicol, C. J. (2008) Leg disorders in broiler chicken: Prevalence, risk factors and prevention. *PLoS One*, vol 3, issue 2, pe1545. DOI:10.1371/journal.pone.0001545

10

SUSTAINABLE PIG PRODUCTION

Finding solutions and making choices

Alistair Lawrence and Emma Baxter

According to the FAO (FAO, 2016) pork is the world's most consumed meat from terrestrial animals and, along with poultry, is the fastest growing livestock sector. This popularity of pig meat is reflected in the global numbers of pigs which are estimated by the FAO to have reached 1 billion in 2015. China dwarfs the rest of the world in having over 500 million pigs compared to, for example, an estimated 150 million pigs in the entire enlarged EU. This recent and substantial increase in global pig numbers has been achieved through the same intensification process that has been applied to other livestock sectors, in particular broiler chickens, involving:

(a) increases in the size of farms, numbers of animals per farm, and stocking density (numbers of animals per unit space) on farms;
(b) development of specialised housing to increase efficiency including significant reductions in the labour required to remove manure and to feed and water the stock;
(c) application of animal science (genetics, nutrition, reproductive biology) to further increase the efficiency of production. See David Fraser's paper on intensification of animal agriculture for more details on all of these aspects.

(Fraser, 2005)

This growth in global production in pigs and the drive to make the farm-end of pig meat supply more efficient has however brought with it a range of concerns over the wider consequences of such a growth in pig farming including in terms of its long-term sustainability and the ethical standards. It is noteworthy that these concerns can increasingly be found voiced in 'mainstream' economics circles. A recent *Economist* article (*The Economist*, 2014) for example pointed to a range of issues emerging from China's growing consumption of pork including animal welfare through environmental and human health concerns. In the first section of this paper we will review briefly some of these wider concerns which of course apply to all intensive pig production systems including in the EU and North America with a focus on animal welfare and ethical concerns about the treatment of pigs in global pig production systems.

Animal welfare

The first concerns to be raised about modern pig production were about pig welfare in Ruth Harrison's (1964) book *Animal Machines*. Harrison focused mainly on the use of close confinement systems to house sows and the heavily stocked and 'barren' environments used for growing pigs. It is worth just briefly painting a picture of the intensive pig farm that Harrison described.

By the 1960s pig farmers had largely adopted a system for housing pregnant female pigs (sows) in narrow crates (sometimes termed stalls) that allowed them to stand and lie but not to turn; the sows generally defecated and urinated onto a slatted floor (literally a floor with long vertical spaces through which the manure or slurry could escape) and were fed and watered from a trough at their head. They were prevented from 'escape' either by being enclosed by the crate itself or by a tether chain that restrained them around the neck. Aside from the very obvious fact that this type of system largely prevented the natural behaviour of sows (see D'Eath and Turner, 2009), close confinement systems for pregnant sows were also accused of causing specific and severe problems. For example, pregnant sows in crates often performed a type of abnormal behaviour known as stereotypic behaviour (repetitive and persistent behaviour patterns, which are often also seen in confined zoo animals, and are generally seen as indicating poor welfare), and they also often developed physical problems such as leg and joint weakness and urinary tract infections. A similar system had also been developed to house sows before and after giving birth (known as farrowing in pigs). Farrowing crates were very similar in design to those used for pregnant sows but had an additional area around the crate to allow the piglets to move around the sow and locate the udder. Farrowing crates were also heavily restrictive of sow behaviour, and this was a particular issue at farrowing because before they give birth sows are strongly motivated to build a nest (in the forest environment where pigs evolved this would be from branches and other materials the sow could gather and carry). The justification for the use of farrowing crates (over and above increasing stocking density and being easier to manage) was that without them the sow was more likely to crush and kill her piglets.

Once sows were weaned from their piglets they would be served by the boar and then returned to the pregnancy crate. The piglets would be placed into systems specialised to provide these young animals with extra hygiene and heat, and also with specialised feeding and watering equipment. After this 'weaner' stage the piglets would be moved onto 'grower' accommodation. Although there was a wide range of systems used, they typically used slatted floors, solid walls and other than providing food and water were generally devoid of other features. Harrison's book emphasised the 'barrenness' of these environments which did not provide the growing pig the opportunities to express behaviours such as exploration that would have been the case in a more natural setting. In addition these systems involved high stocking densities, often with poor light and air quality and proneness for pigs to develop physical problems from being constantly on solid floors (e.g. lameness and leg swelling).

Today, in certain countries, some progress has been made towards implementing systems with less confinement and in countries that have specific animal welfare legislation there is some recognition of an animal's behavioural as well as physical needs (Council of Europe, EU Directive 2008/120/EC, 2008). Regarding sow welfare complete bans of gestation stalls have been in place in the UK, Switzerland, Sweden, Norway and Finland since the 1990s. The wider EU implemented a partial ban in 2013 (sows still permitted to be confined in stalls for up to four weeks after service). The New Zealand and Australian industry voluntarily announced partial stall bans in 2015 and 2017 and in Canada any new pregnancy housing built after 2014 must allow for sows to be grouped, with major retailers committing to stall-free supply chains by 2022. The industry in the United States is facing similar pressure from retailers. However, at present there is no definitive industry action to eliminate the use of gestation stalls. The same is true in China with apparently little pressure by consumers to abolish the system. Thus despite progress in many countries and a growing societal pressure to abolish any restraint system, it is the case that in countries producing the largest amount of pork, pregnant sows are still very commonly housed in gestation stalls.

Regarding farrowing accommodation confinement systems predominate with only Switzerland, Sweden and Norway having in place unilateral bans. However, in Europe the 2013 gestation stall ban appears to have galvanised the farrowing crate debate by placing a spotlight on any confinement system. This has created industry momentum to trial loose housing resulting in the emergence of several alternative free farrowing systems[1] and pledges from large pig producing nations such as Denmark to have 10% of its breeding herd loose farrowing by 2021. In the UK, despite 40% of the breeding herd already farrowing loose under outdoor production systems, the industry stated in their "2020 vision" that they would continue to focus on finding solutions that allow the sow freedom around farrowing. Harrison highlighted confinement systems as the major welfare issue for sows; however, there have since been other issues raised including the practice of having to restrict feed for sows during gestation to 40–60% of their ad libitum intake. The high feed intake capacity of pregnant sows (exacerbated by genetic selection strategies for fast growth rate in their offspring destined for slaughter) means they cannot be fed a conventional diet ad libitum. Such a practice would result in obesity and concomitant damaging effects on health and reproductive efficiency. Thus their whole daily feed allowance is typically given in one or maybe two concentrated meals and is often consumed rapidly, which can result in hunger, as evinced by increased food motivation, increased activity and foraging behaviour, often redirected which can become stereotypic (especially when sows are housed in stalls/crates). Such a welfare issue has not gone unnoticed, not least because evidence suggests it contravenes at least two of FAWC's Five Freedoms (see Webster's chapter in this book) namely: freedom from hunger and thirst and freedom to express normal behaviour. Feeding sows alternative diets with increased roughage content is one way proposed to satisfy the feeding motivation of sows and as such has been reflected in the EU animal welfare policy which requires that sows receive 'a sufficient quantity of bulky or high-fibre food as well as high-energy food' (Council Directive, 2008/120/EC). There is still discussion as to whether or not this would enhance satiety (see D'Eath et al., 2009 for a review), and there continues to be an interaction with housing; regardless of whether or not the sows are provided additional fibre in their concentrate feed, an environment providing substrate to satisfy foraging behaviour is likely to reduce the development of stereotypic behaviour.

The aetiology of the sow hunger issue lies within a much larger animal welfare issue not highlighted by Harrison but a continual challenge for all of our livestock species. That is the wider effects of selective breeding for production traits on health and welfare (Rauw et al., 1998). Striving for ever greater efficiencies has led to genetic selection strategies to get more from less, and in the pig industry a potent example of this is the rise of the super-prolific sow capable of producing very large litter sizes. Such an approach exploits the female pig's natural life-history strategy to produce surplus offspring as an insurance policy against neonatal mortality. The drive for increased litter size is a consequence of the desire to improve production efficiency by increasing the number of slaughter animals produced per sow. This maximises financial gains and also reduces the environmental impact (per kg of product) of pork production. However, super-prolific breeds producing in excess of 16 piglets born alive are becoming commonplace and there are growing concerns that large litter size poses a risk factor for decreased animal welfare in pig production (e.g. Baxter et al., 2013), including increased piglet morbidity and mortality resulting from increased incidences of low birth weight and its associative negative effects as well as increased competition at the udder for vital colostrum and milk. In addition increased production pressure placed on sows bearing large litters may produce health and welfare concerns for the sow. Broadening the breeding goals to incorporate traits that promote piglet survival, growth and vitality is one way to mitigate health and welfare issues associated with large litters and will be discussed in more detail later. Management strategies to optimise sow nutrition and minimise stress could also reduce the impact on both dam and offspring.

When considering whether or not Harrison's view of the growing and finishing stages of pig production has changed, we must first consider other issues that have arisen since her work was published. When discussing the farrowing sow we have already suggested there are concerns with increased mortality and morbidity of neonatal piglets which are exacerbated when selecting for increased litter size. Other issues for piglets include the 'clipping' (i.e. using clippers to remove part) of the teeth and tails in the first seven days of life. Clipping (or grinding) of teeth is performed to prevent piglets damaging each other and the sow when scrambling to get access to the udder. The clipping (known more commonly as docking) of tails helps control the occurrence of tail-biting often performed latterly in the grower-finisher stages of production and involves pigs biting and damaging each other's tails, often causing substantial injuries. It is similar to a number of welfare problems in confined animals including feather-pecking in hens and fin-nibbling in farmed fish, in that it occurs unpredictably and once triggered can escalate very rapidly through a pen, group or tank. There is no single factor underlying tail-biting but the behaviour is generally only found in intensive conditions, probably as a result of a number of factors coming together to trigger the initial exploration and biting of tails (D'Eath et al., 2014). As a result there is no easy solution to this problem and the practice of tail-docking is still widely used to prevent the occurrence of tail-biting despite EU legislation stating that 'neither tail-docking nor reduction of corner teeth must be carried out routinely, only where there is evidence that injuries to sows' teats or to other pigs' ears or tails have occurred'. This latter 'sub-clause' is the likely reason that such procedures remain commonplace as part of pig husbandry. However any mutilation to an animal is an area of great public concern and as such has driven policy changes and recommendations. Very recent EU activity (2016/336) relating to Council Directive 2008/120/EC states that Member States must 'ensure that pigs have permanent access to a sufficient quantity of material to enable proper investigation and manipulation activities, such as straw, hay, wood, sawdust, mushroom compost, peat or a mixture of such ("enrichment material"), which does not compromise the health of those animals'. Additional guidance for auditors of compliance is given in the recommendations and the recognition that the permanent enrichment material should actually fulfil the biological needs of the animals is cause for optimism that progress is being made.

Other challenges for the piglet include the practice of early weaning in order to more quickly encourage the sow back into oestrous. Weaning in commercial pig production is an abrupt process that causes nutritional challenges for the young, slows growth rate and can compromise immune function. There are also possible psychological and long-term consequences of early weaning. Prior to weaning piglets will be conditioned to regular and synchronised feeding patterns, at this stage controlled by the sow delivering a highly nutritious and palatable milk source. Abrupt weaning involves a complete change in the pattern and delivery of food, requiring both behavioural and physiological adaptations by the piglet. The legal minimum weaning age in the EU is 28 days; however as with tail-docking and teeth-clipping, there are sub-clauses which allow earlier weaning (no less than 21 days old) if 'the welfare or health of the dam or the piglet would otherwise be adversely affected'. With the advent of super-prolific breeding programmes and the subsequent use of nurse sow strategies and artificial rearing systems to raise surplus piglets this 'sub-clause' is more common practice and artificially reared piglets may be under-going very early weaning from the dam in order to ensure survival.

Another challenge for pigs in modern production is mixing into new (i.e. non-litter) groups (regrouping), primarily done in order to manage animals at different growth rates. This occurs at weaning as well as at subsequent landmark stages of development or, in the case of sows, after each lactation. One of the welfare issues arises because the social structure of the domestic pig is based on dominance hierarchies. In the wild it is rare that established groups will mix and when they do the integration process is slow and involves very little aggression. In contrast the frequent regrouping occurring on commercial farms leads to dominance hierarchies being formed through vigorous fighting. This is stressful for pigs, resulting in injuries, increased risk of infection and reduced weight gain. Mitigating these effects would involve maintaining stable groups; however regrouping is often unavoidable. Therefore other strategies involve greater consideration of building and pen design which would reduce aggression by allowing animals to display important submissive behaviours, allow escape from aggression and reduce aggressive encounters over limited resources. Genetic selection strategies to reduce aggressiveness are also being researched (Turner, 2011).

A final challenge not specifically highlighted by Harrison but something most animals in livestock production face are the issues relating to transport and slaughter including the animals' responses to transport and slaughter.

Environmental concerns including land use

Animal production is one of the most impactful forms of human activity to affect the environment (Davis et al., 2015). Large amounts of land, water and other natural resources are used in producing livestock and in addition there are significant negative outputs including emissions of 'greenhouse gases' (GHG), eutrophication (man-made enrichment of ecosystems usually resulting from use of man-made fertilisers) and acidification (the decrease in the pH of oceans as a result of man-made release of carbon dioxide). Pig production has to be a significant contributor to these environmental impacts of eating meat, especially given the global increase in this sector already discussed. However, as with poultry, the higher efficiency of pig production means that some of these impacts, for example GHG emissions, will tend to be lower relative to those from ruminants (see later in the chapter and Herrero et al., 2013). Another related and important issue is the 'land-use' competition intrinsic to current pig (and poultry) production, over the use of grains and other plant materials that could be used to feed humans directly but instead are used to produce animal products. Recent calculations indicate that the expansion in animal production (including pigs) to meet growing demand (over and above that required to meet population growth) has come about largely through use of grains and other 'animal feeds' that could have been used directly to feed humans (see Fig. 10.1 (Davis and D'Odorico, 2015). As indicated earlier this shift towards feed-based production has led to substantial increases in the efficiency of livestock production which in turn has reduced the environmental burden per animal calorie (EBC) and the emission of GHG from livestock production. However despite this apparent benefit of intensive production, there are 'hidden' costs in the form of vastly increased use of artificial fertiliser to produce the animal feeds and also a substantial shift towards the use of imported feeds to support countries' livestock production. Davis et al. (2015) estimate that globally,

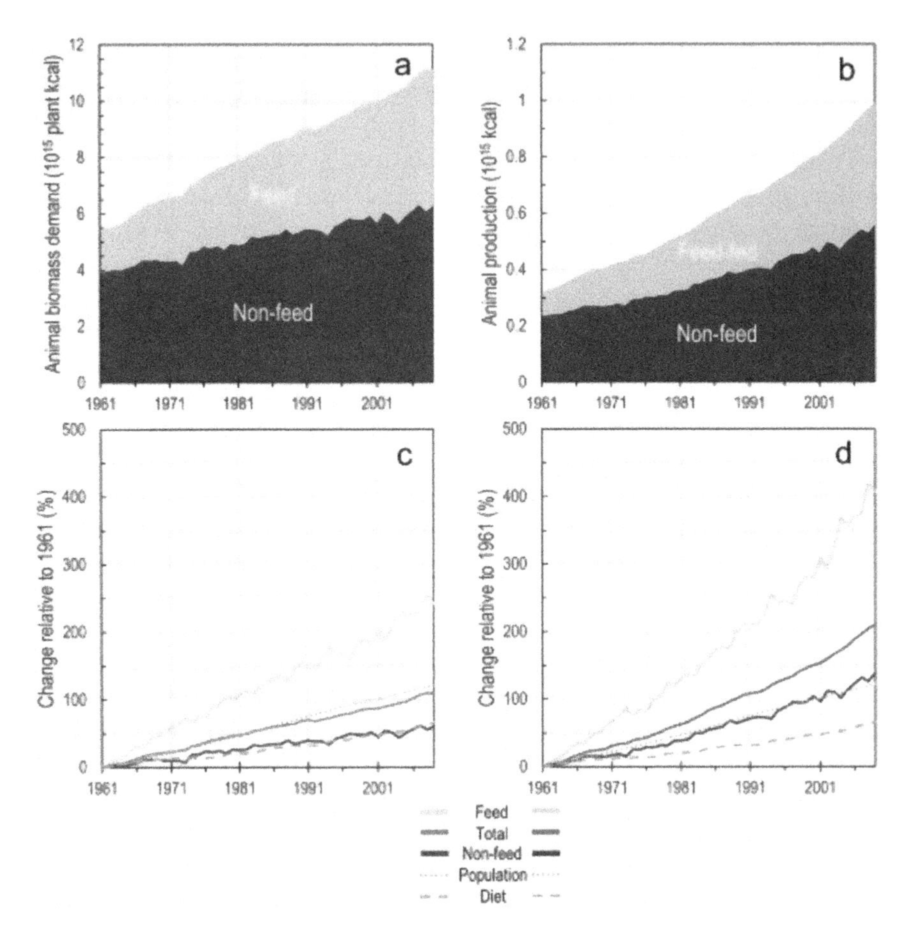

FIGURE 10.1 Taken from Davis and D'Odorico (2015): These graphs summarise relative change in livestock demand and how production has met this demand. Graph (a) shows how calories required by livestock split into Feed (foods that could be used directly by humans) and Non-feed (foods that cannot be used directly by humans) have changed over time illustrating the relatively greater use of Feed in recent years; (b) shows a similar story looking at the production of animal calories from Feed and Non-feed sources; (c) shows how calories required by livestock from Feed and Non-feed sources compare to population growth and dietary demand for animal calories, illustrating that whilst Non-feed use has tracked population growth, use of Feed has greatly exceeded population growth; (d) shows a similar story but from the perspective of production of animal calories produced from Feed and Non-feed sources.

whilst intensive production has reduced EBC by 62% and GHG emissions by 46%, there has been a 188% increased use of nitrogen (artificial fertiliser) with 77% of countries now relying on imported animal feeds. Hence whilst in the short-term intensive approaches can claim to be a benefit, their longer-term sustainability must be questioned.

Human health concerns

Antibiotics are widely used in animal production including in pigs, but actual usage figures are not comprehensively available (Barton, 2014). The risks to human health have been recognised since the mid-1960s when Michael Swann chaired an independent committee into the use of antibiotics in animal production following the discovery of drug-resistant bacteria in the UK, recommending various restrictions to the use of antibiotics in livestock farming (Swann, 1969). In retrospect despite some restrictions being put in place including the EU ban on use of antibiotics as growth promoters, it seems that 'too little was done too late' particularly if you view the issue on a global scale. Within the very recent past there has been renewed concern that multi-resistant strains are resulting from the continued use of antibiotics in livestock farming and most concerning that some bacterial strains are now resistant to a class of antibiotics (polymyxins) usually reserved in humans for use as 'drugs of last resort' (Liu et al., 2016). In a latter-day repeat of the Swann Commission a UK committee (chaired by an economist, Jim O'Neill) is recommending a substantial reduction if not complete cessation of antibiotic use in livestock farming (*The Guardian*, 2015a). UK pig farmers have responded by saying that pig production would be impossible without the use of antibiotics (*The Guardian*, 2015b). This statement is perhaps not surprising given that partly as a result of long-term breeding goals for high productivity modern pigs are more susceptible to stress and disease and may have an increasing difficulty to cope with environmental challenges. The environmental argument to cope with this is to improve environments and remove stressors; the genetic argument is to breed for greater resistance and tolerance to disease and environmental challenges. A step further within genetics would proffer gene editing techniques to engineer resilience.

What has further complicated the arguments over the sustainability of livestock farming including pig production has been the reemergence of concerns over 'food security' and the very real likelihood that there will be food shortages in the future (Environment, Food and Rural Affairs Committee, 2015). The complication here is that the need to feed a growing global population, combined with changes in affluence increasing global demand for meat, could counter the aims of making livestock production more sustainable, not least because of the wider environmental effects of an increase in animal numbers if demand for animal products is unrestrained.

In the second part of this short essay we will look at various strategies to balance (optimise) the various demands for increased sustainability. We will also touch on wider policy areas that will need attention if sustainability goals are to be met in the face of a growing demand for pig meat.

Farm-level innovation

An obvious place to look for solutions that could help improve sustainability of pig production is at farm level. The majority of the welfare issues concerning the public about modern pig production are on-farm, and many of the wider environmental issues also are farmed based (e.g. the majority of the 'carbon-footprint' of livestock production occurs before the animals (or products) leave the farm).

At the simplest level we could look at optimising 'components' of systems to improve sustainability. Piglet mortality is an example of a system-component which remains high at close to 20% including still-births; it is both an important welfare issue as well as an environmental and economic issue as it represents a waste of resources. The welfare issue not only lies with the piglets who may suffer as a result of the predisposing risk factors resulting in the different causes of death (i.e. starvation, chilling, crushing by the sow and disease), but also with the sow because of the restrictive farrowing crate imposed to improve piglet survival. A recent research project aimed to address both issues by breeding for improved piglet survival under loose farrowing conditions on an outdoor commercial breeding unit in Scotland (Welfare Quality, 2009a). Sows and their litters from lines of pigs selected for high survival at weaning were compared with a control population selected for average survival. The results were encouraging with the high-survival lines showing improved piglet survival over two subsequent generations. Important points raised by this work are that:

(a) the lines that were compared had been bred in intensive conditions yet still showed improved survival in a very different (outdoor) environment suggesting that the same characteristics support high survival in both indoor and outdoor conditions. One implication of this is that there should be no need to set up a separate outdoor breeding programme aimed at increasing piglet survival.
(b) one of the traits the high-survival sows showed was greater care when lying hence lessening the risk of crushing their piglets (a major cause of piglet deaths in systems that do not use the farrowing crate to protect piglets).
(c) the findings represent an example where it is possible to align a number of sustainability goals. The use of genetic selection to reduce piglet mortality in a non-crate system is a significant welfare gain and could help in the future to reduce the reliance on the farrowing crate (see also later in the chapter). At the same time increased piglet survival also reduces the environmental impact of pig farming (by reducing waste) and contributes positively to the profitability of the farm business.

Of course not all examples are so clear cut in terms of their sustainability gains. The issue of fighting following regrouping as discussed earlier, which causes injury and stress and results in reduced weight gain, also represents a production and environmental waste. Research has demonstrated the potential of selecting genetically against the aggressive personality types that are at the basis of this problem (Welfare Quality, 2009b). There appear to be few if any negative welfare implications of such a selection, with likely benefits in terms of reducing the amount of fighting and wider impacts (e.g. preventing loss of weight gain) that occurs when pigs are mixed. However, as this approach involves genetic selection to reduce what is effectively a 'natural' (if a potentially damaging) behaviour in pigs, it may raise ethical concerns about breeding for pigs to 'fit the system' as opposed to using a 'system that fits the pigs' (D'Eath et al., 2010).

These sorts of concerns are even more apparent in the issue of tail-biting. There is evidence of a genetic basis to the behaviour; however the use of genetics to resolve a problem that appears to directly reflect keeping pigs under sub-optimal conditions seems even more questionable than in the case of aggressive behaviour at mixing. There are examples of systems where tail-biting is a rarity and tail-docking is not required, and one way forward could be system-level analysis to explore how to optimise conditions to better fit the pigs' needs (and hence reduce the risk of tail-biting). The recent additions (Commission Recommendations C/2016/336) to Council Directive 2008/120/EC include performing such a risk assessment on-farm to identify if the conditions the pigs are kept in and the provisions to meet their behavioural needs are considered 'optimal, sub-optimal or marginal'.

When discussing any farm-level innovation we cannot ignore economics and the widely held notion that improving animal welfare will come at a cost. However it is possible to demonstrate that improving animal welfare can have immediate effects on productivity and hence economic performance. Improving piglet survival is an obvious headline story representing wins for all stakeholders. A tougher 'sell' is observed when discussing adoption of free farrowing because it appears to be incongruent to good piglet survival. However recent research efforts have led to successful development of loose farrowing systems delivering high performance and high welfare without excessive financial trade-offs. Key to success has been recognising that allowing the display of species-typical behaviours contributes to the biological fitness of the behaving animal. Biological fitness encompasses important economic performance indicators including: reproductive potential, number and quality of offspring produced, ability to rear offspring and viability of offspring. The 'PigSAFE' project is an example of a free-farrowing project that demonstrated survival rates equivalent to conventional farrowing crates as well as additional benefits of higher weaning weights and better weaning condition in piglets and sows respectively weaned out of the loose farrowing system (PigSAFE).[2] Higher weaning weights could be reflective of greater milk let down, a behaviour observed by other researchers studying piglet survival factors in free farrowing (Pedersen et al., 2011). Suckling success is key to survival and evidence suggests that plentiful nest-building opportunities for the sow results in greater oxytocin and prolactin levels as well as greater immunoglobulin levels in piglets, a sign of high colostrum intake (Yun et al., 2013). Such benefits have the potential to offset the capital investment of installing a higher welfare system (Guy et al., 2012) and therefore encourage uptake.

Understanding how to achieve multiple sustainability goals

The innovation at farm-level approach has the capacity to improve sustainability but tends to lack understanding of how improvements will specifically improve different elements of sustainability. It is therefore important to also develop approaches and tools to assess multiple sustainability goals, and in recent years there have been a number of studies published looking at pig production from the perspective of how it matches against different sustainability criteria. Despite the importance of this type of work, it would appear there is currently no satisfactory approach to capturing the interactions between different sustainability goals in order to understand how we best optimise pig production for a sustainable future.

As examples of issues with current approaches:

(a) Studies can be narrow or even deficient in their coverage of sustainability goals. For example in a study of the sustainability of Dutch pork production, societal acceptance of pig production methods was scored in relation to antibiotic use and pig mortality rate (Dolman et al., 2012) which are clearly unrepresentative of the range of public concerns including those on animal welfare. On the other hand another study (Stern et al., 2005) looking at sustainable pig production at the whole farm level, developed future scenarios for pig farming that fulfilled different sustainability goals (animal welfare, low environmental impact and product quality and safety) but did not explicitly include or exclude antibiotic use in their assessment.

(b) Studies can have difficulty in combining multiple sustainability goals or finding integrated 'solutions'. For example, Bonneau et al. (2014) developed a complex tool for assessing sustainability of pig production across the EU, but in the estimation of the authors they could not provide an integrated assessment of sustainability. Stern et al. (2005) found that no one scenario fulfilled all sustainability goals: animal welfare was the most economically costly, the economic scenario had potential welfare costs (the pigs being housed indoors to control environmental impacts) and the product-quality scenario had the highest environmental impact.

(c) Studies may be overly constrained by the current context. Most of the current studies with the exception of (Stern et al., 2005) have not looked at scenarios that may emerge in the medium term, such as the impact of phasing out of antibiotics or the application of a cap or tax on consumption of animal products.

There clearly remains much work still to be done in evaluating how variants on pig systems can affect a range of sustainability goals and in many ways the studies which are reported here are just starting points for more detailed analyses to come. The work on system 'components', such as using genetic selection to reduce aggression in pigs, has tended to be conducted by biologists and often there has been no analysis of the wider impacts of such technical approaches. On the other hand the more recent 'systems-level' work needs to be expanded and developed to deal with the 'real-life' complexity of pig production systems and also to include more extreme examples of future scenarios that reflect current concerns such as the use of antibiotics or the competition between humans and animals for foods.

Demand side and the consumer

All the foregoing examples have involved the 'supply-end' of the problem, looking at how farms can become more sustainable and the 'trade-offs' between achieving different sustainability goals. It is of course equally important to consider the 'demand side' of the sustainability issue.

There are two general levels to consider here: (a) the consumer and (b) the citizen and the state. In addition there is the interaction between these most importantly in understanding where 'responsibility' for action should lie between consumers and citizens (or the state). In terms of (a) and (b) there has been an increase in studies of citizen and consumer perceptions and attitudes towards sustainability. Generally the picture that emerges is of a complex set of interconnecting 'factors' that relate to concerns for the environment, animal welfare and food safety (e.g. Worsely et al., 2015). There has been a growing interest in how we could translate animal welfare standards into a labelling scheme that would allow consumers to make more informed choices, and there are increasing examples of 'carbon' labelling on animal products. However there is also evidence that a lack of knowledge is not a major factor lying behind food choices and eating animal products from intensive systems (Weible et al., 2013). That is why some (e.g. Lang and Heasman, 2004) have suggested that we will need more than voluntary shifts in consumer behaviour if we are to seriously address the question of 'what can the planet afford for us to eat'. Other policy levers that have been proposed to change our consumption patterns include fiscal measures (e.g. a tax on animal products) or even some form of food rationing. In support of this studies do find surprisingly large numbers in favour of increased prices in order to achieve sustainability goals such as improved animal welfare standards. Furthermore there a number of clear examples from outside of agriculture that clearly point to the efficacy of governmental imposed 'rules' in terms of shifting our behaviour; these include the imposed use of seat belts, the prevention of smoking in public places and the use of mobile phones whilst driving. It is important to begin to analyse the potential impact of the use of governmental approaches to shift our behaviour towards more sustainable food choices not just in terms of their impact on consumer behaviour, but also on the production base that will still be required to produce animal products into the foreseeable future.

In conclusion pig production systems have developed in a rather piecemeal fashion, largely driven by short-term financial considerations of how to produce more pig meat at least cost. The future will see increasing pressure on pig production to become more aligned with other sustainability goals not least because it will be required to play its part in reducing GHG emissions, reducing the use of antibiotics and in improving animal welfare. We conclude there is much work still to be done in developing integrative modelling to provide a systematic analysis of options, and to help provide a 'road map' to achieving longer-term sustainability targets. Partly the success of this integrative approach will be dependent on there being a much closer alignment of biologists, modellers and social scientists than in the past. The benefits should be a more transparent set of options for policy makers, farmers and retailers on how to best tackle the pressing problems wrapped up in the production of pig meat for our consumption. In addition there is a need to consider the options for governmental imposed 'rules' either governing the supply base (e.g. on limiting use of antibiotics or on the objectives of selective breeding programmes) but as importantly on shifting our behaviour towards more sustainable food choices.

Notes

1 See www.freefarrowing.org for examples of alternative farrowing systems and further information on the subject.
2 For final report of Defra project AW0143 see www.freefarrowing.org/downloads/file/5/pigsafe_project_final_report.

References

Barton, M.D., (2014). Impact of antibiotic use in the swine industry. *Current Opinion in Microbiology*, 19: 9–15.

Baxter, E.M., Rutherford, K.M.D., D'Eath, R.B., Arnott, G., Turner, S.P., Sandøe, P., Moustsen, V.A., Thorup, F., Edwards, S.A. and Lawrence, A.B., (2013). The welfare implications of large litter size in the domestic pig II: Management factors. *Animal Welfare*, 22: 219–238.

Bonneau, M., Klauke, T.N., Gonzalez, J., Rydhmer, L., Ilari-Antoine, E., Dourmad, J.Y., Greef, K. de, Houwers, H.W.J., Cinar, M.U., Fabrega, E., Zimmer, C., Hviid, M., Oever, B. van der and Edwards, S.A., (2014). Evaluation of the sustainability of contrasted pig farming systems: Integrated evaluation. *Animal*, 8: 2058–2068.

Council Directive 2008/120/EC of 18 December, (2008). Laying down minimum standards for the protection of pigs. *Official Journal of the European Communities*, L4, 18.2.2009: 5–13.

Commission Recommendation (EU) 2016/336 of 8 March 2016 on the application of Council Directive 2008/120/EC laying down minimum standards for the protection of pigs as regards measures to reduce the need for tail-docking.

Davis, K. and D'Odorico, P., (2015). Livestock intensification and the influence of dietary change: A calorie-based assessment of competition for crop production. *Science of the Total Environment*, 538: 817–823.

Davis, K., Yu, K., Herrero, M., Havlik, P., Carr, J. and D'Odorico, P., (2015). Historical trade-offs of livestock's environmental impacts. *Environmental Research Letters*, 10 (12): 125013.

D'Eath, R.B., Arnott, G., Turner, S.P., Jensen, T., Lahrmann, H.P., Busch, M.E., Niemi, J.K., Lawrence, A.B. and Sandøe, P., (2014). Injurious tail biting in pigs: How can it be controlled in existing systems without tail docking? *Animal*, 8: 1479–1497.

D'Eath, R.B., Conington, J., Lawrence, A.B., Olsson, I. and Sandøe, P. (2010). Breeding for behavioural change in farm animals: Practical, economic and ethical considerations. *Animal Welfare*, 19: 17–27.

D'Eath, R.B., Tolkamp, B.J., Kyriazakis, I. and Lawrence, A.B., (2009). Freedom from hunger and preventing obesity: The animal welfare implications of reducing food quantity or quality. *Animal Behaviour*, 77: 275–288.

D'Eath, R.B. and Turner, S.P., (2009). The Natural Behaviour of the Pig. In: *The welfare of the pig* (ed.) J. N. Marchant-Forde, Springer Science and Business Media B.V., Netherlands: 13–45.

Dolman, M.A., Vrolijk, H. and Boer, I., (2012). Exploring variation in economic, environmental and societal performance among Dutch fattening pig farms. *Livestock Science*, 149: 143–154.

The Economist, (2014). Empire of the pig. www.economist.com/news/christmas-specials/21636507-chinas-insatiable-appetite-pork-symbol-countrys-rise-it-also

Environment, Food and Rural Affairs Committee, (2015). *Food security: Demand, consumption and waste.* House of Commons, London. www.publications.parliament.uk/pa/cm201415/cmselect/cmenvfru/703/703.pdf

FAO, (2016). Agriculture and Consumer Protection Department. www.fao.org/ag/againfo/themes/en/pigs/home.html

Fraser, D., (2005). *Animal welfare and the intensification of animal production: An alternative interpretation.* FAO, Rome, Italy.

The Guardian, (2015a). Antibiotic use in food fuels resistance to vital drugs – report. www.theguardian.com/society/2015/dec/08/antibiotic-use-food-fuels-humans-resistance-vital-drugs-report

The Guardian, (2015b). Cut use of antibiotics in livestock, veterinary experts tell government. www.theguardian.com/uk-news/2014/jul/07/reduce-antibiotics-farm-animals-resistant-bacteria

Guy, J.H., Cain, P., Baxter, E.M., Seddon, Y. and Edwards, S.A., (2012). Economic evaluation of high welfare indoor farrowing systems for pigs. *Animal Welfare* 21(S1): 19–24.

Harrison, R., (1964). *Animal machines.* Stuart, London.

Herrero, M., Havlik, P., Valin, H., Notenbaert, A., Rufino, M.C., Thornton, P.K., Blummel, M., Weiss, F., Grace, D. and Obersteiner, M., (2013). Biomass use, production, feed efficiencies and greenhouse gas emissions from global livestock systems. *Proceedings of the National Academy of Sciences of the United States of America*, 110: 20888–20893.

Lang, T. and Heasman, M., (2004). *Food wars: The battle for mouths, minds and markets.* Earthscan, London.

Liu, Y.Y., Wang, Y., Walsh, T.R., Yi, L.X., Zhang, R., Spencer, J., Doi, Y., Tian, G.B., Dong, B.L., Huang, X.H., Yu, L.F., Gu, D.X., Ren, H.W., Chen, X.J., Lv, L.C., He, D.D., Zhou, H.W., Liang, Z.S., Liu, J.H. and Shen, J.Z., (2016). Emergence of plasmid-mediated colistin resistance mechanism MCR-1 in animals and human beings in China: A microbiological and molecular biological study. *Lancet Infectious Diseases*, 16: 161–168.

Pedersen, M.L., Moustsen, V.A., Nielsen, M.B.F. and Kristensen, A.R., (2011). Improved udder access prolongs duration of milk letdown and increases piglet weight gain. *Livestock Science* 140: 253–261.

Rauw, W.M., Kanis, E., Noordhuizen-Stassen, E.N. and Grommers, F.J., (1998). Undesirable side effects of selection for high production efficiency in farm animals: A review. *Livestock Production Science*, 56: 15–33.

Stern, S., Sonesson, U., Gunnarsson, S., Oborn, I., Kumm, K.I. and Nybrant, T., (2005). Sustainable development of food production: A case study on scenarios for pig production. *Ambio*, 34: 402–407.

Swann, M.M., 1969. Report, joint committee on the use of antibiotics in animal husbandry and veterinary medicine. HMSO, London.

Turner, S.P., (2011). Breeding against harmful social behaviours in pigs and chickens: State of the art and the way forward. *Applied Animal Behaviour Science*, 134: 1–9.

Weible, D., Christoph-Schulz, I.B. and Salamon, P., (2013). Does the Society Perceive Its Own Responsibility for Modern Pig Production? In: *The ethics consumption: The citizen, the market and the law* (eds.) H. Röcklinsberg and P. Sandin, © Wageningen Academic Publishers, Wagingen, DOI 10.3920/978-90-8686-784-4_62: 386–392.

Welfare Quality® Fact Sheet, (2009a). Improving piglet survival. www.welfarequality.net/everyone/41858/5/0/22

Welfare Quality® Fact Sheet, (2009b). Reducing aggression in pigs through selective breeding. www.welfarequality.net/everyone/41858/5/0/22

Worsley, A., Wang, W. and Burton, M., (2015). Food concerns and support for environmental food policies and purchasing. *Appetite*, 91: 48–55.

Yun, J., Swan, K.-M., Vienola, K., Farmer, C., Oliviero, C., Peltoniemi, O. and Valros, A., (2013). Nest-building in sows: Effects of farrowing housing on hormonal modulation of maternal characteristics. *Applied Animal Behaviour Science*, 148: 77–84

11

ISSUES IN FISHERIES AND AQUACULTURE

Sustainability and fish welfare

Steve Kestin

Part I: Sustainability issues in fisheries

I live close to Newlyn, historically an important fishing port in Cornwall in South-west England. Many old photos show the port crammed with a fleet of sailing luggers loaded to the gunwales with pilchards. Indeed, the abundant pilchard fishery that flourished off the Cornish coast maintained many of the villages here. Now at Newlyn there are a few offshore fishing vessels and a small fleet of day boats. Talk to the fisherman and they speak of landing quotas on most species of fish, size limits for fish landed, limitations on fishing effort, limitations on horsepower and a scarcity of fish generally. Only this year the Bass fishery, traditionally important in Cornwall, has had an 80% reduction in quota, and even recreational anglers are now restricted to one fish per day. This picture is repeated in many fisheries all over the world. Over 1000 species of fish are caught commercially and many of these are seeing a serious decline in fish stocks and fish landings. In short, today they are not being fished sustainably.

The decline of fisheries is a topic very well covered in the media, scientific journals and legislation, yet there are very few fisheries that can be shown to be sustainable. In this chapter I will discuss why this is and some ways that sustainability could be improved. I will discuss wild capture fisheries (finfish and shellfish unless otherwise stated) and aquaculture separately as the main issues are different.

What is sustainability in fisheries?

There are many aspects to sustainability in fisheries, including production of greenhouse gasses, animal welfare and other ethical issues, but there is one main sustainability issue.

Can the fishery be carried out:

1 Indefinitely without prejudice to the fish species ability to maintain its population?
2 Without affecting other species by
   i) Removing their food supply?
   ii) Damaging the environment?
   iii) Accidentally killing them as bycatch, for example?

Note: To understand fisheries statistics, it is important to understand the terms used.

Catch and catches include all the fish of the target species taken from the ocean. **Landings** means that part of the catch of the target species that is 'landed' (processed for sale or used). It does not include bycatch.

Bycatch means any marine organism caught unintentionally while catching a certain target size and species of fish. There are two components to bycatch: undersized or over quota fish of the target species here called **discards** and species different from the target. Here bycatch will refer only to species different from the target. This can include any animal from non-target fish to birds, whales, invertebrates and even coral.

How fisheries develop

Almost all fisheries have developed in a similar manner, starting from small-scale artisanal capture methods based on hook and line, small nets, fish traps or hand gathering. Many of these fisheries were inherently sustainable. They were small scale and inefficient using primitive technologies that made little impact on fish stocks. As demand increased there was pressure to develop more efficient fishing methods/technologies. Competition between individual fishermen, boats and countries has driven a cycle of ever-increasing fishing effort and increasing efficiency of capture. The transition from artisanal to industrial fishing continues until populations of the target species start to be depleted.

At some point, regulation is usually introduced into the system, sometimes voluntarily, sometimes imposed by regulators. If it is introduced early enough, uses a good enough model, is prescriptive enough and is policed well enough, the fishery can become sustainable. But this is rarely the case. In the next section I will discuss examples to indicate how a fishery becomes unsustainable and the problems of regulating a fishery sufficiently rigorously for it to achieve sustainability.

Example 1. Whaling

The rise and fall of the baleen whale fishery provides an excellent illustration of the evolution of a fishery and the drivers that caused the industry's growth and eventual demise. Baleen whales, like blue, fin and right whales, feed by sieving small crustaceans and fish from seawater through baleen plates in their mouth. They weigh 30 to 100 tonnes each and each individual represents a very valuable resource. Whaling for the slow-swimming bowhead and right whales started centuries ago in the North Atlantic. Initially this whale fishery developed close to shore in the Bay of Biscay but, as numbers declined, expanded in the mid-17th century to voyages offshore and to the Arctic where a very profitable fishery developed off Greenland. Whaling voyages were private ventures and the sponsors stood to make large profits if the ventures were successful. The whaling ships were sailing ships and the whales were killed by hand from open boats and processed either ashore or alongside the ships.

The whaling industry grew unregulated for two centuries, marked by a steady expansion in whaling areas as the population of whales reduced. By the start of the 20th century populations of bowhead and right whales in the North Atlantic were so depleted that it was no longer profitable to hunt them and effort was directed towards other species. The populations of bowhead and right whales in the North Atlantic have not recovered and the species remain critically endangered. Numbers are now estimated to be only 300 to 400 individuals (less than 2% of the original population size).

There were large populations of rorqual whales (blue and fin, etc.) inhabiting the same seas as the right whales, but because they swam fast and sank when dead they could not be hunted from open rowing boats with hand harpoons. However, as the bowhead and right whale populations were reduced, rorquals attracted the attention of whalers and drove changes in technology. Initially fast steam-powered vessels and then explosive harpoons were developed, later followed by floating factory ships, ultimately equipped with spotter helicopters. These developments enabled the industry to expand to all oceans and exploit all stocks of whales.

No regulations applied to whaling carried out in international waters, so whalers operated without interference. However in 1946, several whaling nations, conscious of the over-exploitation of whale stocks, formed the International Whaling Commission (IWC) to "provide for the proper conservation of whale stocks and thus make possible the orderly development of the whaling industry" (IWC 1946, p. 1). This organisation has attempted to regulate whaling ever since. However, despite passing regulations to limit catches and protect specific species, by the 1960s populations of all species in all oceans were depleted, some to the point of extinction. In the 1980s a moratorium on commercial whaling was introduced which still applies today. Now the numbers of some species are starting to recover but other species like the iconic blue whale are showing very limited signs of recovery.

Example 2. Grand Banks cod fishery

A similar pattern of over-exploitation has driven the Grand Banks cod fishery to virtual extinction. For five centuries this fishery was very productive. Portuguese fishermen were working the Grand Banks off Newfoundland before Cabot or Columbus discovered the Americas. For decades, about three quarters of a million tonnes of cod were landed every year and the fishery could sustain this level of fishing. But in the 1960s fishing effort started to increase. Landings increased to one and three quarter million tonnes in 1970. The fishery could not sustain this level of depredation and by 1992 the fishery had collapsed and 35,000 workers lost their jobs. Populations of surviving cod were less than 1% of earlier levels (Hamilton and Butler 2001). There has been very limited recovery in cod stocks since.

The reasons cited for the collapse of this fishery are worth reviewing as they provide a typical illustration of the issues. Briefly they were:

1 Introduction and proliferation of new equipment and new technology that increased the volume of landed fish.
2 Large catch of undersize cod and prey species that were discarded dead (discards) – destroying young fish and the food resource.
3 Uncertainty of the size of the cod stock, age class and reproductive rate. Rather catastrophically, the increase in cod landings resulting from (1) above was taken to indicate an increase in cod stocks thus driving increases in quotas!
4 Difficulty in tracking natural fluctuations locally in cod stocks.

In the early 1990s scientists became aware of the decline in stocks and calculated that the total allowable catch should be halved. However Canadian legislators did not reduce the quota due to pressure from countries, companies and individuals involved in the industry. In 1992, the year of the collapse, a quota for cod of almost 200,000 tonnes was set, even though a year before only 130,000 tonnes had been landed due to scarcity of fish (MacDowell 2012). Today, twenty-five years after the collapse there are the first signs that this fishery may eventually recover.

Why have these industries failed, and what are the mechanisms that have led to the destruction of the fishery? In the case of whaling, the answer is clear: the whalers were catching many more whales than were being replaced by reproduction. The Grand Banks story is more complex. Several factors conspired to destroy the fishery: lack of understanding of the dynamics of the fishery leading to inadequate modelling of the population, damage to the ecosystem reducing its carrying capacity and lobbing by interested parties leading to over-generous, unsustainable quotas.

Drivers of unsustainability

In the first edition of this book Colin Tudge neatly summarised the forces that can lead industries to become unsustainable. Simply put, in a capitalist economy, every part of an industry is in a struggle to 'survive economically' by working harder or more efficiently than competitors. In the case of fisheries this is achieved by increasing fishing effort, building bigger more powerful boats, using bigger nets or improved technology (better catching methods, new materials, better fish detection sonar, better predictive models, etc). However this competition is being carried out within a common and *finite* resource. Eventually the catching pressure reaches the point where the stocks can no longer cope and the resource is being mined.

Nothing in this model rewards sustainability. Those who reduce catching effort to preserve stocks for breeding or to feed other species simply leave more fish for a less scrupulous competitor. There are added costs but *no rewards* for fishing carefully so as not to catch undersize fish, bycatch or damage the environment. There is, moreover, positive feedback in the system. As landing of the species starts to decline, fishing effort per unit landed increases and scarcity makes the commodity more valuable. When populations fall to levels where exploitation is no longer profitable, even at elevated prices, fishing effort is transferred to other species, often using similar gear, so that the original species may be further predated, now as bycatch, as the cycle starts over again with the new target species.

The common resource

The main problem is that fishermen, unlike farmers, have no ownership of the resource until they have captured it. When the industry is in its infancy, the resource may appear limitless. There are accounts of whalers harpooning whale calves so that the mother will stay close and be more easily captured. It is still common for fisheries to capture juvenile fish as bycatch and discard them dead. This behaviour is a good example of what is known, rather quaintly, as the 'tragedy of the commons'. Individuals, acting rationally according to their own self-interest, behave contrary to the best interests of the whole by depleting a common resource.

If a fishery is in private ownership, none of the problems of a common resource apply. Management becomes more like that of a terrestrial farm. In private fisheries and most forms of aquaculture, the most basic requirement of sustainability, allowing the species to maintain its population, is always satisfied, though other requirements of sustainability like environmental damage and predator control may not be safeguarded. However, private ownership is really only applicable to small local fisheries. It is clear that if a common fishery is ever to be sustainable, the fishery has to be subject to some form of stringent management and regulation.

Management options

The traditional approach to sustainable management has been to establish a mathematical model to estimate the maximum sustainable catch. At their simplest, these models are based on the reproductive and growth rate of the species, coupled with estimates of mortality and of other losses. The models have become increasingly complex, incorporating uncertainty factors and feedback from catch data and population surveys (Edwards and Dankel 2016). However regulating fisheries using maximum sustainable catch models is fraught with difficulties. Many of the factors are not known with any precision, some are uncontrolled and some are ignored: These include:

Fish stock and fish landing statistics: Gathering good data on stock size and age structure is a major problem. To be reasonably accurate, these assessments need to be independently acquired. The sampling plan needs to be carefully designed and this can consume significant resources. Relying on data for fish landings to estimate stock size is dangerous, as we have seen with the Grand Banks cod fishery. Accurate, detailed knowledge of fish landings is complicated by fish taken from the fishery but not recorded (as discards and blackfish – see later in the chapter). The term *blackfish* is used to describe illegally caught fish that are landed and marked fraudulently on a black market by falsification of records.

A recent paper in *Nature* (Pauly and Zeller 2016) illustrates the inaccuracies in fish landing statistics. The authors carefully reconstructed fish catch data for all world fisheries, critically examining national statistics, and using local knowledge to include data for small-scale fisheries and artisanal fisheries. Importantly, they also included good estimates for the rate of discards and illegal landings for each fishery. They concluded that for 2010, whilst the United Nations Food and Agriculture Organisation (FAO) reported world catches of 77 million tonnes per year, the actual catches were 100 million tonnes per year, i.e. 53% greater than the official estimate.

Uncertainty factors: Fish stocks freely roam the ocean and can be subject to unpredictable events that dramatically change their distribution. The El Niño event is perhaps the best known, but other changes, some thought to be associated with global warming, increase the unpredictability of fish stocks. The North East Atlantic mackerel stock has been moving north in the last few years, extending its range from EU waters into Icelandic waters. This is causing problems for EU fish management planners as they are setting quotas based on historical data for fish that are now being fished by Icelandic boats.

Discarding of target species fish: When fish are sorted after catching, undersize, juvenile and over-quota fish are discarded. High rates of discards are not unusual in many fisheries. This practice makes modelling the maximum sustainable catch problematic because there are no accurate statistics for the scale of discards. Pauly and Zeller (2016) estimated the quantity of fish discarded worldwide at about 10% of the total catch, i.e. about 10 million tons of fish are caught and thrown back into the sea dead. There are moves in some fisheries to require all discarded fish to be landed so that the scale of the problem can be assessed (and the resource utilised). Different fishing techniques vary in their selectivity, with some net-based systems being unselective, and pole- and line-based systems being very selective. Reducing the proportion of discards increases the stock size and thus ultimately its sustainability and/or the maximum sustainable catch of a fishery.

Fraud and the difficulty in policing fisheries: The scale of illegal fish landings worldwide is huge. The International Union for Conservation of Nature estimated illegal fish landings to be 16 million tonnes per year whilst Agnew et al. (2009) estimated it to be between 11 and 26 million tonnes in 2009, or about one fifth of total fish landings. Fishing is a very difficult activity to police. Seventy per cent of the Earth's surface is sea (360 million square kilometers), so monitoring the activities of vessels fishing hundreds of miles from land is virtually impossible. A few examples will illustrate the magnitude of this problem.

In 1993 Russian biologists revealed that the Soviet Union had conducted a vast global campaign of illegal whaling that began in 1948 and lasted for three decades (Yablokov 1994). Revaluation of the catch data showed that they had killed at least 150,000 (82%) more whales of all species, including protected ones, than they declared (Baker et al. 2009). The scale of the falsification is almost unbelievable. For example, they declared 2,700 humpback whales were killed, whereas they had actually killed 48,900. Other countries are also implicated in false reporting and recent DNA surveys of whale meat on sale in shops and restaurants indicates that species of whale protected for decades are still being killed (Baker et al. 2007).

Systematic falsification of paperwork to hide the landing and sale of fish in excess of quota has been reported many times. In 2009 skippers from my local port of Newlyn were fined more than £200,000 for landing blackfish, and in 2012 skippers and fish processing firms in Scotland received fines of £1 million for a fraud involving the illegal landing and sale of quantities of mackerel and herring estimated to be worth £63 million.

Recent studies of fish on sale in several countries, using DNA species identification, have shown that roughly 25% of fish on retail sale were not the species they were claimed to be (Warner et al. 2013). Food fraud of this nature is not uncommon in other industries, but this is a much higher proportion than reported for other meats. A major problem with illegal fishing exists in third world countries which cannot prevent the plundering of fish stocks within their the Exclusive Economic Zone (EEZ) by foreign fishing fleets because they cannot afford to police them.

Damage and degradation of fisheries: In addition to the factors outlined above, there is concern that fisheries are being damaged by other unseen but equally insidious anthropogenic factors. These include widespread pollution from sewage and wastewater discharged into coastal waters. These degrade environments and damage fisheries and, particularly, shell-fisheries. Fisheries themselves are responsible for a lot of unseen environmental damage, the best known being seabed damage from beam trawling. This damages and degrades the ecosystem and reduces its carrying capacity. Industrial waste, dredging and coastal works degrade environments: many coral reefs including the Great Barrier reef are being damaged by sediment from dredging and agricultural runoff, pesticides and heavy metals.

It is estimated that 12.6 million tonnes of plastic waste are dumped in the oceans each year and, as it is virtually non-biodegradable, the quantity circulating is increasing. Plastic directly affects fish and animals that ingest it or get entangled, but micro-particles of plastic that are ingested by zooplankton, deleteriously affecting their digestion and metabolism. In a recent survey Rochman et al. (2015) found 25% of all fish and shellfish examined had plastic or other anthropogenic debris in them.

Approximately 600,000 tonnes of redundant fishing gear are lost or dumped in the oceans each year where it can keep on killing fish, marine mammals and birds even after it is abandoned. Dead fish in the net, hook or trap attract other animals that in turn get entangled and die, continuing the cycle – so-called ghost fishing. There are no estimates for bycatch caught in ghost fishing gear.

The effect of global warming on fisheries should have a chapter in its own right. There are two known ways global warming affects fish. The first concern is the effect of raising water temperatures. Some fish populations may benefit, whilst others are damaged or relocate to cooler seas. A particular current concern is the death of coral reefs, which indicates how susceptible some marine ecosystems are to relatively small changes in the environment. Second, the oceans are acidifying as the level of dissolved CO_2 rises. If current trends continue, the pH of ocean water is predicted to fall from a preindustrial pH of 8.2 to pH 7.8 by 2100 (Caldeira and Wickett 2005). This, in biological terms, is a huge drop and how life forms will cope is not known. However, as the pH of seawater falls, so animals with calcified shells find it increasingly difficult (they need more energy) to secrete aragonite and calcite, the calcium constituents of their shells. Shellfish are therefore expected to be amongst the worst affected (Orr et al. 2005).

Socioeconomic pressure to increase quotas: Whenever quotas are proposed, no matter how lenient, there is always strong lobbying from individuals, businesses and even countries to increase them. In many cases, this pressure results in quotas being set above the maximum sustainable catch. Largely due to pressure from interested parties, Canada set quotas for the Grand Banks cod fishery far in excess of the maximum sustainable catch, with the result that the fishery collapsed.

Where a consortium of nations manages a fishery, the pressure to maximise quota for each nation frequently results in unsustainably large quotas being set. Most of the fisheries in the European Union are managed by the Common Fisheries Policy and scientific opinion is that many EU fisheries are over-exploited (Khaliliana et al. 2010). Interestingly, similar fisheries bordering the EU but under individual nation control, e.g. Norwegian and Icelandic waters, are rigorously managed and appear to be much more sustainable.

Other approaches to achieve sustainability

Recently, other approaches to achieving sustainability have been suggested and are being trialed.

Ecosystem-based fisheries management and Marine Protected Areas (MPAs)

This model seeks to address the serious weakness of models that fail to take into account interactions and interrelationships between fish stocks and the wider ecosystem. The objectives with ecosystem-based fisheries management are to maintain all the components of the ecosystem in a functional and resilient form (Ruckelshaus et al. 2008). These include:

- Critical food webs, including both predators and forage fish.
- Seafloor habitats, as these are important for biodiversity, food and shelter for many species.
- Larger older fish – as these maintain the size structure of the population. (If larger fish are removed from the spawning population, there is evolutionary pressure favoring smaller, earlier maturing fish, and each generation becomes progressively smaller.) Old large female fish are particularly fecund.

The most obvious uptake of the ecological approach is in the adoption of Marine Protected Areas (MPAs). The idea behind MPAs is that they should maintain all the critical factors important to a healthy ecosystem and that overspill fish will continuously repopulate the surrounding area. MPAs are particularly appropriate for spawning grounds of fish and other sensitive habitats. Provided the area of the MPA is of sufficient size and strictly controlled, it should provide a refuge and allow the ecosystem to recover and thrive. The EU is currently requiring member states to establish a network of MPAs representing all appropriate habitats.

The use of MPAs in fisheries management is very new and it is too early to determine how effective they are. Ideally, MPAs need to protect all species and the ecology of the whole area, but due to socioeconomic pressure some only protect a limited range of species. Nevertheless, the evidence is encouraging, with signs are that the protected species are indeed thriving within the protected area, and are spilling over to repopulate the surrounding area (Beukers-Stewart et al. 2005).

Reasonably sized MPAs overcome much of the scientific uncertainty associated with traditional fisheries management based on mathematical models. There is some discussion over the size MPAs need to be in order to be effective, and no consensus has been reached. Currently MPAs tend to be small (if they exist at all) and tucked into odd corners of an ecosystem where they will have least effect on fishing activity. It has been suggested that for maximum benefit, up to one third of the total area should be in the MPA. However large, MPAs will still be as open to abuse and fraud as traditional fisheries and will require strict policing.

Market-driven improvements in sustainability

Awareness of the unsustainable nature of many fisheries has been growing for years, and NGOs, such as the Marine Conservation Society (MCS), have been encouraging people to eat sustainable fish and avoid the most threatened species. One of the ways they achieve this is by publishing guides to which species are threatened and which are not. As part of their campaigns, the MCS and other NGOs also rank the major retailers according to how sustainable the fish they sell is. An early campaign to highlight the bycatch of dolphins in some tuna fisheries encouraged supermarkets to market 'dolphin-friendly tuna'. These campaigns have been quite successful in changing the buying practices of more high-end supermarkets, particularly in developed nations.

Responding to the need to certify fisheries for sustainability, the Marine Stewardships Council (MSC) has developed a brand of MSC-certified sustainable seafood. The MSC set standards for sustainable fishing, fishing companies sign up to these, make the necessary changes to their practices and use the MSC branding to promote their product. Companies are periodically audited to ensure compliance and traceability is checked to help limit fraud. Fish branded with the MSC certification command a premium and sales are claimed to be approaching 10 million tonnes a year, set against total world catch of approximately 100 million tonnes.

If these schemes are to be credible, they need to address certain criteria:

1. Experienced scientists independent of the certification body and the auditing body should set the standards.
2. Fisheries should be audited by competent and experienced people familiar with the operations and alive to the specific rogueries of each industry and possibilities for fraud. They should observe the fishing taking place rather than 'ticking boxes' after examining records, and audits should be carried out at random and unannounced. 'Ethically sourced' fish will be attractive to fisheries fraudsters and it will be important to be aware of this and devise penalties to control it.
3. Particular attention should be paid to the chain of custody to ensure traceability is preserved, as the pressures for fraud in the supply chain will be as severe as any other fishing activity.
4. For each fishery, the scheme should periodically and independently assess fish stocks and review fishing licences and landings to ensure they remain sustainable.
5. The cost of joining particular schemes should to be in line with the income of the businesses and individuals joining. If fees are too high, individuals will be excluded and only companies will be able to afford to join.

Whether these schemes will actually change fishing practices is uncertain. Market-driven improvements could be a powerful way to influence the sustainability of some fisheries if they can maintain credibility, but they are likely to work best in developed countries. However they may simply skim off the limited produce available from fisheries that are still sustainable, leaving the rest for less discerning markets: tuna from fisheries with high dolphin bycatch is still freely available, even in more developed nations.

Fishing methods: environmental damage and bycatch

Different fishing techniques vary in their selectivity and the damage they do to the ecosystem over and above the capture of the target species. Hand lining, pole and line fishing, jigging and hand gathering all score highly for sustainability when applied in a well-managed fishery. Traps and pots also score well on most counts. Fixed nets and long lines and some purse seines are intermediate in impact but can cause high levels of bycatch. Most towed gears like beam trawls and dredges badly affect the seabed and/or have high rates of bycatch. Whilst efforts can be made to improve the more damaging methods of fishing, they are often not popular with fishermen as they can reduce catches of the target species. The MCS provides an excellent table that summarises the impact of many common fishing methods on marine habitats (mainly the seabed), on juveniles that end up as discards and on non-target species bycatch (Marine Conservation Society 2016).

Bottom trawls and particularly beam and scallop dredges cause a lot of damage to the seabed, effectively harrowing the seafloor and destroying a lot of fragile components of the ecosystems. This unseen destruction of the sea bed is being carried out all over the continental shelf on a vast scale.

The worldwide scale of bycatch is not known because there are no central statistics. In some cases the animals are returned to the sea alive, in other cases the animals (usually fish) are landed and sold, but in many cases the animals are dumped back into the sea dead. In a recent publication in *Global Ecology and Conservation*, Norwegian investigators estimated that over 11,000 seabirds (mainly fulmars and guillemots) were caught each year in Norwegian gill net and long line industries (Fangela et al. 2015). The RSPB, a UK NGO, estimates that 55,000 Great Shearwaters are caught off Ireland each year as bycatch. Another study reports that 4,000 common dolphins are killed each year in the Western English Channel. The IWC estimate that 300,000 cetaceans are caught in fishing nets every year worldwide, including the highly threatened North Atlantic right whale.

Bird and cetacean bycatch is only a small proportion of total bycatch. Data are relatively scarce for fish caught as bycatch, but 20,000 tonnes of blue sharks (equalling about 800,000 individuals) are estimated to be caught and discarded dead each year in North Atlantic longline fisheries (Campana et al. 2015, Gallaghera et al. 2014). In 2006 at the Spanish long line fishery for swordfish, sharks caught as bycatch were landed and sold and amounted to 70% of landings by weight, which rather questions which were the target species and which bycatch. Several species of shark are now threatened with extinction because of mortality from bycatch. The survival of quite a few species of turtle, marine birds and marine mammals are also threatened. Clearly the reduction of bycatch has to be incorporated into any consideration of fisheries sustainability.

Other drivers of unsustainable fisheries

Subsidies: Very few fishing fleets from developed countries function without subsidies from governments. Frequently, the scrapping of old fishing vessels is subsidised whilst simultaneously grants are available for the construction of new vessels. Whilst this may lead to more modern and safer vessels, almost invariably the technology in the newer vessels is more efficient, allowing greater exploitation of fish resources. In addition, national fishing fleets often enjoy tax advantages such as tax-free fuel. Subsidies are one of the main elements enabling industrial-scale fleets from developed nations to fish at an unsustainable pace and out-compete smaller operations, often from developing countries. Countries in the EU occupy seven of the top ten places in the league for subsidising their fish fleet. Perversely, the Spanish fleet, in top place, receives fuel subsidies of €976 million each year for a catch worth €2388 million (Willson et al. 2011). Subsidies have led to and are sustaining overcapacity in fishing fleets.

Poor data: The state of many world fisheries is not known because accurate data for fish landings, let alone for fish stocks, is not available. The Food and Agriculture Organisation (FAO) of the United Nations, which complies yearly statistics for fish landings, calculated that world fisheries production reached a maximum of

86 million tonnes in 1996 and has since declined at a rate of –0.38 million tonnes per year (FAO 2012). However Pauly and Zeller (2016) reassessed world catches after critically examining reported landing statistics, correcting omissions and including discards that are not part of FAO statistics and calculated that catches peaked at 130 million tons in 1996 (52% higher than the FAO total) and were declining at a rate of –1.22 million tonnes per year, a decline more than three times faster than the FAO statistic. The poor quality of the data produced by FAO is wholly reminiscent of the whaling industry and the Grand Banks cod fishery during their decline.

Summary

Apart from a few surviving artisanal fisheries, most modern fishing practices are a long way away from achieving sustainability. The pressure on fishermen to compete, the international nature of fisheries, unselective fishing gear, bycatch and discards, difficulty in policing fisheries and the scope for fraud and misreporting all make achieving sustainability very difficult. Moreover very poor recording of fishery statistics makes determining what is actually going on in most fisheries, in terms of effects on target species, bycatch species, habitats, fraudulent landing, etc., very difficult to determine. Fisheries have a mountain to climb to achieve sustainability. Fisheries management during the 20th and 21st centuries has been weak. Going forward, management will need to be much more robust. Well-policed and large-scale Marine Protected Areas may be the best hope for fisheries to become sustainable. Unless this is achieved very soon, the recent predictions such as those published in the leading scientific journals *Nature* and *Science* (Pauly et al. 2003), that all major fisheries will have collapsed by about 2050, will come true (Worm et al. 2006).

Part II: Sustainability and welfare issues in aquaculture

Introduction

Fish have been farmed in the Far East and Europe for hundreds of years. Early aquaculture was based on species like carp farmed on a small scale. Carp are largely herbivorous and, when farmed in ponds on a small scale, often as part of a polyculture system, are inherently sustainable. Some of these systems are still practised in the Far East where polyculture of pigs, chickens and fish are practised in a vertical system; the faeces of the pigs and chickens feed the fish in the ponds below. The output from these farms is surprisingly large and when practised on a small scale must make one of the most sustainable farming systems available.

However as with all agricultural systems, fish farming is becoming industrialised. Industrial aquaculture started before the Second World War, and has expanded rapidly since the mid-1950s. Aquaculture is now a major provider of world food supplies. To put it in context, in 2012, farmed fish production was in excess of 65 million tonnes and growing at 6% per annum. This compares with the world poultry production of 83 million tonnes in 2012 with an annual growth of 1.6%, and wild fisheries catches (not landings) of 100 million tonnes a year, declining by 1.22% per year. Aquaculture is predicted to become the largest animal farming enterprise worldwide by 2020 when it will outstrip pork production, currently the largest meat production industry. With increasing global demand for food, and reducing catches of wild fish, aquaculture has a very large part to play in global food supplies.

Land-based animal farming utilises only a few species (pigs, sheep, cattle and chickens are the big four) and during domestication genetic selection within species has developed many breeds fitted for different purposes. With farmed fish, almost no genetic selection has occurred so no breeds exist, but a diverse range of species of fish fills that role. Fish species farmed in 2016 included such diverse species as tuna, lumpsuckers, sturgeon, catfish, salmon, prawns, octopuses, mussels and oysters. There are different requirements and sustainability issues for each species and a book would be required to discuss them all, but sustainability issues fall into two general groups:

- Those arising from impacts on the environment.
- Those arising from fish welfare.

Sustainability issues arising from impacts on the environment

Environmental degradation

Fish farming has been blamed for many types of environmental damage and destruction. One of the most damaging activities is the destruction of wetlands, both coastal and inland. For example, low-lying coastal salt marshes and mangrove swamps are particularly suitable for constructing ponds for aquaculture for sea bass, sea bream and shrimp (prawns). An estimated 3 million hectares has been destroyed to establish tropical shrimps farms alone. All wetlands are biodiverse habitats and some of the destroyed wetlands were mangrove swamps inhabited by a particularly diverse range of species. Many prawn farms are being built in developing countries where environmental regulation is lax. Similar loss of coastal salt marshes has occurred where sea bass and sea bream farms are established and freshwater wetlands are destroyed to construct catfish and carp farms.

Unless the fish are farmed in closed-cycle recirculation systems, large amounts of concentrated waste in the form of uneaten food, faeces and excretion products like ammonia and carbon dioxide enter the aquatic environment directly. In lakes, non-tidal and shallow seas the solid waste settles on the lake or sea bed immediately adjacent to the farm. In tidal areas the waste is spread more widely. If the waste builds up it smothers the normal benthic fauna and flora, decays anaerobically, releasing toxic gasses, and adds to eutrophication. In 2000, the WWF estimated that Scotland's salmon farms released nitrogen wastes equal to more than 3 million people and phosphorus wastes equal to 11 million people (MacGarvin 2000) (Scotland's human population is slightly over 5 million people). Production has expanded considerably since then.

The very word *farming* implies environment modification to enhance a particular output. The question for aquaculture is how much environment modification is acceptable before an activity becomes unsustainable.

Fish diseases and chemicals used to treat them

High densities of any animal promote the development and transmission of diseases and parasites, and fish farming is no exception. Some diseases of farmed fish (particularly salmonids) can be controlled by the use of vaccines but many require treatment with chemicals and pharmaceuticals including antibiotics and anti-parasitics. All of these have potential to damage the environment. Antibiotics and particularly antiparasitics are biologically active even when very dilute and can affect the ecology some distance from the farms.

Sea lice, a copepod exoparasite of salmon, widely affect farmed salmon and can severely debilitate the fish unless controlled. Several chemicals based on avermectin, a class of drug used to control invertebrate parasites in animals and man, are used to control sea lice. Farmed salmon are fed the antiparasitic drug in their feed. The drug enters the fishes' circulation and is absorbed by sea lice attached to the fish, eventually ending up in the sea. The avermectins work by disrupting nerves and affect many classes of invertebrate including crustaceans such as prawns, crabs and lobsters. Because of this, there is considerable concern about the release into the sea of these (and other) chemicals used to control sea lice. The industry is using protocols to attempt to limit releases but how effective these are is not known.

With antibiotics, the concern is the development of strains of microorganism resistant to antibiotics. In aquaculture, antimicrobials are added to the feed, which is then fed to fish, or in some cases, antimicrobials may be added directly to the water as a bath treatment. Like the antiparasitics, a wide variety of non-target bacteria are exposed to the antibiotic when it enters the environment. A real concern is that the widespread use of antibiotics in agriculture and aquaculture is leading to bacteria becoming resistant to antibiotics and that this resistance can be transferred to bacteria pathogenic to humans.

The particular concern with aquaculture is the way the antibiotics enter the environment. Bacteria experiencing a 'sub-lethal' dose of antibiotic are exposed to a strong selection pressure for resistance to that antibiotic. A concentration gradient of antibiotic will develop around a fish farm using antibiotics and a sub-lethal concentration will exist somewhere along the gradient: the ideal environment for the development of resistance. It's difficult to think of a more effective way for generating resistance in bacterial populations.

There is widespread use and abuse of antibiotics in aquaculture. For example, in a 2003 study of shrimp farms in Thailand, 74% were using antibiotics in the ponds, mostly prophylactically, and thirteen different antibiotics were in use including

Tetracyclines, Quinolones and Chloramphenicol (Holmstrom et al. 2003). There are obvious public health implications for the development of resistance bacteria from this sort of use, as well as implications for adjacent ecosystems.

Diseases of farmed fish have the capacity to transfer from the farmed population into wild fish. A widespread crash in the numbers of wild salmon and sea trout has been blamed on wild fish becoming infested with sea lice from salmon farms on their migration from their spawning river to their feeding grounds at sea. This parasite is indigenous to the North Atlantic and has coexisted with wild salmon for millennia. However the wild fish can receive a very high challenge dose of sea lice as they pass the farms and this is debilitating and killing them. Farmed fish can be treated with chemicals, pharmaceuticals, and cleaner fish (fish such as wrasse that are introduced to the salmon cage and pick off and eat the sea lice infesting the salmon), but the wild population has to take its chance. Vaccines against sea lice are being trialled and may eventually help to control the parasite load on farmed fish and thus the challenge to wild fish.

The transport of farmed fish from one area to another other spreads diseases and exposes wild populations to new diseases to which they have no natural immunity. Salmon anaemia virus, Bonamia parasite of flat oysters, Oyster herpes virus and white spot virus of shrimps are all serious diseases that have been spread widely by fish farming and are now causing mortality, sometimes very serious, in wild fish populations. Effective biosecurity with fish movements is being encouraged, but diseases are still spreading.

Escapees and the introduction of invasive non-native species

Fish are being farmed in areas where they are not indigenous and there is concern that escapees can establish viable populations and become invasive and damaging to the biodiversity of local ecosystems. There are many examples of this. In the UK the signal crayfish, indigenous to the US, escaped from farms and is now widely established in fresh waterways causing the local extinction of the indigenous white-clawed crayfish. Wild populations of Pacific oysters, indigenous to the Pacific, are now found around the coast of England and other countries bordering the English Channel and southern North Sea. In the US there are more than five species of non-native fish in Florida alone that have escaped from farming and established breeding populations. Non-native species can out-compete native species because they are often not constrained by pathogens and predators, whereas native species are. Ecosystems that have unique indigenous populations of fish can be particularly sensitive to the invasion of non-native species.

Using wild juveniles as farming stock

Some farm species of fish are not yet routinely bred in captivity and the juveniles for farming are captured from the wild. This particularly applies to tuna and European eels. Stocks of both these fish are seriously depleted in the wild and taking juveniles depletes them further. Trout and salmon were amongst the first species to be bred in captivity on a large scale. The reproduction of these fish is now closed-cycle (meaning each new generation of fry comes from captive bred fish – no wild stock are needed to maintain the breeding programme). Selective breeding has started in these species. One of the reasons salmon and trout were amongst the first to be bred in captivity is they have large ova and thus large fry able to eat artificial diets straight from hatching. On the other hand, fish with very small ova have very small fry or even a planktonic larval stage first. The breeding of these species in captivity presents a particular challenge: brood stock have to be brought to maturity, successfully spawned, either naturally or by hand, the ova collected and incubated under the right conditions and the planktonic larvae fed on live feed such as algae and rotifers. Some economically important species such as turbot and bream have been bred successfully for a few decades, and a lot of research effort is being devoted to other species. This has been partially successful on a laboratory scale for both blue fin tuna (a very high-value species) and European eel. But the large-scale production of viable juveniles of some species is still long way off and unsustainable wild capture continues.

Fish food

Many of the high-value fish farmed, including salmon, trout, bass/bream and shrimp/prawns are carnivorous. They require feed containing high-quality protein and oils. For many years the main source of protein and oil in carnivorous fish feed has been fishmeal and fish oil.

For years the fishmeal industry has been based around catching small pelagic fish like anchovies, sand eels and caplin and rendering them down into meal. A large proportion of the fish caught for fishmeal production comes from the seas off Peru and Chile where vast shoals of small pelagic fish live just offshore in the Humboldt current. Worldwide, between 12 and 29 million tonnes of fish are caught each year and processed into fishmeal, and a further 5 million tonnes of fish waste is processed to produce fishmeal. (Note that El Niño events are responsible for some of the variation in feed fish landings.) In an average year, 4 million tonnes of fishmeal and 900,000 thousand tonnes of fish oil are produced. Fishmeal contains between 60% and 72% of very good quality protein and fish oil is a very good source of omega-3 fatty acids, making both products valuable commodities.

Aquaculture is the main user of both fishmeal and fish oil. In 2010 aquaculture was using 71% of global production of fishmeal and 73% of fish oil. Developing fish diets less reliant on fishmeal and fish oil has been a priority of the fish feed industry as fishmeal is both expensive and likely to become limiting. Considerable progress has been made with carefully balanced plant substitutes. Salmonid diets contained about 55% fishmeal and 28% fish oil in the 1990s compared to 25% and 18% respectively now. Producing fishmeal and oil from waste fish is clearly highly sustainable, but catching wild fish for meal production is questionable. The Marine Ingredients Organisation (the industry body representing fishmeal producers) claims 40% of global production of fishmeal and fish oil is responsibly sourced. If the 25% of fishmeal made from fish waste is deducted, then only 15% of fishmeal from wild sources is sustainable. The criterion for 'responsibly sourced' relates to catch limits and whether the fishery can be sustained in the long term, but as we have seen in Part 1 of this chapter, calculating meaningful maximum sustainable catches is fraught with problems. No account is taken of environmental damage, bycatch or the removal of fish that would be feed for other species. It is difficult to see how many millions of tonnes of fish can be removed from the oceans without having major effects on food webs. This may be illustrated by the decline of diving birds in the North Sea. One million tonnes of sand eels were caught in the North Sea each year for fishmeal production until 2002 when the fishery collapsed. Almost simultaneously steep declines in the populations of Arctic terns, kittiwakes and puffins were reported. Similar declines in sea bird populations in the important fishmeal production areas off Chile and Peru have also been reported. These effects on seabirds are likely to be only the tip of the iceberg, with effects on marine mammals and predatory fish being less obvious.

Fish are widely quoted to have very good feed conversion ratios and values of approaching 1:1 are mentioned, which make them appear very efficient. However, these figures are a little misleading since they refer to the conversion of a *dry* (10% moisture) diet into whole animals, with a moisture content of 70%. A more meaningful comparison is the conversion of feed protein into food protein for us. In this case, the most efficient fish (cod, trout, salmon, halibut, etc.) have a protein conversion ratio of 4–5:1. High-yielding laying hens achieve 2.6:1, the dairy cow 3.9:1 and broiler poultry 4.7:1. It is worth remembering that the dairy cow in particular is fed very low-grade protein whilst the fish are being fed a very high-grade protein, one which could be fed directly to humans. Omnivorous fish like carp and catfish achieve 9–12:1 and prawns/shrimp 18:1, compared with sheep at 14:1 and beef at 20:1 (Tilman and Clark 2014). Fish are thus similar to comparable land-based farm animals, but not dramatically better, as widely believed.

Shore-based recirculation systems

Some of the more unsustainable aspects of aquaculture can be overcome by rearing the fish in shore-based containment facilities, ideally with closed-cycle recirculation. Facilities like this are costly to construct and run. Water is pumped through the system, being reconditioned at each pass with mechanical and biological filters, and frequently pasteurised with UV or ozone. Although expensive, these systems have the advantage that the conditions can be closely controlled and some of the environmental impacts reduced.

Sustainability issues arising from fish welfare

Fish welfare – why bother?

It is worth briefly reviewing the reasons why many people consider we (humans) should care about animal welfare. Jeremy Bentham, in the 17th century, eloquently argued that concern for animal welfare and the need to prevent suffering in animals depended not on how may legs they had, whether they could talk or on their ability to reason, but more on their ability to experience suffering. He questioned why the law should refuse protection to any sensitive being (*sentient being* is the phrase we would use now). The animal welfare movement still holds this tenet at its heart today and preventing animal suffering is at the centre of animal welfare legislation. In the UK it is an offence to cause 'unnecessary suffering'. (In my view, we should focus on preventing *avoidable suffering*.) Then the debate is: what is unavoidable, and how hard should we, as the fish's carers, work to prevent suffering. In animal welfare science, how hard an animal will work to avoid suffering is a very good index of how aversive it finds it.

Considering the apparently barbaric procedures found in many wild capture fisheries, such as the gutting of live fish (live evisceration), fish farmers might well question why they should be concerned about fish welfare. The argument is: wild fish roam freely without direct interference from man and are able to satisfy their needs themselves and largely avoid suffering induced by man (until capture and death). Farmed fish, by their nature, are captive and not able to satisfy many of their own needs. Man then has a duty of care to them, not only to provide their most basic needs like food, but also to prevent suffering. This view is increasingly accepted in developed and developing countries. Buyers from major food retailers are now demanding their farmed fish comes from farms that have been audited and certified by animal welfare NGOs such as the Royal Society for the Prevention of Cruelty to Animals who have developed a 'RSPCA Assured' brand of high welfare products, including farmed fish.

What then does 'suffering' mean? The Oxford English Dictionary definition is: "To experience or be subjected to something bad or unpleasant". An expanded definition would be "an experience of unpleasantness and aversion associated with physical harm, the perception of harm or threat of harm in an individual".

Why do we believe fish are capable of suffering?

For an animal to suffer, it needs to be capable of detecting aversive stimuli and sentient enough to perceive them and be troubled by them. The investigation of sentience, suffering and fish welfare is relatively recent. Practical steps to improve fish welfare have started with practices such as slaughter or chronic injury where, from experience with mammals, we know pain and fear can be caused. Because pain and fear are sensations and emotions and there is no direct way of measuring them, we infer whether animals perceive and suffer them in a similar way to humans by comparison with humans.

Four areas are being investigated:

1. Neuro-anatomical and neuro-pharmacological comparison with mammals.
2. Behavioural indicators of pain and fear including learning and motivation.
3. Pharmaco-manipulation of pain and fear.
4. Behavioural and physiological indicators of stress.

Neuro-anatomical comparisons

Higher fish like the bony teleosts have pain-detecting nerves (nociceptors) in their skin, lips and mouth. These nerves respond to noxious stimuli and conduct the impulses to the brain via the central nervous system in just the same way as in mammals. Whilst the fish's brain is organised slightly differently to mammals, with different regions responding to noxious stimuli, it mediates and coordinates pain information in a similar way. In man and higher mammals, a neocortex is important in pain perception, and the telencephalon appears to perform this function in fish. It has been argued that the absence of a neocortex means that fish cannot experience suffering. But it is flawed logic to suggest that different brain structures cannot perform similar functions. Fish don't have a visual cortex, the part of the human brain processing vision, but seem to be able to see perfectly satisfactorily.

Higher fish have similar neurotransmitters to mammals and similar endogenous opioid systems that modify the actions of neurotransmitters in the central nervous system. In mammals for example, they down-regulate the sensation of pain when the animal is fearful and trying to escape. Tellingly, many analgesics and anxiolytics used in humans and other mammals are effective in fish (Bastos-Ramos et al. 1998, Sneddon 2003). Behavioural responses of many species of fish to noxious stimuli are moderated by opioid analgesics such as morphine and Tramadol (a synthetic opioid drug) in just the same way as in man (Sneddon 2012). Naloxone, an opioid antagonist that stops morphine working in man by blocking the opioid receptors, works in a similar way in fish and makes them more aware of painful stimuli (Wolkers 2013 et al.). We must conclude that fish show a remarkable similarity with mammals in the way their central nervous system senses and processes noxious stimuli.

Indicators of pain and fear

How then do noxious stimuli affect their behaviour, and what does that say about sentience and suffering? At the most basic level, in many species of vertebrate including man, noxious stimuli increase heart and ventilation rate, raise the circulating levels of the stress hormone cortisol and the animal attempts to move away from the stimulus. If escape is impossible, they change their behaviour by, for example, sparing an injured limb, freezing or hiding. Man, when experiencing pain, will seek analgesics such as paracetamol. Fish behave in a remarkably similar way. They try to avoid noxious stimuli, change their behaviour to reduce the effects of the stimuli by, for example, shaking the head or rubbing the mouth on surfaces to try to remove the source of pain. Fish learn quickly to avoid noxious stimuli, and after only one hooking experience with a particular bait become more difficult to catch on that bait (Verheijen and Buwalda 1988). Of course, hooking involves pain and fear, a doubly motivating experience. Specific bait avoidance like this is known to last months or years. Further evidence of the level of sentience in fish comes from observational learning studies which show that fish can interpret the experiences of conspecifics and modify their behaviour and responses accordingly (Brown and Laland 2003).

A classic demonstration that pain is important to animals is that they will self-select analgesics when experiencing pain and will 'work' to access them. Self-selection of analgesics by animals in pain has been demonstrated in mammals, birds and recently fish (Sneddon 2013). When experiencing painful stimuli, fish select a less preferred environment if analgesia is available, whereas fish not experiencing painful stimuli do not. Most of the above studies have been done in teleost fish like carp and trout. More primitive fish like sharks and rays have not been investigated in such detail, but there is nothing so far to suggest they do not experience suffering.

In summary, fish demonstrate remarkable similarity with mammals in the decisions they make and the way they behave when experiencing pain or fear. Their ability to learn and adapt to situations imply cognitive processes that are complex and as sophisticated as many other vertebrates and show all the accepted signs of sentience and suffering (Bateson 1991).

Fear in animals is a far less well-studied emotion than pain. I believe this is because in modern man, pain is a common and regularly experienced sensation by all of us, whilst fear is seldom experienced with any intensity or duration, and certainly nothing like the experience of a prey animal in full flight from a predator. We therefore do not assign it as much importance as pain in our hierarchy of unpleasant emotions. However, in animals it is probably at least as important as pain and probably more so. When animals are exposed to situations that are simultaneously painful and fearful, they will often inflict apparently painful mutilations on themselves to try to escape from fear. A whale, with a 30 kg harpoon embedded in its musculature will tow a 300-ton catching vessel whilst attempting to escape, rather than lying still to prevent further painful tissue damage. Similarly, when held and caught in a leg-hold trap, some species of animal (mainly predators) will chew off their foot to escape. In these situations, the apparently painful sensations from self-mutilation may be down-regulated by the release of endogenous opiods. This implies that in the hierarchy of emotions, evolution has prioritised escape from fear rather than escape from pain. Interestingly humans show similar behaviour. There are well-authenticated cases of humans amputating their own hand or arm to escape from seemingly inescapable entrapment. In this case, fear of death is overriding the painful experience of self-mutilation. Anxiolytics like fluoxetine (Prozac) and diazepam (Valium), both commonly used in human medicine, are effective anxiolytics in fish, reducing the stress response and behavioural indicators of stress a manner similar to humans (Richendrfer et al. 2011).

Stress in fish

All higher animals have a stress response enabling the animal to adapt to changing circumstances or challenges, and fish are no exception. It is a coping strategy mediated by neuro-endocrine, physiological and behavioural responses. When a fish is stressed by any of a number of disagreeable experiences, there is a cascade of responses helping them to cope. If the stressor is a short-term stress, then if it is possible, fish adapt behaviourally by moving away. If the stressor is longer term or unavoidable, physiological and neuro-endocrine responses occur. Where welfare is concerned, it is the long-term, chronic or inescapable stressors that are of concern. The standard physiological indicator of stress in vertebrates is increased ventilation and heart rate. The main neuro-endocrine response is the secretion of cortisol in the blood. In fish, cortisol performs in exactly the same way as in mammals and birds. It is elevated in cases where fish are obviously undergoing aversive experiences, whether they are related to poor water quality, agonistic interaction, chronic fear or chronic pain (Pottinger 2008). It is thus as useful an indicator of chronic stress in fish as it is in mammals and birds. For further reading on pain, fear, stress, sentience and cognition in fish see Chandroo et al. (2004), Sneddon (2006) and Pottinger (2008).

Where do we go from here?

If we accept that fish are sentient and capable of suffering, then several farming practices could expose them to suffering. These include:

1. Practices where man is indirectly the cause of suffering, often centring on stocking density, water quality and disease.
2. Practices where man has direct contact with fish, for example handling for vaccination, mutilations such as fin clipping, handling, transport and killing.

The welfare of farmed fish has received much less study than that of the traditional farm animals. We do not understand yet how farming disrupts normal behaviour and if this causes suffering, or how stressful is hunger from, for example, pre-slaughter fasting. But we do have good evidence for suffering resulting from some of the more obviously stressful farming practices.

Water quality, stocking density and disease

High stocking density is not necessarily stressful to all species of fish but stocking density and water quality are interrelated and poor water quality is stressful. Each species of fish is adapted to a set of water quality conditions – salinity, temperature, pH, oxygen levels and suspended solids, etc. High stocking densities lead to poor water quality. Some fish species such as eels and catfish appear to tolerate poor water quality and do not exhibit stress as indicated by cortisol and behavioural markers at high stocking densities (up to 150 kg per m^3). However both species are capable of air breathing and gulp air from the surface when conditions are poor. Trout, which are not capable of air breathing, become stressed by poor water quality at stocking densities above 40 kg per m^3. High stocking densities bring fish into intimate contact with each other and disease and conditions such as fin erosion can be exacerbated. If high stocking densities can only be maintained by oxygenation or aeration, equipment breakdowns can lead very quickly to low oxygen levels, high stress levels followed by mass mortality, economic loss and serious abuse of fish welfare.

Handling, transport and slaughter

In most species handling, where the fish is removed from water, elicits a maximal stress response with vigorous escape activity and elevation in blood cortisol, all indications that fish find the process very aversive. From this evidence, handling should be kept to an absolute minimum, even if the fish is to be killed at the end of the process. Killing fish should be as stress-free as possible, with the fish being rendered insensible immediately. Percussive and electrical stunning can both achieve this in fish. There are a number of pre-slaughter handling processes and slaughter methods such as so-called CO_2 stunning, that are highly aversive to fish and should not be employed. Humane slaughter of fish is one of key areas that major retailers look for when assessing the welfare and sustainability of fish they buy. In recent years there have been worthwhile advances in identifying and mechanising humane slaughter methods (Lines and Spence 2014) and some branches of the industry are now adopting them on a wide scale.

Transport of live fish is frequently undertaken, as hatcheries tend to be separate from rearing farms. It can be potentially very stressful for the fish, particularly because stocking densities tend to be high or very high, meaning that water quality needs to be closely monitored and maintained.

A section on fish welfare would not be complete without briefly reviewing the welfare of wild fish at capture. Based on widely accepted principles of animal welfare, once an animal is captured and is our responsibility, it is beholden on us to prevent unavoidable suffering. Since we know that taking a fish out of water is very stressful, we should kill it rapidly if it is to be retained (the ideal is to quickly render it irreversibly insensible). If it is bycatch and to be discarded, we should endeavour to release it as quickly and as unharmed as possible.

There is little published research reviewing how long fish suffer before dying. In a preliminary study, Lambooija et al. (2012) found that cod and haddock retained brain function indicative of consciousness for more than two hours after landing. During a one-week research cruise on a trawler in the North Sea (in December!), my observations were that a large percentage of fish are alive when discharged on deck of the trawler and that fish retain responsiveness to stimulation for some time after landing; typically five minutes in the case of herring and mackerel, two hours for cod and three hours for flat fish like Dover sole. We must conclude that these fish were suffering for a long time. If they were mammals or birds this would be considered completely unacceptable. A further concern (for me) was that many of the larger fish like cod and haddock were processed by gutting whilst still alive. This is normal practice on commercial fishing boats.

Number of fish killed in wild capture fisheries and aquaculture

The numbers of fish killed each year for food by man amounts to approximately 80 billion fish from aquaculture and 1 to 3 trillion from wild capture fisheries (Mood and Brooke 2010, 2012). If we apply the widely recognised criteria for evaluating the magnitude of animal welfare problems – the severity of suffering, its duration and the numbers of animals affected – abuses to fish welfare need to be addressed as a matter of priority.

Fantasy sustainable aquaculture

Based on the issues outlined above, we can conjure to mind the perfect sustainable aquaculture enterprise. This would take no juveniles from the wild, use no artificial feed based on fishmeal, use no chemicals or pharmaceuticals, discharge nothing to the sea, recycle all components, destroy no habitat or wild life and farm a species that is not sentient. Ideally it should create a biodiverse habitat, remove carbon dioxide from the atmosphere and reduce eutrophication.

This is in fact what happens with suspended culture of bivalve molluscs. When the farm is first set up, natural spat (spat are very young shellfish that develop from a floating planktonic larval stage) settle on the recycled culture ropes from the vast cloud present in the plankton. Once the farm is established it releases more spat than the farm can possibly use. The small mussels feed on phytoplankton in the water drifting by, thus reducing eutrophication, no chemicals or pharmaceuticals are used and all the apparatus of the farm is recycled or reused. No marine habitat or wildlife should be destroyed if the farm is appropriately sited, and mussels show almost no signs of sentience. Mussel farms create a biodiverse habitat, as attractive to fish as a Fish Aggregation Device (floating rafts used to attract fish so that they can be caught). In addition, mussels capture carbon and lock it away in their shells. For every ten tonnes of mussels harvested, three tonnes of carbon dioxide is locked up in the form of calcium carbonate. There are not many farming enterprises that can claim to be so environmentally benign.

Aquaculture summary

Aquaculture is producing a high-value product; fish are a good source of quality protein, rich in essential amino acids and polyunsaturated fatty acids. Production from aquaculture now equals landings from wild fisheries. Small-scale artisanal fish production systems from the Far East, some based on polyculture, are inherently sustainable. Several aspects of industrial aquaculture are not sustainable, but the industry is still at an early stage of development and is intensifying and industrialising rapidly.

To move towards a more sustainable future, industrial aquaculture needs to:

- Stop using wild-caught juveniles.
- Source fishmeal and fish oil–based feeds from sustainable sources, such as oil from processing of fish waste.

- Replace fishmeal and fish oil with plant-based feeds from sustainable sources.
- Farm species indigenous to the area or contain them in land-based systems.
- Reduce environmental impacts from:
  - Discharges and effluents.
  - Destruction of habitats.
  - Destruction of wildlife.
  - Abuse and discharge of pharmaceuticals.
- Use husbandry practices that minimise stress and disease.
- Use husbandry practices that respect the welfare of the animal and do not expose them to unavoidable or prolonged pain, fear or stress.

General conclusions

Having been associated with aquaculture and fisheries for many years, I was aware how some fisheries had been over-exploited and had collapsed in the past. What I had not appreciated before gathering the information for this chapter was that so many fish stocks are now fully or over-exploited and heading towards collapse. The prediction that all major wild fisheries could collapse by 2050 is not fanciful but based on good science (Worm et al. 2006). Clearly current tools used to manage fisheries are inadequate and open to abuse. Models are based on poor-quality data, political decision makers pander to socioeconomic pressure and increase quotas and illegal fishing is rife. However the main issue that management fails to address is the 'tragedy of the commons', where no fishermen has ownership of the resource and there is no pressure or reward to husband or preserve any part of the resource. All pressure on the system is to over-exploit it for short-term gain.

We urgently need a new paradigm for managing fisheries, easier to police and with the precautionary principle at its heart. Some practices need to be curtailed, such as discarding undersize fish back into the sea dead and the use of unselective or environmentally damaging fishing gear. Above all, we need to address the effects of the 'tragedy of the commons'. Experience from Iceland and Norway shows when they expanded their Exclusive Economic Zone (EEZ) to 200 miles and imposed strict management stocks recovered relatively rapidly (Matthíasson 2003). Expansion of EEZs and the establishment of large-scale Marine Protected Areas, provided they are adequately policed should enable fisheries to recover, although, being realistic, I doubt whether they can be introduced in international waters. Whatever management policy is adopted, measures must be taken to reduce the vast tonnage of bycatch. Irrespective of the discards issue, the toll on wildlife is not acceptable. Killing 300,000 cetaceans, 100,000 albatrosses and 400,000 turtles each year is not sustainable nor is it morally acceptable.

Aquaculture has a different set of sustainability issues to address. Some of the currently unsustainable aspects of aquaculture reflect its relative infancy. The use of wild-caught juveniles and the excessive use of medications should reduce as we understand how to farm fish better. Some local environmental modification/degradation/destruction is inevitable, but this needs to be controlled and limited. Whilst progress will be made in reducing the inclusion rate of fishmeal in fish diets, the steady growth in aquaculture will mean continued pressure on fishmeal and oil supplies. Increasing the tonnage of herbivorous farmed fish (including that of bivalve molluscs) could play a significant part in improving the sustainability of aquaculture.

Looking into the future I see no reason why aquaculture production should not continue to grow substantially over the next fifty years. Fishmeal will continue to be an important ingredient. If wild fisheries have collapsed, this will be prepared from jellyfish and plankton, which is all that Daniel Pauly predicts will be left to fish (Pauly et al. 2003). This will be balanced with proteins and oils from many other plant and by-product sources. Aquaculture will have destroyed more habitats and there will be more discharges of effluents and more disease spread just as there will be in land-based agriculture. The main question with wild fisheries is, will we respond quickly enough and with enough force to prevent many from collapse? This I doubt. My prediction is that some fisheries within the EEZs of some developed countries will be sustainable, whilst the vast majority of offshore and third world fisheries will have collapsed. This collapse will necessitate a completely new management structure so that by 2116 sustainable global fisheries may once again become a reality.

References

Agnew, D.J., Pearce, J., Pramod, G., Peatman, T., Watson, R., Beddington, J.R. and Pilcher, T.J. (2009) Estimating the worldwide extent of illegal fishing. *PLoS One*, Vol 4, Issue 2: Available here: http://dx.doi.org/10.1371/journal.pone.0004570

Baker, C.S., Cooke, J.G., Laverly, S., Dalebout, M.L., Ma, Y.-U., Funahashi, N., Carraher, C. and Brownell, R.L. (2007) Estimating the number of whales entering trade using DNA profiling and capture-recapture analysis of market products. *Molecular Ecology*, Vol 16, Issue 13, pp 2617–2626.

Baker, C.S., Ivashchenko, V. and Brownell, R.L. (2009) Catches of humpback whales by the Soviet Union and other nations in the Southern Ocean, 1947–1973. *Marine Fisheries Review*, Vol 71, Issue 1, pp 39–43.

Bastos-Ramos, W.P., Gonçalves, N.M.F.M. and Bacila, M. (1998) Anasthesia and analgesia in Antarctic fish: And experimental approach. *Archives of Veterinary Science*, Vol 3, Issue 1, pp 95–100.

Bateson, P. (1991) Assessment of pain in animals. *Animal Behaviour*, Vol 42, pp 827–839.

Beukers-Stewart, B.D., Vause, B.J., Mosley, M.W.J., Rossetti, H.L. and Brand, A.R. (2005) Benefits of closed area protection for a population of scallops. *Marine Ecology-Progress Series*, Vol. 298, pp 89–204.

Brown, C. and Laland, K.N. (2003) Social learning in fishes: A review. *Fish and Fisheries*, Vol 4, Issue 3, pp 280–288.

Caldeira, K. and Wickett, M.E. (2005) Ocean model predictions of chemistry changes from carbon dioxide emissions to the atmosphere and ocean. *Journal of Geophysical Research*, Vol 110, Issues C9, pp 1–12.

Campana, S.E., Fowler, M., Houlihan, D., Joyce, W., Showell, M., Miri, C. and Simpson, M. (2015) Current Status and Threats to the North Atlantic Blue Shark (Prionace Glauca) Population in Atlantic Canada. Research Document 2015/026. Canadian Science Advisory Secretariat 200 Kent Street Ottawa ON K1A 0E6. Available here: www.dfo-mpo.gc.ca/csas-sccs/publications/resdocs-docrech/2015/2015_026-eng.pdf

Chandroo, K.P., Duncan, I.J.H. and Moccia, R.D. (2004) Can fish suffer? Perspectives on sentience, pain, fear and stress. *Applied Animal Behavioural Science*, Vol 86, Issues 3–4, pp 225–250.

Edwards, C.T.T. and Dankel, D.J. eds. (2016) *Management Science in Fisheries: An Introduction to Simulation-Based Methods*. Routledge, Abbingdon, UK. ISBN-10: 1138806803.

Fangela, K., Aasa, Ø., Vølstadb, J.H., Bæruma, K.M., Christensen-Dalsgaardc, S., Nedreaasb, K., Overvikd, M., Wolda, L.C. and Anker-Nilssenc, T. (2015) Assessing incidental bycatch of seabirds in Norwegian coastal commercial fisheries: Empirical and methodological lessons. *Global Ecology and Conservation*, Vol 4, pp 127–136.

FAO (2012) The state of Worlds Fisheries and Aquaculture 2012 Food and Agriculture Organisation of the United Nations Fisheries and Aquaculture Department. Available here: www.fao.org/docrep/016/i2727e/i2727e.pdf ISBN 978-92-5-107225-7

Gallaghera, A.J., Orbesenc, E.S., Hammerschlaga, N. and Serafyc, J.E. (2014) Vulnerability of oceanic sharks as pelagic longline bycatch. *Global Ecology and Conservation*, Vol 1, pp 50–59.

Hamilton, L. and Butler, M. (2001) Outport adaptations: Social indicators through Newfoundland's cod crisis. *Human Ecology Review*, Vol 8, Issue 2, pp 1–11. Available here: www.humanecologyreview.org/pastissues/her82/82hamiltonbutler.pdf

Holmström, K., Gräslund, S., Wahlström, A., Poungshompoo, S., Bengtsson, B.-E. and Kautsky, N. (2003) Antibiotic use in shrimp farming and implications for environmental impacts and human health. *International Journal of Food Science and Technology*, Vol 38, Issue 3, pp 255–266.

IWC (1946). *International Convention for the Regulation of Whaling*. Washington. 2 December 1946. Available here: http://web.archive.org/web/20140407095822/ www.iwcoffice.org/private/downloads/1r2jdhu5xtuswws0ocw04wgcw/convention.pdf

Khaliliana, S., Froeseb, R., Proelssc, A. and Requated, T. (2010) Designed for failure: A critique of the Common Fisheries Policy of the European Union. *Marine Policy*, Vol 34, Issue 6, pp 1178–1182.

Lambooija, E.H., Digreb, H., Reimerta, H.G.M., Aursandb, I.G.L., Grimsmob, L. and Vis, J.W. van de (2012) Effects of on-board storage and electrical stunning of wild cod (Gadus morhua) and haddock (Melanogrammus aeglefinus) on brain and heart activity. *Fisheries Research*, Vols 127–128, pp 1–8.

Lines, J.A. and Spence, J. (2014) Humane harvesting and slaughter of farmed fish. *Scientific and Technical Review of the Office International des Epizooties (Paris)*, Vol 33, Issue 1, pp 255–264.

MacDowell, L.S. (2012) *An Environmental History of Canada*. 332 pp. UBC Press, Vancouver. ISBN: 9780774821025.

MacGarvin, M. (2000) *Report: Scotland's Secret? Aquaculture, Nutrient Pollution Eutrophication and Toxic Blooms*. WWF, Scotland, The Tun, 4 Jackson's Entry, Holyrood Road, Edinburgh, EH8 8P. Available here: www.wwf.org.uk/filelibrary/pdf/secret.pdf

Marine Conservation Society (2016) Available here: www.mcsuk.org/downloads/fisheries/Most%20sustainable%20fishing%20methods.pdf

Matthíasson, T. (2003) Closing the open sea: Development of fishery management in four Icelandic fisheries. *Natural Resources Forum*, Vol 27, Issue 1, pp 1–18.

Mood, A. and Brooke, P. (2010) Estimating the Number of Fish Caught in Global Fishing Each Year. Available here: http://fishcount.org.uk/published/std/fishcountstudy.pdf

Mood, A. and Brooke, P. (2012) Estimating the Number of Farmed Fish Killed in Global Aquaculture Each Year. Available here: http://fishcount.org.uk/published/std/fishcount study2.pdf

Orr, J.C., Fabry, V.J., Aumont, A., Bopp, L., Doney, S.C., Feely, R.A., Gnanadesikan, A., Gruber, N., Ishida, A., Joos, F., Key, R.M., Lindsay, K., Maier-Reimer, E., Matear, R.,

Monfray, P., Mouchet, A., Najjar, R.G., Plattner, G.-K., Rodgers, K.B., Sabine, C.L., Sarmiento, J.L., Schlitzer, R., Slater, R.D., Totterdell, I.J., Weirig, M.F., Yamanaka, Y. and Yool, A. (2005) Anthropogenic ocean acidification over the twenty-first century and its impact on calcifying organisms. *Nature*, Vol 437, pp 681–686.

Pauly, D., Christensen, V. and Dalsgaard, J. (2003) Counting the Last Fish. *Scientific American*, Vol 289, pp 42–47.

Pauly, D. and Zeller, D. (2016) *Catch Reconstructions Reveal That Global Marine Fisheries Catches Are Higher Than Reported and Declining.* Nature Communications, 7. 10244. Available here: www.nature.com/ncomms/2016/160119/ncomms10244/full/ncomms10244.html

Pottinger, T.G. (2008) The Stress Response in Fish – Mechanisms, Effects and Measurement. In: Branson, E.J. ed. *Fish Welfare.* Wiley-Blackwell Publishing Ltd, UK, pp. 32–48. ISBN: 978-1-4051-4629-6.

Richendrfer, H., Pelkowski, S.D., Colwill, R.M. and Creton, R. (2011) On the edge: Pharmacological evidence for anxiety-related behavior in zebrafish larvae. *Behavioural Brain Research*, Vol 228, Issue 1, pp 99–106.

Rochman, C.M., Tahir, A., Williams, S.L., Baxa, D.V., Lam, R., Miller, J.T., Teh, F.-C., Werorilangi, S. and Teh, S.J. (2015). Anthropogenic debris in seafood: Plastic debris and fibers from textiles in fish and bivalves sold for human consumption. *Scientific Reports*, Vol 5, p 14340. PMC Available here: www.ncbi.nlm.nih.gov/pmc/articles/PMC4585829/

Ruckelshaus, M., Klinger, T., Knowlton, N. and Demaster, D.R. (2008) Marine ecosystem-based management in practice: Scientific, and governance challenges. *Bioscience*, Vol 58, pp 53–63.

Sneddon, L.U. (2003) The evidence for pain in fish: The use of morphine as an analgesic. *Applied Animal Behaviour Science*, Vol 83, Issue 2, pp 153–162.

Sneddon, L.U. (2006) Ethics and welfare: Pain perception in fish. *Bulletin of the European Association of Fish Pathologists*, Vol 26, Issue 1, pp 6–10.

Sneddon, L.U. (2012) Clinical anesthesia and analgesia in fish. *Journal of Exotic Pet Medicine*, Vol 21, Issue 1, pp 32–43.

Sneddon, L.U. (2013) Do painful sensations and fear exist in fish. In: Kemp, T.A. van der and Lachance, M. eds. *Animal Suffering: From Science to Law, International Symposium.* Carswell, Toronto, pp 93–112. ISBN/ISSN/Product Number: 978-2-89635-919-6.

Tilman, D. and Clark, M. (2014) Global diets link environmental sustainability and human health. *Nature*, Vol 515, pp 518–522. Available here: www.nature.com/nature/journal/v515/n7528/fig_tab/nature13959_ST7.html

Verheijen, F.J. and Buwalda, R.J.A. (1988) Do Pain and Fear Make a Hooked Carp in Play Suffer. Report of the Department of Comparative Physiology, University of Utrecht. pp. 1–4. ISBN 90–9002167–1.

Warner, K., Timme, W., Lowell, B. and Hirshfield, M. (2013) Oceana Study Reveals Seafood Fraud Nationwide. Report from Oceana, 1350 Connecticut Ave., NW 5th Floor Washington, DC 20036 USA. Available here: http://oceana.org/sites/default/files/reports/National_Seafood_Fraud_Testing_Results_FINAL.pdf

Willson, K., Cabra, M. and Garcia Rey, M. (2011) *€6 billion in subsidies fuel Spain's ravenous fleet.* Report The International Consortium of Investigative Journalists. 910 17th Street NW Suite 700 Washington, DC 20006 USA October 2011 Available here: www.publicintegrity.org/2011/10/02/6733/nearly-6-billion-subsidies-fuel-spain-s-ravenous-fleet

Wolkers, C.P.B., Junior, B.A., Menescal-de-Oliveira, L. and Hoffmann, A. (2013) Stress-induced antinociception in fish reversed by naloxone. *PLoS ONE*, Vol 8, Issue 7, pp e71175. Available here: http://journals.plos.org/plosone/article?id=10.1371/journal.pone.0071175

Worm, B., Barbier, E.B., Beaumont, N., Duffy, J.E., Folke, C., Halpern, B.S., Jackson, J.B.C., Lotze, H.K., Micheli, F., Palumbi, S.R., Sala, E., Selkoe, K.A., Stachowicz, J.J. and Watson, R. (2006) Impacts of biodiversity loss on Ocean ecosystem services. *Science*, Vol. 314, Issue 5800, pp 787–790.

Yablokov, A.V. (1994) Validity of whaling data. *Nature*, Vol 367, p 108.

PART III

The implications of meat production for human health

12

INDUSTRIAL ANIMAL AGRICULTURE'S ROLE IN THE EMERGENCE AND SPREAD OF DISEASE

Michael Greger

The first major period of disease since the beginning of human evolution probably started approximately 10,000 years ago with the domestication of farm animals (Armelagos et al., 1996). Human measles, for example, which has killed roughly 200 million people over the last 150 years, probably arose from a rinderpest-like virus of sheep and goats (Weiss, 2001). Smallpox may have resulted from camel domestication (Gubser et al., 2004), and whooping cough may have jumped to us from sheep or pigs (Weiss, 2001). Leprosy may have originated in water buffalo (McMichael, 2001) and human influenza may have only started about 4,500 years ago with the domestication of waterfowl (Shortridge, 2003). Rhinovirus, the cause of the human cold, may have come from cattle (Rodrigo and Dopazo, 1995). Indeed, before domestication, the common cold may have been common only to them.

Over the last few decades, there has been a dramatic resurgence in emerging infectious diseases, approximately three quarters of which are thought to have come from the animal kingdom (Woolhouse and Gowtage-Sequeria, 2005). It is estimated that over 1 billion cases of human zoonotic disease occur every year (Johnson et al., 2015). The World Health Organization defined the term 'zoonoses' to describe this phenomenon (Mantovani, 2001), from the Greek *zoion* for 'animal' and *nosos* for 'disease'. This trend of increasing zoonotic disease emergence is expected to continue (WHO/FAO/OIE, 2004), and the US Institute of Medicine suggests that without appropriate policies and actions, the future could bring a 'catastrophic storm of microbial threats' (Smolinski et al., 2003).

Animals were domesticated thousands of years ago, though. What new changes are taking place at the human/animal interface that may be responsible for this resurgence of zoonotic disease in recent decades?

In 2004, a joint consultation was convened by the World Health Organization, the Food and Agriculture Organization of the United Nations and the World Organization for Animal Health to elucidate the major drivers of zoonotic disease emergence (WHO/FAO/OIE, 2004). A common theme of primary risk factors for both the emergence and spread of zoonoses was 'increasing demand for animal protein', associated with the expansion and intensification of animal agriculture.

Strep. suis

In 2005, China, the world's largest producer of pork (RaboBank International, 2003), suffered an unprecedented outbreak in scope and lethality of *Streptococcus suis*, a newly emerging zoonotic pig pathogen (Gosline, 2005). *Strep. suis* is a common cause of meningitis in intensively farmed pigs worldwide and presents most often as meningitis in people as well (Huang et al., 2005), particularly those who butcher infected pigs or later handle infected pork products (Gosline, 2005). Due to the involvement of the auditory nerves connecting the inner ears to the brain, half of the human survivors become deaf (Altman, 2005).

The WHO reported that it had never seen such a virulent strain (Nolan, 2005) and blamed intensive confinement conditions as a predisposing factor in its sudden emergence, given the stress-induced suppression of farmed pigs' immune systems (WHO, 2005). The US Department of Agriculture explains that these bacteria can exist as a harmless component of a pig's normal bacterial flora, but stress due to factors such as crowding and poor ventilation can drop the animal's defences long enough for the bacteria to become invasive and cause disease (USDA and Animal and Plant Health Inspection Service, 2005). China's Assistant Minister of Commerce admitted that the disease was 'found to have direct links with the foul environment for raising pigs' (China View, 2005). The disease can spread through respiratory droplets or directly via contact with contaminated blood on improperly sterilized castration scalpels, tooth-cutting pliers or tail-docking knives (Du, 2005). China boasts an estimated 14,000 confined animal feeding operations (CAFOs) (Nierenberg, 2005), colloquially known as factory farms, which tend to have stocking densities conducive to the emergence and spread of disease (Arends et al., 1984). Recent reports of Ebola virus infection in pigs may underscore this point (Barrette et al., 2009).

Nipah virus

This *Strep. suis* outbreak followed years after the emergence of the Nipah virus on an intensive industrial pig farm in Malaysia. Nipah turned out to be one of the deadliest of human pathogens, killing 40 per cent of those infected, a toll that propelled it on to the US list of potential bioterrorism agents (Fritsch, 2003). This virus is also noted for its 'intriguing ability' to cause relapsing brain infections in some survivors (Wong et al., 2002) many months after initial exposure (Wong et al., 2001). Even more concerning, a 2004 resurgence of Nipah virus in Bangladesh showed a case fatality rate on par with some strains of Ebola – 75 per cent – and showed evidence of human-to-human transmission (Harcourt et al., 2004). The Nipah virus, like all contagious respiratory diseases, is a density-dependent pathogen (US CIA, 2006). 'Without these large, intensively managed pig farms in Malaysia', the director of the Consortium for Conservation Medicine said, 'it would have been extremely difficult for the virus to emerge' (Nierenberg, 2005, p44).

Bovine spongiform encephalopathy

Global public health experts have identified specific 'dubious practices used in modern animal husbandry' beyond the inherent overstocking, stress and unhygienic conditions that have directly or indirectly launched deadly new diseases (Phua and Lee, 2005). One such 'misguided' practice was the feeding of slaughterhouse waste, blood and excrement to farm animals to save on feed costs (Stapp, 2004).

A leading theory on the origin of BSE, also known as mad cow disease, is that cattle (naturally herbivores) became infected by eating diseased sheep (Kimberlin, 1992). Corporate agribusiness fed protein concentrates (or 'meat and bone meal', euphemistic descriptions of 'trimmings that originate on the killing floor, inedible parts and organs, cleaned entrails, foetuses') (Ensminger, 1990) to dairy cows to increase milk production (Flaherty, 1993), as well as to most other farm animals (*Economist*, 1990). According to the WHO, nearly 10 million metric tons of slaughterhouse waste was fed to farm animals every year (WHO/OIE, 1999). The recycling of the remains of infected cattle into cattle feed was likely what led to the British mad cow epidemic's explosive spread (Collee, 1993) to nearly two dozen countries around the world in the subsequent 20 years (USDA and Animal and Plant Health Inspection Service, 2005). Dairy producers could have used only corn or soybeans as a protein feed supplement, but slaughter plant by-products can be cheaper (Albert, 2000). Though only a few hundred people have died of the human variant of mad cow disease, the presence of the infectious agent in appendixes removed during routine surgery suggests a small percentage of the population may currently still be incubating the disease (Diack et al., 2014).

Multidrug-resistant bacteria

Another risky industrial practice is the mass feeding of antibiotics to farm animals. The Union of Concerned Scientists estimate that up to 80 per cent of antimicrobials used in the US are utilized as feed additives for chickens, pigs and cattle for non-therapeutic purposes (Hollis and Ahmed, 2014). Indeed, the use of growth-promoting antibiotics in industrial animal agriculture may be responsible for the majority of the increases in antibiotic-resistant human bacterial illness (Tollefson et al., 1999), the emergence of which is increasingly being recognized as a public health problem of global significance (Moore et al., 2006). The worldwide spread of a multidrug-resistant strain of *Salmonella* has been blamed on the use of antibiotics in global fish farming (Angulo and Griffin, 2000). With an estimated 80 per cent of the antibiotics used in US fish farms being released into the environment, there is a buildup of antibiotics in aquatic systems, increased residues in fish, plus evidence that wild fish living in proximity to treated fish farms contained quinolone residues (Hollis and Ahmed, 2014).

Alarmingly high rates of methicillin-resistant *Staphylococcus aureus* (MRSA) detection in farm animals and retail meat in Europe, for example, have led to increased scrutiny of the agricultural use of antibiotics. The former Dutch Agriculture, Nature and Food Standards Minister, Cees Veerman, was reported as saying that 'the high usage of antibiotics in livestock farming is the most important factor in the development of antibiotic resistance, a consequence of which is the spread of resistant microorganisms (MRSA included) in animal populations' (Soil Association, 2007). The recent discovery of MRSA in a significant proportion of pigs tested in North America suggests the potential public health risk attributed to farm animal–associated MRSA may be a global phenomenon (Goldburg et al., 2008; Smith et al., 2009a). Long-distance live animal transport and antibiotic use in pigs have both been considered factors in the emergence and spread of livestock associated MRSA (Wulf and Voss, 2008).

Bird flu

The dozens of emerging zoonotic disease threats must be put into context. SARS, which emerged from the live animal meat markets of Asia (Lee and Krilov, 2005), infected thousands of humans and killed hundreds. Nipah infected hundreds and killed scores. *Strep. suis* infected scores and killed dozens. AIDS, which arose from the slaughter and consumption of chimpanzees (Hahn et al., 2000), has infected millions, but only one virus is known to be able to infect billions – influenza.

Influenza, once called the 'last great plague of man' (Kaplan and Webster, 1977), is the only known pathogen capable of a truly global catastrophe (Silverstein, 1981). Unlike other devastating infections like malaria, which is confined equatorially, or HIV, which is only fluid-borne, influenza is considered by Keiji Fukuda, of the US Centers for Disease Control and Prevention, to be the only pathogen carrying the potential to 'infect a huge percentage of the world's population inside the space of a year' (Davies, 1999). In its 4,500 years of infecting humans since the first domestication of wild waterbirds, influenza has always been one of the most contagious pathogens (Taylor, 2005). Only since 1997, with the emergence of the highly pathogenic strain H5N1, has it also emerged as one of the deadliest.

H5N1 has so far only killed a few hundred people (WHO, 2016). In a world in which millions die of diseases like malaria, tuberculosis and AIDS, why is there so much concern about bird flu?

The risk of a widespread influenza pandemic is dire and real because it has happened before. An influenza pandemic in 1918 became the deadliest plague in human history, killing up to 100 million people around the world (Johnson and Mueller, 2002), and the 1918 flu virus was probably a bird flu virus (Belshe, 2005) that made more than one quarter of the world's population ill and killed more people in 25 weeks than AIDS has killed in 25 years (Barry, 2004). Despite the harrowing effects of that influenza nearly a century ago, the case mortality rate was less than 5 per cent (Frist, 2005). H5N1, in comparison, has so far officially killed just over half of its human victims (WHO, 2016).

Free-ranging flocks and wild birds have been blamed for the recent emergence of H5N1, but people have kept chickens in their backyards for thousands of years, and birds have been migrating for millions. What has changed in recent years that led us to this current crisis? According to Dr Robert Webster, the 'godfather of flu research', it is because

> Farming practices have changed. Previously, we had backyard poultry. . . . Now we put millions of chickens into a chicken factory next door to a pig factory, and this virus has the opportunity to get into one of these chicken factories and make billions and billions of these mutations continuously. And so what we've changed is the way we raise animals. . . . That's what's changed.
>
> *(Council on Foreign Relations, 2005)*

The United Nations specifically calls on governments to fight what they call 'factory farming':

> Governments, local authorities, and international agencies need to take a greatly increased role in combating the role of factory farming, which [combined with live bird markets] provide ideal conditions for the virus to spread and mutate into a more dangerous form.
>
> *(UN, 2005)*

Factory farms can be thought of as incubators for the original emergence of dangerous strains of the influenza virus.

Swine flu

The H1N1 swine flu virus has infected millions of people and killed thousands (Centers for Disease Control and Prevention, 2009). Pregnant women and young people are among the hardest hit. Where did this virus come from, and what can be done to help prevent the emergence of flu pandemics in the future?

The genetic fingerprint of the H1N1 swine flu virus confirms that the main ancestor of the 2009 pandemic virus is the triple hybrid human/pig/bird flu virus that emerged and spread throughout factory farms in the United States more than a decade ago (Smith et al., 2009b). Swine flu emerged in 1918 and remained stable for 80 years in North America until August 1998, when our first hybrid swine flu virus was detected on a factory farm in Sampson County, North Carolina (Wuethrich, 2003), the county with the single highest pig population in the country, confining more than 2 million pigs (Sampson County Health Department, 2007).

The factory farm in which the virus was first found was a breeding facility confining thousands of sows in sow stalls, metal cages so small the pigs can't even turn around. These instruments of extreme confinement have not only been criticized as inhumane, but may pose a public health threat, as crated sows have been reported to have higher stress levels and impaired immune systems (Siegel, 1983).

Other factors that make intensive farms such breeding grounds for disease include the sheer numbers of animals (Poljak et al., 2008), the overcrowding (Maes et al., 2000), the millions of gallons of excrement, which releases ammonia that burns the animals' lungs (Donham, 1991) and the lack of adequate fresh air and sunlight. The ultraviolet (UV) rays in sunlight are actually quite effective in destroying these viruses. Just 30 minutes in direct sunlight completely inactivates the flu virus, but it can last for days in the shade and weeks in moist manure (Songserm et al., 2006). Overcrowding thousands of animals snout to snout into stressful filthy football-field sized sheds may create a Perfect Storm environment for the emergence and spread of new 'superstrains' of influenza (Greger, 2007a).

The public health community has been warning about the human health risks posed by factory farms for years. In 2003, the American Public Health Association, the largest affiliation of public health professionals in the world, called for a moratorium on factory farms (American Public Health Association, 2003). In 2008, the Pew Commission on Industrial Farm Animal Production released its final report and concluded that industrialized animal agriculture posed 'unacceptable' public health risks (Pew Commission on Industrial Farm Animal Production, 2008a). The Pew Commission was a prestigious, independent panel chaired by a former Kansas Governor and including a former US Secretary of Agriculture, former Assistant Surgeon General, and the Dean of the University of Iowa College of Public Health. The Commission recommended that gestation crates be banned, noting that '[p]ractices that restrict natural motion, such as sow gestation crates, induce high levels of stress in the animals and threaten their health, which in turn may threaten our health' (Pew Commission on Industrial Farm Animal Production, 2008b, p13).

The worst case scenario might be if the H1N1 swine flu virus combined with the highly pathogenic H5N1 bird flu virus, both of which have been found infecting pigs. If a single pig in parts of Asia or Africa where bird flu has become endemic becomes co-infected with both the new swine flu and bird flu, the concern is that it could theoretically produce a virus with the human transmissibility of swine flu, but also with the human lethality of bird flu (NN, 2009).

Michael Osterholm, the director of the US Center for Infectious Disease Research and Policy and an associate director within the US Department of Homeland Security, tried to describe what an H5N1-type pandemic could look like in one of the leading US public policy journals, *Foreign Affairs*. Osterholm suggested policy makers consider the devastation of the 2004 tsunami in South Asia: 'Duplicate it in every major urban centre and rural community around the planet simultaneously, add in the paralyzing fear and panic of contagion, and we begin to get some sense of the potential of pandemic influenza' (Kennedy, 2005, pA1). 'An influenza pandemic of even moderate impact', Osterholm continued, 'will result in the biggest single human disaster ever – far greater than AIDS, 9/11, all wars in the 20th century and the recent tsunami combined. It has the potential to redirect world history as the Black Death redirected European history in the 14th century' (Kennedy, 2005, pA1).

Interestingly, the UK government declares that because A(H1N1)pdm09 has been circulating in the population each flu season since 2009, it is now regarded as one of the seasonal flu strains (Pebody, 2016).

Hopefully, the world will move away from raising animals by the billions under intensive confinement, thus potentially lowering the risk of us ever being in this same precarious situation in the future.

Conclusion

H1N1 swine flu is not the first virus whose emergence has been linked to factory farms, and it won't be the last unless significant changes are made in the way animals are raised: measures as simple as providing straw bedding so these animals don't have the immune-suppressive stress of lying on bare concrete their whole lives (André and Tuyttens, 2005) have been shown to significantly decrease swine flu transmission rates (Ewald et al., 1994). Such a simple measure, yet we deny these animals even this modicum of mercy – both to their detriment and potentially to ours as well.

In addition to phasing out extreme confinement, the replacement of long-distance live animal transport with a carcass-only trade (Greger, 2007b), intensive farms with smaller-scale production with lower densities of animals (Maillard and Gonzalez, 2006) and an overall reduction in the number of animals intensively confined and raised for food (Benatar, 2007) have all been suggested as ways to reduce the emergence of zoonotic infectious diseases.

'The bottom line', according to a spokesperson for the WHO, 'is that humans have to think about how they treat their animals, how they farm them, and how they market them – basically the whole relationship between the animal kingdom and the human kingdom is coming under stress' (Torrey and Yolken, 2005, p112). Along with human culpability, though, comes hope. If changes in human behaviour can cause new plagues, changes in human behaviour may prevent them in the future.

References

Albert, D. (2000) 'EU meat meal industry wants handout to survive ban', *Reuters World Report*, 5 December.

Altman, L. K. (2005) 'Pig disease in China worries UN', *New York Times*, available at www.iht.com/bin/print_ipub.php?file=/articles/2005/08/05/news/pig.php, last accessed 5 August 2009.

American Public Health Association (2003) 'Precautionary moratorium on new concentrated animal feed operations', available at www.apha.org/advocacy/policy/policysearch/default.htm?id=1243, last accessed 18 November 2009.

André, F. and Tuyttens, M. (2005) 'The importance of straw for pig and cattle welfare: A review', *Applied Animal Behaviour Science*, vol 92, pp261–282.

Angulo, F. J. and Griffin, P. M. (2000) 'Changes in antimicrobial resistance in *Salmonella enterica* serovar Typhimurium', *Emerging Infectious Diseases*, vol 6, no 4, pp436–437.

Arends, J. P., Hartwig, N., Rudolphy, M. and Zanen, H. C. (1984) 'Carrier rate of *Streptococcus suis* capsular type 2 in palatine tonsils of slaughtered pigs', *Journal of Clinical Microbiology*, vol 20, no 5, pp945–947.

Armelagos, G. J., Barnes, K. C. and Lin, J. (1996) 'Disease in human evolution: The re-emergence of infectious disease in the third epidemiological transition', *National Museum of Natural History Bulletin for Teachers*, vol 18, no 3, pp7–22.

Barrette, R. W., Metwally, S. A., Rowland, J. M., Xu, L., Zaki, S. R., Nichol, S. T., Rollin, P. E., Towner, J. S., Shieh, W., Batten, B., Sealy, T. K., Carrillo, C., Moran, K. E., Bracht, A. J., Mayr, G. A., Sirios-Cruz, M., Catbagan, D. P., Lautner, E. A., Ksiazek, T. G., White, W. R. and McIntosh, M. T. (2009) 'Discovery of swine as a host for the Reston ebolavirus', *Science*, vol 325, pp204–206.

Barry, J. M. (2004) 'Viruses of mass destruction', *Fortune*, 1 November.

Belshe, R. B. (2005) 'The origins of pandemic influenza – lessons from the 1918 virus', *New England Journal of Medicine*, vol 353, no 21, pp2209–2211.

Benatar, D. (2007) 'The chickens come home to roost', *American Journal of Public Health*, vol 97, pp1545–1546.

Centers for Disease Control and Prevention (2009) 'CDC estimates of 2009 H1N1 influenza cases, hospitalizations and deaths in the United States, April – October 17, 2009', available at www.cdc.gov/h1n1flu/estimates_2009_h1n1.htm, last accessed 12 November 2009.

China View (2005) 'China drafts, revises laws to safeguard animal welfare', available at http://news.xinhuanet.com/english/2005-11/04/content_3729580.htm, last accessed 4 November 2009.

Collee, G. (1993) 'BSE stocktaking 1993', *Lancet*, vol 342, no 8874, pp790–793, available at www.cyber-dyne.com/~tom/essay_collee.html, last accessed 9 December 2009.

Council on Foreign Relations (2005) 'Session 1: Avian flu – where do we stand?', *Conference on the Global Threat of Pandemic Influenza*, available at http://cfr.org/publication/9230/council_on_foreign_relations_conference_on_the_global_threat_of_pandemic_influenza_session_1.html, last accessed 16 November 2009.

Davies, P. (1999) 'The plague in waiting', *Guardian*, available at http://guardian.co.uk/birdflu/story/0,,1131473,00.html, last accessed 7 August 2009.

Diack, A. B., Head, M. W., McCutcheon, S., Boyle, A., Knight, R., Ironside, J.W., Manson, J.C. and Will, R.G. (2014) 'Variant CJD. 18 years of research and surveillance', *Prion*, vol 8, pp286–295.

Donham, K. J. (1991) 'Association of environmental air contaminants with disease and productivity in swine', *American Journal of Veterinary Research*, vol 52, pp1723–1730.

Du, W. (2005) *Streptococcus Suis, (S. Suis) Pork Production and Safety*, Ontario Ministry of Agriculture, Food and Rural Affairs, Ontario, Canada.

Economist (1990) 'Mad, bad and dangerous to eat?', February, pp89–90.

Ensminger, M. E. (1990) *Feeds and Nutrition*, Ensminger Publishing Co., Clovis, CA.

Ewald, C., Heer, A. and Havenith, U. (1994) 'Factors associated with the occurrence of influenza a virus infections in fattening swine', *Berliner und Münchener tierärztliche Wochenschrift*, vol 107, pp256–262.

Flaherty, M. (1993) 'Mad cow disease dispute: UW conference poses frightening questions', *Wisconsin State Journal*, 26 September, p1C.

Frist, B. (2005) *Manhattan Project for the 21st Century*, Harvard Medical School Health Care Policy Seidman Lecture, available at http://frist.senate.gov/_files/060105manhattan.pdf, last accessed 1 June 2009.

Fritsch, P. (2003) 'Containing the outbreak: Scientists search for human hand behind outbreak of jungle virus', *Wall Street Journal*, 19 June.

Goldburg, R., Roach, S., Wallinga, D. and Mellon, M. (2008) 'The risks of pigging out on antibiotics', *Science*, vol 321, no 5894, p1294.

Gosline, A. (2005) 'Mysterious disease outbreak in China baffles WHO', available at www.newscientist.com/article.ns?id=dn7740, last accessed 9 December 2009.

Greger, M. (2007a) 'The human/animal interface: Emergence and resurgence of zoonotic infectious diseases', *Critical Reviews in Microbiology*, vol 33, pp243–299.

Greger, M. (2007b) 'The long haul: The risks of livestock transport', *Biosecurity and Bioterrorism*, vol 5, pp301–311.

Gubser, C., Hué, S., Kellam, P. and Smith, G. L. (2004) 'Poxvirus genomes: A phylogenetic analysis', *Journal of General Virology*, vol 85, pp105–117.

Hahn, B. H., Shaw, G. M., De Cock, K. M. and Sharp, P. M. (2000) 'AIDS as a zoonosis: Scientific and public health implications', *Science*, vol 287, pp607–614.

Harcourt, B. H., Lowe, L., Tamin, A., Liu, X., Bankamp, B., Bowden, N., Rollin, P. E., Comer, J. A., Ksiazek, T. G., Hossain, M. J., Gurley, E. S., Breiman, R. F., Bellini, W. J., and Rota, P. A. (2004) 'Genetic characterization of Nipah virus, Bangladesh, 2004: Centers for disease control and prevention', *Emerging Infectious Diseases*, vol 11, no 10, available at www.cdc.gov/ncidod/EID/vol11no10/05-0513.htm, last accessed 9 December 2009.

Hollis, A. and Ahmed, Z. (2014) 'The path of least resistance: Paying for antibiotics in non-human uses', *Health Policy*, vol 118, no 2, November, pp264–270.

Huang, Y. T., Teng, L. J., Ho, S. W. and Hsueh, P. R. (2005) '*Streptococcus suis* infection', *Journal of Microbiology, Immunology and Infection*, vol 38, pp306–313, available at http://jmii.org/content/abstracts/v38n5p306.php, last accessed 9 December 2009.

Johnson, C. K., Hitchens, P. L., Evans, T. S., Goldstein, T., Thomas, K., Clements, A., Joly, D. O., Wolfe, N. D., Daszak, P., Karesh, W.B. and Mazet, J. K. (2015) 'Spillover and pandemic properties of zoonotic viruses with high host plasticity', *Nature Reviews*, Scientific Reports 5, Article number: 14830, doi:10.1038/srep14830.

Johnson, N. P. A. S. and Mueller, J. (2002) 'Updating the accounts: Global mortality of the 1918–1920 "Spanish" influenza pandemic', *Bulletin of the History of Medicine*, vol 76, pp105–115.

Kaplan, M. M. and Webster, R. G. (1977) 'The epidemiology of influenza', *Scientific American*, vol 237, pp88–106.

Kennedy, M. (2005) 'Bird flu could kill millions: Global pandemic warning from WHO. "We're not crying wolf: There is a wolf: We just don't know when it's coming"', *Gazette* (Montreal), 9 March, pA1.

Kimberlin, R. H. (1992) 'Human spongiform encephalopathies and BSE', *Medical Laboratory Sciences*, vol 49, pp216–217.

Lee, P. J. and Krilov, L. R. (2005) 'When animal viruses attack: SARS and avian influenza', *Pediatric Annals*, vol 34, no. 1, pp43–52.

McMichael, T. (2001) *Human Frontiers, Environments and Disease*, Cambridge University Press, Cambridge.

Maes, D., Deluyker, H., Verdonck, M., Castryck, F., Miry, C., Vrijens, B. and Kruif, A. de (2000) 'Herd factors associated with the seroprevalences of four major respiratory pathogens in slaughter pigs from farrow-to-finish pig herds', *Veterinary Research*, vol 31, pp313–327.

Maillard, J. C. and Gonzalez, J. P. (2006) 'Biodiversity and emerging diseases', *Annals of the New York Academy of Sciences*, vol 1081, pp1–16.

Mantovani, A. (2001) *Notes on the Development of the Concept of Zoonoses*, WHO Mediterranean Zoonoses Control Centre Information Circular 51, available at www.mzcp-zoonoses.gr/pdfen/circ_51.pdf, last accessed 9 December 2009.

Moore, J. E., Barton, M. D., Blair, I. A., Corcoran, D., Dooley, J. S. G., Fanning, S., Kempf, I., Lastovica, A. J., Lowery, C. J., Matsuda, M., McDowell, D. A., McMahon, A., Millar, B. C., Rao, J. R., Rooney, P. J., Seal, B. S., Snelling, W. J. and Tolba, O. (2006) 'The epidemiology of antibiotic resistance in Campylobacter', *Microbes and Infection*, vol 8, pp1955–1966.

Nierenberg, D. (2005) 'Happier meals: Rethinking the global meat industry', *World-watch Paper 171*, available at http://www.worldwatch.org/system/files/WP171.pdf, last accessed 29 April 2017.

NN (2009) 'Exclusive: SARS sleuth tracks swine flu, attacks WHO,' *ScienceInsider*, 4 May, available at http://blogs.sciencemag.org/scienceinsider/2009/05/exclusive-meet.html, last accessed 9 December 2009.

Nolan, T. (2005) '40 people die from pig-borne bacteria', available at www.abc.net.au/am/content/2005/s1441324.htm, last accessed 9 December 2009.

Pebody, R. (2016) 'Why "swine flu" is now considered a normal, seasonal flu strain', *Public Health England*, https://publichealthmatters.blog.gov.uk/2016/01/28/why-swine-flu-is-now-considered-a-normal-seasonal-flu-strain/.

Pew Commission on Industrial Farm Animal Production (2008a) 'Expert panel highlights serious public health threats from industrial animal agriculture', available at www.pewtrusts.org/news_room_detail.aspx?id=37968, last accessed 11 April 2009.

Pew Commission on Industrial Farm Animal Production (2008b) 'Putting meat on the table: Industrial farm animal production in America', *Executive Summary*, p13, available at www.ncifap.org/_images/PCIFAPSmry.pdf, last accessed 9 December 2009.

Phua, K. and Lee, L. K. (2005) 'Meeting the challenges of epidemic infectious disease outbreaks: An agenda for research', *Journal of Public Health Policy*, vol 26, pp122–132.

Poljak, Z., Dewey, C. E., Martin, S. W., Christensen, J., Carman, S. and Friendship, R. M. (2008) 'Prevalence of and risk factors for influenza in southern Ontario swine herds in 2001 and 2003', *Canadian Journal of Veterinary Research*, vol 72, pp7–17.

RaboBank International (2003) 'China's meat industry overview: Quietly moving towards industrialization', *Food and Agribusiness Research*, May, pp1–12.

Rodrigo, M. J., and Dopazo, J. (1995) 'Evolutionary analysis of the Picornavirus family', *Journal of Molecular Evolution*, vol 40, pp362–371.

Sampson County Health Department (2007) 'Community health assessment: Sampson county', available at www.sampsonnc.com/HealthAssessment.pdf, last accessed 9 December 2009.

Shortridge, K. F. (2003) 'Severe acute respiratory syndrome and influenza', *American Journal of Critical Care and Respiratory Medicine*, vol 168, pp1416–1420.

Siegel, H. S. (1983) 'Effects of intensive production methods on livestock health', *Agro-Ecosystems*, vol 8, pp215–230.

Silverstein, A. M. (1981) *Pure Politics and Impure Science, the Swine Flu Affair*, Johns Hopkins University Press, Baltimore, MA, pp129–131.

Smith, G. J., Vijaykrishna, D., Bahl, J., Lycett, S. J., Worobey, M., Pybus, O. G., Ma, S. K., Cheung, C. L., Raghwani, J., Bhatt, S., Peiris, J. S. M., Guan, Y. and Rambaut, A. (2009b) 'Origins and evolutionary genomics of the 2009 swine-origin H1N1 influenza a epidemic', *Nature*, vol 459, pp1122–1125.

Smith, T. C., Male, M. J., Harper, A. L., Kroeger, J. S., Tinkler, G. P., Moritz, E. D., Capuano, A. W., Herwaldt, L. A. and Diekema, D. J. (2009a) 'Methicillin-resistant *Staphylococcus aureus* (MRSA) strain ST398 is present in midwestern US swine and swine workers', *PLoS One*, vol 4, e4258.

Smolinksi, M. S., Hamburg, M. A. and Lederberg, J. (2003) *Microbial Threats to Health: Emergence, Detection and Response*, National Academies Press, Washington, DC.

Soil Association (2007) 'MRSA in farm animals and meat', available at www.soilassociation.org/LinkClick.aspx?fileticket=%2bmWBoFr348s%3d&tabid=385, last accessed 9 December 2009.

Songserm, T., Jam-On, R., Sae-Heng, N. and Meemak, N. (2006) 'Survival and stability of HPAI H5N1 in different environments and susceptibility to disinfectants', in Schudel, A. and Lombard, M. (eds) *Proceedings of the OIE/FAO International Scientific Conference on Avian Influenza*, vol 124, International Association for Biologicals, Karger, Switzerland.

Stapp, K. (2004) 'Scientists warn of fast-spreading global viruses', *IPS-Inter Press Service*, 23 February.

Taylor, M. (2005) 'Is there a plague on the way?', *Farm Journal*, 10 March.

Tollefson, L., Fedorka-Cray, P. J. and Angulo, F. J. (1999) 'Public health aspects of antibiotic resistance monitoring in the USA', *ACTA Veterinaria Scandinavica Supplement*, vol 92, pp67–75.

Torrey, E. F. and Yolken, R. H. (2005) *Beasts of the Earth: Animals, Humans, and Disease*, Rutgers University Press, New Jersey.

UN (2005) 'UN task forces battle misconceptions of avian flu, mount Indonesian campaign', *UN News Centre*, available at www.un.org/apps/news/story.asp?NewsID=16342&Cr=bird&Cr1=flu, last accessed 24 October 2009.

US CIA (2006) *CIA World Fact Book*, Malaysia, available at http://cia.gov/cia/publications/factbook/geos/my.html, last accessed 29 March 2009.

USDA and Animal and Plant Health Inspection Service (2005) *List of USDA-Recognized Animal Health Status of Countries/Areas Regarding Specific Livestock or Poultry Diseases*, USDA and Animal and Plant Health Inspection Service, Riversdale, MD.

USDA, Veterinary Services, Center for Emerging Issues (2005) '*Streptococcus suis* outbreak, swine and human, China: Emerging disease notice', available at www.aphis.usda.gov/vs/ceah/cei/taf/emergingdiseasenotice_files/strep_suis_china.htm, last accessed 9 December 2009.

Weiss, R. A. (2001) 'Animal origins of human infectious disease, the Leeuwenhoek Lecture', *Philosophical Transactions of the Royal Society of London, Series B, Biological Sciences*, vol 356, pp957–977.

WHO (2005) 'Streptococcus suis fact sheet', available at www.wpro.who.int/media_centre/fact_sheets/fs_20050802.htm, last accessed 10 December 2009.

WHO (2016) 'Cumulative number of confirmed human cases for avian influenza a (H5N1) reported to WHO, 2003–2016,' available at www.who.int/influenza/human_animal_interface/EN_GIP_20160509cumulativenumberH5N1cases.pdf, last accessed 11 July 2016.

WHO/FAO/OIE (2004) 'Report of the WHO/FAO/OIE joint consultation on emerging zoonotic diseases', available at www.whqlibdoc.who.int/hq/2004/WHO_CDS_CPE_ZFK_2004.9.pdf, last accessed 10 December 2009.

WHO/OIE (1999) WHO Consultation on Public Health and Animal Transmissible Spongiform Encephalopathies: Epidemiology, Risk and Research Requirements, 1–31 December, World Health Organization, Geneva, Switzerland.

Wong, K. T., Shieh, W. J., Zaki, S. R. and Tan, C. T. (2002) 'Nipah virus infection, an emerging paramyxoviral zoonosis', *Springer Seminars in Immunopathology*, vol 24, pp215–228.

Wong, S. C., Ooi, M. H., Wong, M. N. L., Tio, P. H., Solomon, T. and Cardosa, M. J. (2001) 'Late presentation of Nipah virus encephalitis and kinetics of the humoral immune response', *Journal of Neurology, Neurosurgery & Psychiatry*, vol 71, pp552–554.

Woolhouse, M. E. and Gowtage-Sequeria, S. (2005) 'Host range and emerging and reemerging pathogens', *Emerging Infectious Diseases*, vol 11, pp1842–1847.

Wuethrich, B. (2003) 'Infectious disease: Chasing the fickle swine flu', *Science*, vol 299, pp1502–1505.

Wulf, M. and Voss, A. (2008) 'MRSA in livestock animals – an epidemic waiting to happen?', *Clinical Microbiology and Infection*, vol 14, pp519–521.

13

ANTIBIOTIC USE IN FARM ANIMALS

The global threat

Cóilín Nunan

In 2015, scientists at the South China Agricultural University carrying out routine surveillance of E. coli bacteria from farm animals noticed a major increase in resistance to a little-known and highly toxic antibiotic called colistin. They decided to investigate what was happening, suspecting that a new type of resistance might have emerged, one which could prove particularly difficult to control because of its ability to jump from one bacterium to another.

What they found was to stun the scientific world and lead to headlines around the world about how modern medicine was losing its most precious resource – antibiotics – due in part to irresponsible practices in intensive livestock farming.

As the Chinese scientists had feared, the E. coli, which could no longer be killed by colistin, had a new gene which was carried on a small piece of DNA in the bacteria, called a plasmid. The plasmid could replicate inside the bacteria, and copies could be passed from one E. coli to another, and even to other species of bacteria like Salmonella. They called the new gene "mobile colistin resistance 1", or mcr-1, and further testing showed that it was present in over a fifth of pigs, in 15% of pig and poultry meat and in 1% of human infections (Liu et al. 2015).

Colistin is not used in people in China but is widely used in animal feed, so the scientists thought it was very likely that the plasmid carrying the resistance was spreading from farms to people, particularly since they found much higher numbers of resistant bacteria in the animals than in the human infections.

As soon as the discovery was announced, surveillance laboratories in other countries began examining their own archives of bacteria collected from humans, animals and food. Within a few weeks of the Chinese scientists reporting their discovery, there were a number of studies published reporting that the mcr-1 gene was present in European, Asian, North American and African countries too. Just before Christmas, UK government scientists reported that they had found the gene in human E. coli and Salmonella infections, and in pigs from two separate farms.

But why all the concern about colistin resistance? After all, colistin is very toxic to people's kidneys, and is therefore best avoided as a treatment option in most cases. And for many years this is what happened: although colistin had been licensed in 1959, doctors usually did not use it because far better, and less dangerous, antibiotics were available. Unfortunately, as the better antibiotics were used, and overused, in both human and veterinary medicine, resistance to these antibiotics increased. Worse still, for bacteria like E. coli, there had been no discoveries of genuinely new antibiotics in over 30 years.

As a result, in the last decade, colistin has become a last-resort antibiotic, used for serious and highly resistant infections that most other antibiotics would be unable to treat. After colistin, the cupboard is bare, with no new antibiotics in the pipeline for treating serious E. coli infections.

Once our last-resort antibiotics fail, it's the beginning of the post-antibiotic era, when minor injuries could once again lead to fatal infections. Yet, despite colistin's recent elevation to the status of a life-saving drug, in 2012 over 500 times more colistin was used in Europe's farm animals than in human medicine (ECDC et al. 2015).

The Lancet Infectious Diseases Commission has warned that if current trends towards increasing antibiotic resistance continue, medical treatments such as surgery and cancer chemotherapy, treatments which often involve the preventative use of antibiotics, could be seriously undermined. The Commission says, "Within just a few years, we might be faced with dire setbacks, medically, socially, and economically, unless real and unprecedented global coordinated actions are immediately taken" (Laxminarayan et al. 2013, p1057).

So how did we get to this point, and what has been the role played by the overuse of antibiotics in intensive livestock farming?

Accidental discoveries

The birth of intensive livestock farming owes much to accidental scientific discoveries in the field of antibiotics. In 1928, Alexander Fleming made his famous, fortuitous discovery that a mould which had contaminated one of his laboratory petri dishes was killing staphylococcus bacteria he had been cultivating. He soon realised this was because the mould was producing an antibacterial substance, which he called penicillin. However, because he was only to produce penicillin in very small quantities from the mould, he only ever envisaged using it as an antiseptic or as a diagnostic tool.

It wasn't until the early 1940s that methods were developed in Oxford, by Ernst Chain and Howard Florey, and subsequently improved in the United States, which enabled the large-scale production of penicillin by extracting and purifying it from big tanks growing the mould. The new techniques finally enabled penicillin to be developed as a life-saving medicine, and soon a massive search for further substances being produced by micro-organisms yielded a large number of new antibiotics.

By the late 1940s, scientists at American Cyanamid who had developed the antibiotic aureomycin made a second critical accidental discovery. The poultry industry had begun to feed its birds soybean meal as a cheaper substitute for fishmeal. But the new meal lacked a vitamin which the poultry required. The Cyanamid scientists reasoned that the bacteria which produced aureomycin were likely to contain the vitamin and experimented with feeding it to chickens. They found it had a large growth-promoting effect, much larger than expected.

They soon realised that it was due to the presence of the antibiotic, rather than the vitamin. Even when they fed the waste product of the aureomycin fermentation process, with most of the antibiotic having being extracted but very low concentrations remaining, they still found a significant growth-promoting effect. Similar results were also found with pigs.

The New York Times hailed the discovery on its front page with the headline "Wonder drug aureomycin found to spur growth 50%", welcoming the promise of increased meat production. The article reported that Cyanamid was even looking into whether the antibiotic could also be used to increase growth rates in undernourished children and concluded by saying that "no undesirable side effects have been observed, it is said" (Lawrence 1950, p1).

Fleming seemed unimpressed, saying, "I can't predict that feeding penicillin to babies will do society much good" (Kennedy 2014, pSR1). Fleming, and other scientists, already had evidence that misusing antibiotics could lead to resistance, and that the challenge therefore was to use the drugs as strategically and appropriately as possible. As early as 1945, in his acceptance speech for his Nobel Prize, which he received jointly with Chain and Florey, Fleming warned, "There is the danger that the ignorant man may easily under-dose himself and by exposing his microbes to non-lethal quantities of the drug make them resistant".

Fortunately, despite the technological optimism of the age, the suggestion that children should be dosed with antibiotics never really took off, but in farming the outcome was very different. Antibiotic growth promoters were legalised in the US by the Food and Drug Administration in 1951, and in 1953 the Therapeutic Substances Prevention of Misuse Act also made them legal in the UK. Soon enough, antibiotic growth promoters became the norm worldwide, with Iceland the only country to buck the trend by refusing to legalise the practice.

The growth of intensive farming and of antibiotic resistance

Adding low, subtherapeutic doses of antibiotics to animal feed, or drinking water, didn't just make the animals grow faster. It had another effect too: it enabled farm animals to be farmed much more intensively. Certain livestock, particularly pigs and poultry, could now be raised entirely indoors, in conditions which were often cramped and unhygienic, with the inevitable bacterial infections being kept under control by routine dosing with antibiotics.

Ruminant animals, like cattle and sheep, do not generally respond as well to oral dosing with antibiotics because it inhibits digestion and thereby growth rate. This is particularly the case for sheep, and as a result these are usually the least intensively farmed of the major species. However, calves raised for white veal are fed on predominantly liquid diets that do not permit development of the normal processes of microbial fermentation of fibrous feeds in the rumen, and these animals are often routinely dosed with antibiotics and kept in highly intensive conditions.

In addition to the use of antibiotics for growth promotion, which required no prescription, vets could also prescribe slightly higher doses of antibiotics for added disease prevention, and higher doses still when disease outbreaks nevertheless occurred.

The new tool was essential in enabling the establishment of truly intensive indoor farming, where costs were lowered because of reduced need for land and for labour. The advent of cheap meat led to huge increases in consumption and production, with average growth rates of pig and poultry consumption in the rich, developed countries where the faming was most intensive, of 5–7% per year from the 1960s onwards (Alexandratos and Bruinsma 2012).

Unfortunately, much as Fleming had warned, the emergence of antibiotic resistance in farm animals occurred almost as soon as the antibiotics began being used. In 1951, American scientists reported that turkeys fed antibiotics developed resistant E. coli (Starr and Reynolds 1951), and very soon similar reports for pigs and poultry were being published in the UK (Smith and Crabb 1958) and elsewhere. As a result, vets started reporting that they were having increasing difficulties in treating sick animals, but perhaps even more significantly evidence was found that the resistant bacteria were transmitting to humans and causing resistant infections.

In the 1960s, a major outbreak of antibiotic-resistant Salmonella in the UK was traced to the use of growth promoters in calves, and the government established an independent advisory committee to investigate the possible consequences for human and animal health of continuing to use antibiotic growth promoters. The Swann Committee reported in 1969, with the main recommendation that drugs from the penicillin family (the beta-lactams) and tetracycline family of antibiotics should no longer be used as growth promoters, but that other apparently less important antibiotics in human medicine could continue to be used in that way. Beta-lactams and tetracyclines now needed a veterinary prescription, but commenting on the report in 1970, Ernst Chain was not optimistic that it would make much difference at all, saying, "The Swann report has changed nothing essential. . . . The farmers can get hold of exactly the same antibiotics as before, only it is more expensive now as you need a vet's prescription. Of course, in all probability more antibiotics will be used" (Mennie 1970, p52). Chain's forecast was unfortunately to prove prescient: in 2015 the total use of beta-lactams and tetracyclines had increased by nearly seven times (see Table 13.1) (House of Commons 1969) (VMD 2015).

The reason for the increase was straightforward: although prescriptions for beta-lactams and tetracyclines were now required, there was no requirement that any disease be diagnosed before a vet could write a prescription, and with farmers now accustomed to routinely adding antibiotics to feed, nor was there any expectation that antibiotic treatment be limited to sick animals only.

Despite the ultimate failure of the Swann recommendations, the principles of Swann have remained influential, and most international regulatory action since

TABLE 13.1 Use of veterinary antibiotics (tonnes active ingredient) in 2014 compared with pre-Swann use

	1966 (Swann report)	*2015*
Total antibiotics	151	404
Beta-lactam antibiotics	16.8	80
Tetracycline antibiotics	19.6	166

then has also focused on banning growth promotion, rather than reducing overall use levels. Since 2006, all antibiotics have been banned for growth promotion in the European Union, and in December 2013 the US Food and Drug Administration announced it was implementing a voluntary plan with industry to phase out growth promotion within three years. The EU ban on growth promotion unsurprisingly had little effect on antibiotic use levels as farmers switched to using more antibiotics under veterinary prescription. A 2012 study of the Belgian pig industry showed just how routinely antibiotics continue to be prescribed in the absence of any disease diagnosis: the survey found that 93% of group treatments on intensive pig farms were purely preventative, with no pigs having being diagnosed with any disease (Callens et al. 2012). Total use of antibiotics remains extremely high in most European countries: data published in 2015 showed that total veterinary use of antibiotics in 26 European countries was approximately twice total human use (ECDC et al. 2015).

A small number of European countries do not allow routine preventative use of antibiotics: the five Nordic countries – Denmark, Finland, Iceland, Norway and Sweden – as well as the Netherlands, and in all of these countries the use of antibiotics in the most intensively farmed animals, pigs and poultry, is several times lower per animal than it is in countries like the UK (DANMAP 2015, EMA 2015, SDa 2015, VMD 2015). Their success in reducing farm use has led to the European Union as a whole reviewing its own policies, and in March 2016 the European Parliament voted to ban routine preventative use. However, the vote doesn't necessarily result in new legislation, as agreement is needed from the Council of Ministers and the European Commission. Negotiations on new legislation are not due to begin until the autumn of 2017, with the outcome as yet uncertain.

The remarkably slow rate of progress since the Swann report was published nearly 50 years ago and the lack of urgency from politicians and regulators for dealing with the problem can partly be explained by the large number of antibiotics that had been discovered by the time the report was published. The "golden age" of antibiotic discovery lasted from 1945 to 1965 (Livermore 2011), with about 20 antibiotic classes being discovered in this time period. This meant that for many years concerns about antibiotic resistance were alleviated by the knowledge that if one antibiotic was lost, there were many more still available that had been kept in reserve. Many scientists and regulators also expected that the future would be much like the past, and that many more antibiotic substances would be discovered. Unfortunately, those expectations have not been fulfilled, and since the 1980s no genuinely new classes of antibiotics have been discovered and introduced to human medicine. The lack of new antibiotics is a particularly acute problem for many bacteria which can be transmitted to humans from food animals, like E. coli, Salmonella and Campylobacter. The result has been that treatment of serious infections now sometimes relies on toxic antibiotics like colistin, which was discovered as long ago as 1951.

Antibiotic resistance in human infections is linked to farm use

Although human antibiotic use is widely recognised as the main cause of antibiotic resistance in most human infections, the extent to which antibiotic use in livestock can also result in resistance in human infections has long been controversial. There are two main reasons for this, one scientific, the other having more to do with the influence of vested interests.

First we need to understand how resistance arises and how it spreads. When antibiotics are used, they kill or stop the growth of bacteria which are "susceptible" to it. However, some of the bacteria may be resistant to the antibiotic, and when the antibiotic is used, susceptible bacteria are killed or prevented from reproducing, leaving the resistant ones to proliferate. Many of these resistant bacteria live in the intestines, and when animals are slaughtered and eviscerated at the abattoir, contamination of the carcasses can occur, and some bacteria end up on the meat – other bacteria live naturally on skin, and so their presence on retail meat is to be expected. If the meat is cooked properly, most or all of the bacteria will be killed, but handling of raw meat and eating undercooked meat can allow the bacteria to be transferred to humans. If the bacteria directly cause a human infection which is antibiotic resistant, the resistance will have been due to farm antibiotic use.

However, a further complication is that certain farm-animal bacteria, like some strains of E. coli, may not actually cause an infection in humans, but they can nevertheless be transferred to humans and live for some time in the human gut. There, they have an ability to share resistance genes by a process called "horizontal gene transfer" with other bacteria in the gut. Bacteria which are resistant to a particular antibiotic usually have a gene (or genes) which enables them to resist the effects of the antibiotic, and sometimes the bacteria can produce copies of this gene and pass these copies on to other bacteria which then also become resistant. It has been known for decades that resistant E. coli of farm-animal origin on meat can pass on copies of their resistance genes to human E. coli in the human gut (Smith 1969). If those human E. coli subsequently cause an infection, such as a urinary tract infection, the E. coli may be of human origin, but the resistance is of farm-animal origin.

The spread of resistance to colistin appears to be occurring partly this way, and resistance to other critically important antibiotics is also known to be spreading by horizontal gene transfer. This complicated way of resistance spreading does however make it challenging to determine how much of the problem is of farm-animal origin and how much of human origin.

Disagreement and confusion has, unfortunately, also occurred as a result of lobbying by vested interests, with scientists employed or funded by the pharmaceutical industry, and occasionally organisations representing vets or farmers, seeking to downplay, or even at times to totally deny, the impact of farm antibiotic use on human medicine. The effect has often been inaction from politicians and regulators who frequently call for more research to be done and further data to be collected before any decisive actions are taken. Even in situations where clear scientific evidence shows that human treatments are being undermined by unnecessary farm use, lobbying has been used to delay or prevent the appropriate bans or reductions from being implemented (ASOA 2016).

The importance of vested interests was highlighted in a report published in late 2015 by the Review on Antimicrobial Resistance, which had been commissioned by the UK Prime Minister, David Cameron, and chaired by economist Jim O'Neill (Review on Antimicrobial Resistance 2015). The review found "compelling" evidence of a link between veterinary antibiotic use and resistance in human medicine, which the authors said warranted a global reduction in farm antibiotic use to analyse the resistance problem. However, one of the review's most interesting findings, not widely reported, was that it discovered a clear distinction in the scientific literature between the conclusions of academic scientists and those of scientists affiliated to the government or pharmaceutical or animal-health industries. Whereas 72% of papers by academics found evidence of a link between the farm use of antibiotics and resistance in human medicine, this fell to just 26% for government/industry scientists. Furthermore, a majority of studies opposing a reduction of farm antibiotic use were authored by scientists affiliated to either governments or industry.

Overall, as the O'Neill report found, there is a broad scientific consensus that farm antibiotic use does contribute significantly to resistance in human infections. For certain human infections like Salmonella and Campylobacter which directly cause infections when they are transferred to humans in sufficient numbers, we know that most resistance in human infections is actually of farm origin. Organisations like the European Food Safety Authority and the World Health Organisation have come to this conclusion in their own reviews of the science. For some other infections, like E. coli and enterococcal infections, many scientists believe that farm-animal antibiotic use is also a significant contributor to resistance, but the exact extent of the link is still being debated as horizontal gene transfer is known to play an important role (ASOA 2015).

Furthermore, in recent years, the emergence of new types of superbugs in farm animals, such as MRSA (methicillin-resistant Staphylococcus aureus), Clostridium difficile, a new type of highly resistant E. coli, called ESBL E. coli, and some highly resistant Klebsiella, as well as the appearance of identical or very similar strains of all of these bacteria in humans has led some scientists to argue that the impact on human health from farm antibiotic use is likely larger than has been previously assumed (Aarestrup 2015).

Another area where scientific assessments may have underestimated the impact on human health of farm antibiotic use relates to antibiotic residues in food. Up until recently, residues in food have been thought to be relatively irrelevant to the resistance story, unlike the transfer of resistant bacteria on food, as described earlier. This is because the overwhelming majority of residues are at concentrations that are too low to kill any bacteria in the human gut, and therefore scientists assumed they couldn't be selecting for resistance since both sensitive and resistant bacteria survive these concentrations.

However, numerous recent studies have shown that extremely low concentrations of antibiotics can nevertheless have an effect: these low concentrations don't kill the sensitive bacteria or prevent them from reproducing as higher doses would do, but they do slow their growth and allow the resistant bacteria to grow faster. The lowest dose at which this selection can occur is now called the "minimum selective concentration", and it can be up to 200 times lower than the lowest dose that actually kills or stops the growth of sensitive bacteria. According to a review article published in *Nature*, this means that residues in food could be favouring the growth of resistant bacteria in the human gut: "the consumption of meat or milk that has been contaminated with antibiotics in quantities that are below the detection limit, could result in antibiotic concentrations in the body that are above the minimal selective concentration, which could lead to the enrichment of resistant bacteria" (Andersson and Hughes 2014, p486). However, these new findings, which have been replicated in several studies, have not yet been assessed properly by regulators, who continue to assume that residues well above these concentrations have no impact on the amounts of resistant bacteria in the human intestine.

Resistance isn't the only problem

While the science showing that low doses of antibiotics in food could be having an impact on resistance is relatively new, another problem associated with the overuse of antibiotics, also largely ignored by regulators, has been known about for decades. This is the fact that the oral use of antibiotics can kill off beneficial bacteria in the animals' intestines and allow pathogenic bacteria to proliferate. The effect depends on the antibiotic used and can occur for several types of pathogens, but is particularly clear for Salmonella.

The outbreaks of antibiotic-resistant Salmonella in the 1960s UK which had led to the setting up of the Swann committee also focused subsequent scientific research on this bacterium, and numerous studies carried out in the 1970s, 1980s and early 1990s confirmed that farm animals fed certain antibiotics orally, particularly those used for growth promotion, had far greater numbers of Salmonella in their intestines (Smith and Tucker 1978). Again, the findings were challenged by scientists funded by the pharmaceutical industry (Gustafson et al. 1981), which ultimately led to regulators failing to act. More Salmonella in farm animals ultimately led to more cases of Salmonella in people too, and it wasn't until growth promoters were phased out in Europe that Salmonella levels began to fall (the introduction of some new vaccines also helped reduce the incidence of Salmonella). Of course some of the growth promoters remain available for use as prophylactic antibiotics, so while Salmonella food poisoning is not as large a problem as it was in the 1990s, it remains much more common than it was in the pre-antibiotic era.

Regulation of antibiotics won't be enough – we need to change farming too

So what can be done to reduce farm antibiotic use and to limit the dangers to human health? Clearly the proposed EU ban on the routine preventative use of antibiotics would be a major step forward. In addition, even greater restrictions on the use of the most critically important antibiotics will also be required, and in some cases, as with colistin, total bans on the farm use seems the only sensible option. Experiences in the Nordic countries and in the Netherlands has shown that regulations along these lines, and voluntary initiatives taken by farmers, can have a major impact. It is likely that in the next few years we will see the introduction of some new regulations along these lines, but it can also be expected that there will be significant resistance to change and an unwillingness on behalf of regulators to be as decisive as is needed. We were given an example of this approach in May 2016, when the European Medicines Agency recommended that the continued use of colistin for mass medication in pigs and poultry be permitted, even though the EMA accepted that transmission of resistance from farm animals to humans is "likely" (EMA 2016).

In the United States, progress is even slower. Data for 2015, the second year of the three-year period during which the use of growth promoters are being voluntarily phased out and when the FDA expected sales to fall, shows that sales of medically important farm antibiotics was 5% higher than in 2013, and 26% higher than 2009, the first year for which sales data are available (FDA 2016). Farms account for about 75% of total use of medically important antibiotics, with human use only accounting for about 25% (FDA 2012, FDA 2016,). If growth promoters are being phased out (the data don't say one way or the other), these figures suggest that they are simply being replaced with increased use of preventative antibiotics. Since the beginning of 2017, growth promoters have been phased out and all farm antibiotic use in the US requires a veterinary prescription, which is a step in the right direction, but Europe has already had a decade to prove that routine use doesn't stop even when prescriptions are required.

In much of the rest of the world, farm antibiotic use is even less well regulated. The World Organisation for Animal Health (OIE) says that 110 countries have little or no regulations governing farm antibiotic use (OIE 2015). The OIE also says that approximately 50% of the countries in the world have banned growth promotion, but many poorer countries don't have the regulatory resources to implement the ban in practice. While many poorer countries still have less intensive livestock production, and antibiotic use is therefore likely to be lower, no data is available on usage levels for most of these countries. However, if livestock farming continues to intensify, it is likely that consumption will continue to increase. In fact, a study carried out for the OECD has forecast that by 2030, global farm antibiotic use may increase by 67%, and nearly double in middle-income "BRIC" countries Brazil, Russia, India and China, due to extensive farming practices being replaced by "large-scale intensive farming operations" (Van Boeckel et al. 2015).

This forecast strongly suggests that improved and more restrictive regulation of antibiotic use alone is unlikely to deliver the global reductions in use that are now urgently needed. An approach focused merely on antibiotic use, rather than also considering farming methods, also runs the risk of creating animal welfare problems, if the fear of using antibiotics too often means that sick animals end up being denied appropriate treatment. That is why we also need to rethink the way we farm animals, particularly pigs and poultry, so that the risk of disease is minimised, as well as the levels of antibiotic use. And there is overwhelming evidence that by far the lowest levels of antibiotic use are achieved in extensive systems, where animals have full access to the outdoors.

In the UK, about 90% of farm antibiotics are used in intensively farmed pigs and poultry, even though often extensively farmed sheep and cattle have much larger populations (in terms of the EU's livestock units), and it is no surprise that so many problem resistant bacteria (E. coli, Campylobacter, Salmonella, MRSA) appear to mainly associated with pigs and poultry (VMD 2015). In Denmark, antibiotic consumption in pigs is probably about four or five times lower per animal than in most other European countries even though the pigs are still farmed intensively, but Danish government statistics show that use in Danish organic pigs is another ten times lower again (Ministry of Environment and Food of Denmark 2014). Of course cattle too can be farmed very intensively, and when they are, the amounts of antibiotics used can be exceptionally high: a recent Belgian study found that intensively farmed veal calves receive over 25 times more antibiotics than more extensively farmed cattle, and that the levels of resistance are many times higher in the intensively farmed animals (Catry et al. 2016).

If farming is to move towards more extensive systems, based on access to pasture, then the era of very cheap pig and poultry meat will come to an end as production costs will inevitably go up. This may mean that if we want to truly save our antibiotics, will we need to accept eating less but higher-quality and healthier meat.

References

Aarestrup F., 2015. The livestock reservoir for antimicrobial resistance: A personal view on changing patterns of risks, effects of interventions and the way forward, *Philosophical Transactions B*, **370**.

Alexandratos N. and Bruinsma J., 2012. World agriculture towards 2030/2050, *Food and Agriculture Organization of the United Nations*. ESA Working Paper No. 12-03

Andersson D. and Hughes D., 2014. Microbiological effects of sublethal levels of antibiotics, *Nature Review Microbiology*, **12**: 465–78.

ASOA, 2015. Antimicrobial resistance – Why the irresponsible use of antibiotics in agriculture must stop: A briefing from the Alliance to Save Our Antibiotics, www.saveouranti biotics.org/media/1466/antibiotics-alliance-40pp-report-2015-final-artwork-1.pdf

ASOA, 2016. Why the use of fluoroquinolone antibiotics in poultry should be banned, A briefing from the Alliance to Save Our Antibiotics, http://www.saveourantibiotics.org/media/1495/why-the-use-of-fluoroquinolone-antibiotics-in-poultry-must-be-banned-alliance-to-save-our-antibiotics-july-2016.pdf

Callens B., Persoons D., Maes D., Laanen M., Postma M., Boyen F., Haesebrouck F., Butaye P., Catry B. and Dewulf J., 2012. Prophylactic and metaphylactic antimicrobial use in Belgian fattening pig herds, *Preventive Veterinary Medicine*, **106**: 53–6.

Catry B., Dewulf J., Maes D., Pardon B., Callens B., Vanrobaeys M., Opsomer G., de Kruif A. and Haesebrouck F., 2016. Effect of antimicrobial consumption and production type on antibacterial resistance in the bovine respiratory and digestive tract, *PLoS One*, **11.**

DANMAP, 2015. DANMAP 2014: Use of antimicrobial agents and occurrence of antimicrobial resistance in bacteria from food animals, food and humans in Denmark, www.danmap.org/~/media/Projekt%20sites/Danmap/DANMAP%20reports/DANMAP%20%202015/DANMAP%202015.ashx

ECDC et al., 2015. ECDC/EFSA/EMA first joint report on the integrated analysis of the consumption of antimicrobial agents and occurrence of antimicrobial resistance in bacteria from humans and food-producing animals, *EFSA Journal*, **13**: 4006, http://ecdc.europa.eu/en/publications/Publications/antimicrobial-resistance-JIACRA-report.pdf

EMA, 2015. Sales of veterinary antimicrobial agents in 26 EU/EEA countries in 2013, Fifth ESVAC report, www.ema.europa.eu/ema/pages/includes/document/open_document.jsp?webContentId=WC500195687

EMA, 2016. Updated advice on the use of colistin products in animals 4 within the European Union: Development of resistance 5 and possible impact on human and animal health, 26 May, www.ema.europa.eu/docs/en_GB/document_library/Scientific_guideline/2016/07/WC500211080.pdf

FDA, 2012. Antibacterial drug use analysis, Drug use review, Department of Health and Human Services Public Health Service, Food and Drug Administration, Center for Drug Evaluation and Research, Office of Surveillance and Epidemiology, Food and Drug Administration, www.fda.gov/downloads/drugs/drugsafety/informationbydrugclass/ucm319435.pdf

FDA, 2016. 2015 Summary report on: Antimicrobials sold or distributed for use in Food-producing animals, Center for Veterinary Medicine, Food and Drug Administration, www.fda.gov/downloads/ForIndustry/UserFees/AnimalDrugUserFeeActADUFA/UCM534243.pdf

Gustafson R.H., Beck J.R. and Kobland J.D. 1981. The influence of avoparcin on the establishment of Salmonella in chickens, *Zentralblatt fur Veterinarmedizin*, **29**: 119–28.

House of Commons, 1969. Report of the joint committee on the use of antibiotics in animal husbandry and veterinary medicine, London, Her Majesty's Stationery Office.

Kennedy P., 2014. The fat drug, *New York Times*, March 8, pSR1

Lawrence W., 1950. 'Wonder drug' aureomycin found to spur growth 50%, *New York Times*, April 10, p1

Laxminarayan R., Duse A., Wattal C., Zaidi A.K., Wertheim H.F., Sumpradit N., Vlieghe E., Hara G.L., Gould I.M., Goossens H., Greko C., So A.D., Bigdeli M., Tomson G., Woodhouse W., Ombaka E., Peralta A.Q., Qamar F.N., Mir F., Kariuki S., Bhutta Z.A., Coates A., Bergstrom R., Wright G.D., Brown E.D. and Cars O. 2013. Antibiotic resistance – The need for global solutions, *Lancet Infectious Diseases*, **13**: 1057–98.

Liu Y.Y., Wang Y., Walsh T.R., Yi L.X., Zhang R., Spencer J., Doi Y., Tian G., Dong B., Huang X., Yu L.F., Gu D., Ren H., Chen X., Lv L., He D., Zhou H., Liang Z., Liu J.H. and Shen J., 2015. Emergence of plasmid-mediated colistin resistance mechanism MCR-1 in animals and human beings in China: A microbiological and molecular biological study, *Lancet Infectious Diseases*, **62**: 161–8.

Livermore D., 2011. Discovery research: The scientific challenge of finding new antibiotics, *Journal of Antimicrobial Chemotherapy*, **66**: 1941–4.

Mennie A.T., 1970. Report of the proceedings of the symposium at the Royal Society of Medicine, sponsored by Cyanamid of Great Britain Limited, Aspects of Infective Drug Resistance

Ministry of Environment and Food of Denmark, 2014. *Answer to Question from Per Clausen*, 28 August.

OIE 2015. *Towards better surveillance of antibiotic use in animal health*, World Organisation for Animal Health, press release, www.oie.int/for-the-media/press-releases/detail/article/towards-better-surveillance-of-antibiotic-use-in-animal-health/

Review on Antimicrobial Resistance, 2015. Antimicrobials in agriculture and the environment: Reducing unnecessary use and waste, The Review on Antimicrobial Resistance Chaired by Jim O'Neill, https://amr-review.org/sites/default/files/Antimicrobials%20in%20agriculture%20and%20the%20environment%20-%20Reducing%20unnecessary%20use%20and%20waste.pdf

SDa, 2015. Usage of antibiotics in agricultural livestock in the Netherlands in 2014, Netherlands Veterinary Medicines Authority, www.autoriteitdiergeneesmiddelen.nl/Userfiles/Eng%20rapport%20AB%20gebruik%202015/engels-rapportage-2015---geheel-rapport-13122016.pdf

Smith H., 1969, Transfer of antibiotic resistance from animal and human strains of escherichia coli to resident E. coli in the alimentary tract of man, *Lancet*, **1**: 1174–6.

Smith H. and Crabb W., 1958. The effect of the continuous administration of diets containing low levels of tetracyclines on the incidence of drug-resistant bacterium coli in the faeces of pigs and chickens: The sensitivity of bacterium coli to other chemotherapeutic agents, *Veterinary Record*, **70**: 749–54.

Smith H. and Tucker J., 1978. The effect of antimicrobial feed additives on the colonization of the alimentary tract of chickens by Salmonella typhimurium, *Journal of Hygiene*, **80**: 217–31.

Starr M. and Reynolds D., 1951. Streptomycin resistance of coliform bacteria from turkeys fed streptomycin, *American Journal of Public Health and of the Nations Health*, **41**: 1375–80.

Van Boeckel T.P., Brower C., Gilbert M., Grenfell B.T., Levin S.A., Robinson T.P., Teillant A. and Laxminarayan R.., 2015. Global trends in antimicrobial use in food animals, *PNAS*, **112**: 5649–54.

VMD, 2016. UK veterinary antibiotic resistance and sales surveillance report UK-VARSS 2015, Veterinary Medicines Directorate, www.gov.uk/government/uploads/system/uploads/attachment_data/file/582341/1051728-v53-UK-VARSS_2015.pdf

14

HOW MUCH MEAT AND MILK IS OPTIMAL FOR HEALTH?

Mike Rayner and Peter Scarborough

Introduction

Meat and dairy products (MDPs) have long been regarded as good for health (Fiddes, 1991) but this assumption is increasingly being called into question. It has come to be recognized that vegetarians are generally as healthy as non-vegetarians and sometimes healthier. This has led some to question whether MDPs are necessary for a healthy diet and even whether diets would be healthier if people ate less MDPs than they currently do. The debate about MDPs and health is particularly intense in industrialized countries, where people have diets that are relatively high in MDPs and where it has come to be realized that the production of MDPs – at least as generally practised – has detrimental effects on the environment (see chapters by Bernués, D'Silva, Hoekstra and Young in this book).

This chapter aims to summarize where the debate about the health benefits (and otherwise) of MDPs has reached. First, we look briefly at what we mean by 'meat and dairy products'. Second, we look at why MDPs have until relatively recently generally been thought to be good for health. Third, we look at some of the recent research that questions the view that MDPs are good for health. As part of the examination we look at trends in meat and dairy consumption, particularly in the UK (as an example of an industrialized country) and the health effects of these trends. Fourth, we look at what official bodies are precisely saying about MDP consumption. In concluding we look at how we might resolve the answer to the question that is the title for this chapter: 'How much meat and milk is optimal for health?' but also the equally important question: 'What type of MDPs are optimal for health?' and finally and briefly we look at the even more important question 'How much and what type of MDP is optimal for our health *but also that of the planet*?'

What are meat and dairy products?

By 'MDPs' we mean all edible products derived from mammals or birds. So by 'meat' we mean all types of red meat (e.g. from cows, sheep and pigs), white meat (e.g. from chicken), processed meat and offal, but we do not include fish or shellfish. By 'dairy products' we mean milk, cream and processed dairy products such as butter, cheese and yoghurt. Within 'MDPs' we include eggs. 'MDPs' therefore include a large number of different types of foods with different nutritional properties and hence different effects on health.

The animals that end up being consumed as meat or that are the source of dairy products and eggs are fed and kept in different ways. Some have suggested that the ways animals are farmed have important effects on the healthiness of their products and we look briefly at this issue later in the chapter. Moreover MDPs can be subject to extensive processing and this too can have a major impact on their health-related properties. Again this is something we examine later. This means that as well as the question 'How much meat and dairy is optimal for health?', we also need to ask: 'What types of MDPs are optimal for health?'

Perceptions of the health benefits of MDPs

The idea that MDPs are basically good for our health, has, until recently, been deeply entrenched within the culture of most countries. Meat – for many people – has had to be a part of their main meal of the day. In a study carried out in the UK in the mid-1980s, 200 women were asked what the family needs to eat properly and the researchers found that 'meat was mentioned by the women more frequently than any other food. In fact only five women thought meat was not an important item of the family diet' (Kerr and Charles, 1986, cited in Fiddes, 1991). Dairy products, particularly milk, have also been generally considered to be an essential part of a healthy diet, perhaps even more so than meat. As a *Times* (of London) editorial of 1936 put it: 'Milk makes you sleep o'nights, gives you a milky complexion, makes muscle, gives you a healthy old age, and makes the toddler king of the castle. What more can men and women want?' (quoted in McKee, 1997). Attitudes to the relationship between MDPs and health are probably changing, but if so these changes are gradual and vary between countries as illustrated by trends in MDP consumption (see Figure 14.2).

The popular belief that MDPs are good for health has, until relatively recently, been supported by most nutritionists. The primary justification for this has been that meat is relatively high in protein, minerals such as iron and zinc and vitamins such as vitamin B12 and that milk and dairy products are high in protein and calcium.

Protein – like other nutrients within foods – is essential for the normal growth and development of the human body. But protein is often regarded as the most important of these nutrients. The very word 'protein' comes from the Greek word πρωτειος (*proteios*), meaning 'primary'.

The recognition that protein is essential for normal growth and development has led – not particularly logically – to the belief that there is a need for large quantities of protein in the human diet. This is sometimes known as the 'protein myth'. This myth/belief can be traced back at least as far back as the work of Baron Justus von Liebig – the 19th-century German chemist. In *Animal Chemistry* (1846) and *Researches on the Chemistry of Food* (1847), von Liebig glorified meat at the essential source of material to replenish muscular strength lost during physical activity. He believed (wrongly as it turns out) that the more physically active a person, the more protein they need. The doctrines of von Liebig were expanded upon by his many followers including Lyon Playfair in the UK, Carlo von Voit and Max Ruber in Germany and Wilbur Atwater in the US, all of whom made estimates of human protein requirements that were accepted as the basis of many governments' food policy until well into the 20th century (Cannon, 2003). These estimates were based largely not on what people needed, but on what the average healthy person at that time consumed and so tended to overestimate people's actual requirements for protein. Since then estimates of requirements have become more sophisticated and are now based more closely on need.

So today, for example, the UK Government estimates that the average women requires 36g of protein per day and the average man 44g (Department of Health, 1991). However, average protein intakes are currently around 65g for an adult woman and 85g for an adult man, in other words nearly twice as much as 'required' (NatCen Social Research et al., 2015). Moreover these high average intake levels mean that virtually no one in the UK suffers from a protein deficiency. Note, however, that older people and women who are pregnant or breastfeeding need more protein than the average person when measured as a percentage of energy intake (WHO, 2007).

Perhaps surprisingly the health effects of eating less protein than deemed essential are poorly understood. This is because low-protein diets tend to be generally nutrient-poor, deficient to varying degrees in a range of other nutrients, and also often associated with other environmental factors that can adversely influence health (WHO, 2007).

The health effects of very high – or even moderately high – protein intakes are even less clear. What is clear is that high-protein diets promote the growth of young children so that as adults they are much taller than they would otherwise be. It seems likely that the steady increase in average height in most developed countries over the 20th century (in many cases starting well before that) has been mainly due to increasing protein intakes. Furthermore differences in protein intakes are largely responsible for the differences in heights between nationalities. But faster growing and taller is not necessarily healthier and some have argued that high-protein diets have led to all sorts of health and other social problems (Cannon, 2003).

While most foods contain some protein, MDPs tend to be relatively high in protein compared with plant-based foods. This means that MDPs are the biggest source of protein in the UK diet: meat providing 38 per cent and dairy products 13 per cent (NatCen Social Research et al., 2015). This does not mean that plant-based foods could not provide enough protein if people ate less MDPs. In fact the average person is already getting about 25g a day of protein from cereals, fruit, vegetables (including potatoes) and nuts, and if we assume that official recommendations are right and the average person needs about 40g a day, then we don't need to eat much more of these foods to meet the recommendation.

Protein from MDPs is sometimes considered to be of 'higher quality' than protein from plant sources for two reasons. First, the protein in meat and dairy protein is said to provide a 'better balance' of the amino acids that make up proteins. Some amino acids are essential in that they cannot be made within the human body. Meat, and to a lesser extent dairy products, tend to have all these essential amino acids in fairly high and similar amounts while plant-based foods may not. However plant-based diets (provided that they are varied enough) can provide all the essential amino acids the body needs. Second, the protein in MDPs is thought to be more digestible than protein from plant-based sources, although not much more (Millward and Garnett, 2010).

It's not just protein that is found in high levels in MDPs but also other nutrients – particularly minerals and vitamins – that are essential for growth and for the maintenance of normal metabolic functions. MDPs are good sources of zinc, calcium, iodine, iron, vitamins A and B12, riboflavin and niacin (see Table 14.1).

The vitamins and minerals that are present in high levels in MDPs all have different functions. For example iron is an essential component of haemoglobin, which transports oxygen around the body in the blood stream. Calcium is an essential component of bone. Vitamin B12 is needed for normal neural development and so on.

However, in many instances, the precise relationship between these minerals and vitamins and health is still not well understood. It is clear that extremely low levels of the nutrients lead to disease. For example a very low iron intake leads to anaemia, which produces fatigue and impaired performance in adults, reduced motor skills in children and even death. But the effects of moderately low levels are less clear.

TABLE 14.1 Most important of the vitamins and minerals provided by MDPs in the UK diet

Nutrient	*% total intake from meat*	*% of UK population below LRNI*	*Nutrient*	*% total intake from dairy*	*% of UK population below LRNI*
Niacin	36	0	Calcium	36	7
Zinc	35	6	Iodine	33	2
Vitamin B12	29	1	Vitamin B12	33	1
Iron	21	11	Riboflavin	28	8
Vitamin A	16	7	Zinc	15	6

Note: LRNI: the government's 'lower reference nutrient intake'.

Source: NatCen Social Research et al. (2015)

In the UK the Government has published what it considers to be adequate levels for mineral and vitamin intakes in the population (Department of Health, 1991) These adequate levels (lower reference nutrient intakes) are set relative to what is considered desirable (estimated average requirements). Table 14.1 shows that there are very few people in the UK who have inadequate levels of the minerals and vitamins that are present in high levels in MDPs, the exception being iron where there is a particular problem with girls and young women (NatCen Social Research et al., 2015).

As with protein it is unclear to what extent the average intakes of the vitamins and minerals found in high levels in MDPs are higher or lower than necessary for optimal health. It is clear that there are some people in the UK who have less than desirable or even adequate levels of these minerals and vitamins but the precise health effects of this do not seem to be large (Institute for Health Metrics and Evaluation, 2015).

Recent research questioning the health benefits of MDPs

The mid-20th century consensus that MDPs were good for health because they were high in protein and essential minerals and vitamins began to break down in the 1960s and 1970s with the recognition that the high and increasing rates of many chronic diseases in developed countries were partly diet related.

Cardiovascular disease

One of the first studies in this area was carried out in the late 1970s and early 1980s by the pioneering American epidemiologist Ancel Keys, who, by comparing rates of cardiovascular disease (CVD) (that is, coronary heart disease (CHD) and stroke) in seven different countries, showed that there was a strong association between average CVD rates and average blood cholesterol levels. Average blood cholesterol levels were in turn found to be positively associated with average levels of dietary cholesterol and of saturated fat and possibly negatively associated with average levels of unsaturated fat (though this was less clear).

The results of this cross-country comparison were quickly augmented by observational studies on individuals and more latterly by experimental studies (including randomized controlled trials) and thereby relationships were shown to be causal and not just associations (Skeaff and Miller, 2009, Souza et al., 2015, Hooper et al., 2015).

Whereas almost all of the fat in plant-based foods is unsaturated (either monounsaturated or polyunsaturated) most of the fat in MDPs is saturated. At least 60 per cent of saturated fat in the UK diet comes from MDPs (NatCen Social Research et al., 2015). Furthermore it is only animal-derived products that contain dietary cholesterol. Therefore, consumption of MDPs – particularly MDPs high in saturated fat – came to be linked with an increased risk of CVD.

Research carried out since the early 1980s on the relationship between fat intake and risk of CVD has shown it to be more complicated than previously thought. First, it very quickly turned out that saturated fat was more important than dietary cholesterol in raising risk of blood cholesterol and then CVD. Then, more recently, different studies have generated confusing results about the importance of high intakes of saturated fat as opposed to low intakes of monounsaturated and/or polyunsaturated fat. It was also shown that different types of saturated fat (and indeed polyunsaturated fats) were more important than others in their impact on risk of CVD.

The polyunsaturated fat story has become particularly complicated. Some polyunsaturated fats (linoleic acid and α-linolenic acid) cannot be formed in the body and thus it is 'essential' that the diet supplies enough of them. The UK Government therefore recommends a minimum intake of 1 per cent of energy from linoleic and similar n-6 (polyunsaturated) fats and 0.2 per cent of energy from α-linolenic and similar long-chain n-3 (polyunsaturated) fats (Department of Health, 1991). But since the 1960s and 1970s the evidence has grown that higher levels of both n-3 polyunsaturated fats (found in large amounts in fish but also in vegetable oils such as rapeseed oil) and n-6 polyunsaturated fats (found in large amounts in vegetable oils such as sunflower and corn oils) reduce the risk of CVD in different ways and particularly when replacing saturated fats (Skeaff and Miller, 2009, Souza et al., 2015, Hooper et al., 2015).

Since the 1980s evidence has also grown that trans-fats formed from unsaturated fats ultimately derived from plant sources either in animal rumens (which then find their way into MDPs) or industrially by the process known as hydrogenation, are particularly toxic in relation to risk of CVD (Mozaffarian et al., 2006). Ruminant trans-fats and industrially produced trans-fats have similar metabolic effects, but it has generally been thought that the latter can be more easily removed from the food supply than the former.

Despite all this recent research the basic story has remained essentially the same for around the last 20 or 30 years. High intakes of saturated fat increase the risk of CVD, particularly if coupled with high levels of sugar and other refined carbohydrates in the diet, and a reduction in average saturated fat intake in most countries would generate substantial health benefits. We calculate that reducing current average intakes from approximately 14 per cent of energy (as at present) to 10 per cent of energy (the UK Government's recommended goal) would save over 4,000 lives a year in the UK all from CVD (Scarborough et al., 2012). This is not as big as the 15,000 lives that would be saved from increasing fruit and vegetable consumption to at least five portions per day but it is still substantial.

Given that MDPs are the main source of saturated fat and that the health benefits of the current high intakes of MDPs uncertain there would seem – on this basis alone – to be an obvious case for reducing meat and dairy intake. However, many nutritionists have been reluctant to draw such a conclusion, arguing that it is only those MDPs that are high in saturated fat that constitute the risk, not high MDP consumption as such.

There has also been a tendency for all the research into the relationship between different types of fats and CVD to obscure the basic story. There is currently some debate about whether the fat composition of MDPs can be enhanced in relation to its effects on health by different feeding practices. For example it is certainly the case that n-3 polyunsaturated fat levels in beef can be increased by high forage-based diets (Givens, 2005). This is likely to mean that the meat from grass-fed cattle will be slightly healthier than from non-grass-fed cattle. However, it seems unlikely that the slightly improved fat composition of beef from grass-fed animals (compared for example with beef produced more intensively) will have any major impact on the health of its consumers.

Research on the relationships between different types of dietary fat, blood cholesterol levels and risk of CVD has been accompanied by research on the relationship between diet, blood pressure levels and risk of CVD. Even before it became clear that a raised blood cholesterol level increased the risk of CVD, it was known that raised blood pressure did so, and it was suspected that raised blood pressure was partly diet related. The clearest dietary cause of high blood pressure has turned out to be high salt intakes (Aburto et al., 2013).

Only a small amount of salt (more precisely sodium) is required for normal body function and this can be obtained easily enough through its natural occurrence in many foods including meat, fish, eggs, fruits and vegetables. However, salt is used as a preservative and flavour enhancer in most processed foods and consumption of these processed foods can lead to excessive consumption of sodium. Much of the MDP consumption in the UK comes in the form of processed foods (cheese, bacon, ham, sausages, ready meals, etc.), and 38 per cent of the salt in the UK diet comes from such MDPs (NatCen Social Research et al., 2015). We estimate that reducing average salt intakes in the UK from current levels at around 9g per day to the recommended 6g per day would save about 8,000 lives a year (the vast majority from CVD) (Scarborough et al., 2012).

An important systematic review of the evidence for the direct relationship between red and processed meat consumption and the risk of CVD has recently been updated (Micha et al., 2012). It suggests that the effects of red meat consumption on risk of coronary heart disease (CHD) vary depending on processing. In meta-analyses of prospective studies, higher risk of CHD is seen with processed meat consumption but a smaller increase or no risk is seen with unprocessed meat consumption. Differences in sodium content (~400 per cent higher in processed meat in the reviewed studies) appear to account for about two-thirds of this risk difference. A similar meta-analysis shows that consumption of processed red meat as well as fresh red meat, to a lesser extent, is associated with increased risk of stroke (Kaluza et al., 2012).

The strong association between processed meat consumption and cardiovascular health found in these meta-analyses is mirrored in a dose-response meta-analysis of nine prospective cohort studies with all-cause mortality as an outcome (Larsson and Orsini, 2014). The researchers found increased risk of all-cause mortality for processed meat consumption and total red meat consumption, and a non-significant increased risk associated with non-processed red meat consumption. Whereas previous meta-analyses had compared health risks in groups categorized as 'high' or 'low' meat consumers, Larsson and Orsini quantified meat consumption in the included studies and considered how risk changes at different consumption levels. They found that all-cause mortality increases at all levels of processed meat consumption, and they found a very low threshold (10g/d) at which risk begins to increase for total red meat consumption.

The direct relationship between dairy products and risk of CVD is complicated because of the positive benefits of some of the components of dairy products such as calcium and the negative effects of others – particularly saturated fat and salt. The systematic reviews are fairly equivocal on the matter (e.g. Alexander et al., 2016) but most agree that if there are any benefits of dairy products these are limited to those that are low in saturated fat.

Cancer

As with relationship between diet and CVD, the relationship between diet and cancer has become increasingly clear over the last few decades – due particularly to the work of the World Cancer Research Fund (WCRF) which has systematically reviewed all the available studies and published two seminal reports in 1997 and 2007 and propose to publish a further report in 2017 (WCRF/AICR, 1997, 2007).

In their review process researchers at the WCRF have examined all possible relationships between MDP consumption and cancer. The one relationship that the WCRF describes as 'convincing' is the relationship between red and processed meat intake and colorectal cancer. A number of potential mechanisms have been suggested, including the formation of carcinogens in the high temperature cooking of meat, and the potential damage to cells in the gut of free radicals associated with the haem iron component of red meat. At present, these mechanisms are not well established.

After reviewing the accumulated scientific literature the International Agency for Research on Cancer (IARC) has similarly concluded recently that red meat is 'probably carcinogenic to humans' and that the association between red meat consumption and cancer is clearest for colorectal cancer, but associations were also seen for pancreatic cancer and prostate cancer. IARC also classified processed meat as definitely 'carcinogenic to humans' based on sufficient evidence that consumption of processed meat causes colorectal cancer (Bouvard et al., 2015). Colorectal cancer kills about 16,500 people each year in the UK (Townsend et al., 2015). The Global Burden of Disease Study estimates that 3,300 of these could be prevented by completely eliminating processed meat from the diet and cutting red meat consumption to less than one serving a week (Institute for Health Metrics and Evaluation, 2015): quite some way short of the 11,000 deaths from CVD that could be avoided by reducing saturated fat and salt levels to government recommended levels (Scarborough et al., 2012).

Obesity and diabetes

It is well known that obesity is increasing almost everywhere in the world with serious adverse health consequences including increasing rates of diabetes. Some have suggested that this is somehow associated with the high and increasing consumption of MDPs, particularly meat. However, there is little evidence for any direct relationship. Some MDPs are energy dense and the WCRF suggests that the evidence linking the consumption of large amounts of energy-dense foods with overweight and obesity is 'probable'. But the WCRF also indicates that the evidence linking MDP consumption with overweight and obesity is 'limited and inconclusive' (WCRF/AICR, 2007). On the other hand there is growing evidence that red meat consumption may be associated with increased risk of diabetes, with, yet again, higher risks for processed red meats (Micha et al., 2012) although this unlikely to be through its effects on obesity.

Vegetarianism and veganism

Given the negative consequences of MDP consumption and the relatively few and uncertain benefits of a high consumption as described above, it is perhaps not surprising that vegetarians and vegans are often healthier than the general population (Key et al., 1999; Mann, 2009). And it is also clear from this that MDPs are not essential elements of a healthy diet for all individuals. However, a note of caution is needed here. Vegetarians and vegans tend to be more health conscious than the general population, which may explain some of the differences in health outcomes between the two groups. For example as well as eating fewer MDPs, they eat more fruits and vegetables, they smoke less and do more physical activity. Although many people have no problem living healthily on vegan and vegetarian diets, others have found these diets more difficult to maintain.

Trends in MDP consumption

It is an assumption of this chapter that diet is an important determinant of health. Estimates vary but we find that around 30,000 deaths a year could be avoided (or at least delayed) if people in the UK met government recommendations for foods and nutrients (Scarborough et al., 2012). The recent Global Burden of Disease Study estimates that 88,000 per year – 15 per cent of all deaths – are attributable to poor diets in the UK (Institute for Health Metrics and Evaluation, 2015). This figure is higher than the 30,000 deaths that we estimate could be avoided by meeting government recommendations because these recommendations are pragmatic rather than ideal goals. MDPs provide a major source of calories to the average diet in many countries. So on this basis alone MDP consumption is likely to have important effects on various aspects of health (both positive and negative).

This is borne out by recent studies of health trends in different countries including the UK. Figures 14.1 and 14.2 show trends in meat and dairy consumption over the last 40 years. Over this period there has been little change in overall death rates from cancer, but there has been a significant fall in deaths from CVD. For example CVD death rates in adults aged under 75 have fallen by over 79 per cent between 1973 and 2013 (Townsend et al., 2015). This has been partly due to changes in diet

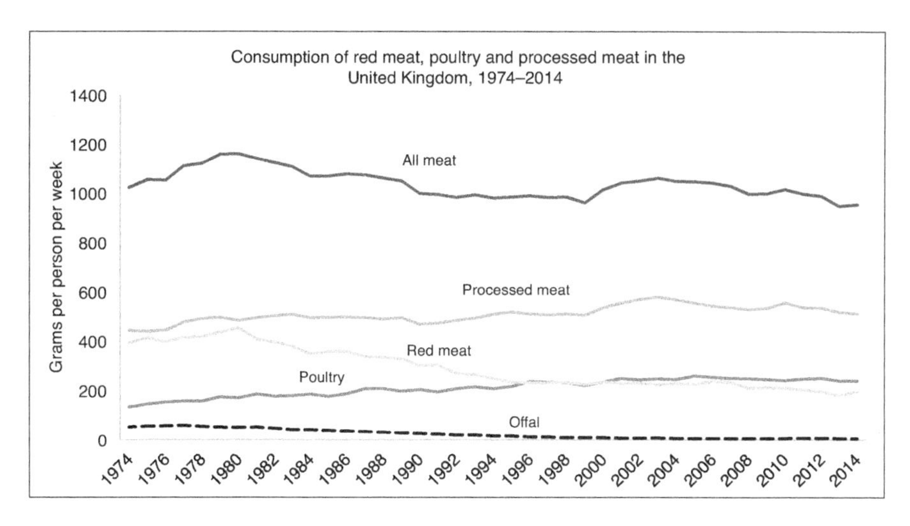

FIGURE 14.1 Consumption of red meat, poultry and processed meat in the United Kingdom, 1972–2014

Source: Department for Environment, Food and Rural Affairs (2016)

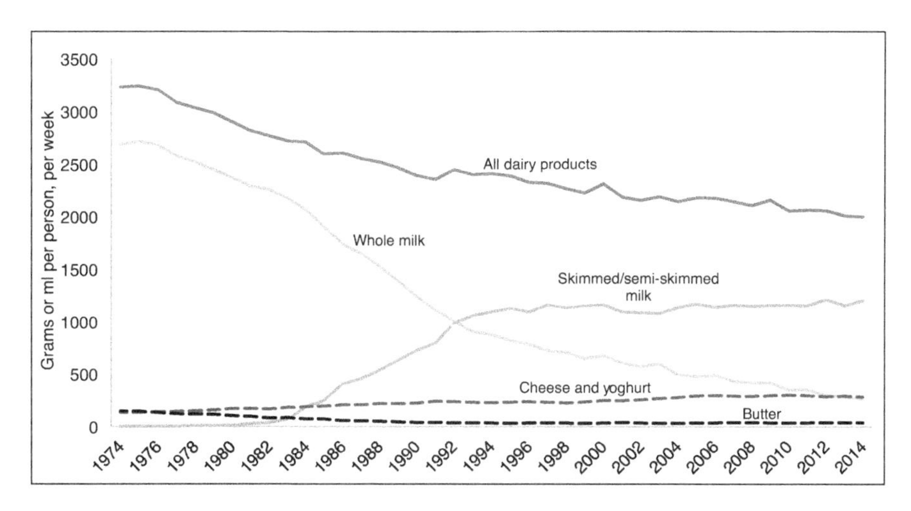

FIGURE 14.2 Consumption of whole milk, semi-skimmed milk, skimmed milk and processed dairy products in the United Kingdom, 1972–2014

Source: Department for Environment, Food and Rural Affairs (2016)

and in particular the reduced consumption of high-fat dairy products – principally whole milk and butter. People have switched from whole milk to semi-skimmed milk (Figure 14.2) and from butter to polyunsaturated spreads. Both of these 'switches' have led to a decline in saturated fat intake from 19 per cent to 14 per cent of total energy since 1975 (Townsend et al., 2015).

It is difficult to quantify exactly the contribution of these changes in MDP consumption to the decline in CVD mortality in the UK, but the contribution is likely to have been considerable. Changes in consumption of MDPs have had similar effects on CVD rates in other countries such as Finland, Norway, the Czech Republic and Poland. In Finland, where it has been possible to compare the contribution of both improvements in treatment for CHD and changes in diet and other lifestyle factors that affect the incidence of CHD, it has been shown that 33 per cent of the decline in CHD mortality observed there can be attributed to a decline in blood cholesterol levels, in turn largely associated with changes in MDP intake (Laatikainen et al., 2005).

Precisely what official bodies are saying about meat and dairy consumption

Despite the changing consensus around the health consequences of MDP consumption, it is only comparatively recently that official government departments and agencies have begun to suggest that MDP consumption is anything other than good for health. Moreover advice about MDP consumption has tended to be about switching from those products that are very high in saturated fat or salt to those that are less high, rather than to cut down on MDPs themselves.

However, very recently it has begun to be suggested that a reduction in MDP consumption, particularly meat, might be advisable. This has generally been in the context of an examination of what constitutes a diet that would be good for the environment as well as health. So for example in 2009 the Swedish Government recommended that people should eat less meat for environmental reasons noting, 'From a health perspective, there is also no reason to eat as much meat as we do today' (National Food Administration and Swedish Environmental Protection Agency, 2009). But despite growing awareness of the impact of food production and therefore consumption on environmental sustainability, authorities have been slow to follow the Swedish Government's example. A recent report from the Food Climate Research Network (FCRN) and the Food and Agriculture Organization (FAO) points out that only four countries have so far included sustainability as an objective of their food-based dietary guidelines: Brazil, Sweden, Qatar and Germany (Gonzalez Fischer and Garnett, 2016). Two countries (the US and Australia) have seen attempts to incorporate environmental considerations reach an advanced stage but have not achieved government endorsement. A few others discuss aspects of sustainability in accompanying supporting information and this now includes the UK (Public Health England, 2016).

An international collaboration of scientists supported by a consortium of funding bodies coordinated by the Wellcome Trust (whose findings were published in the *Lancet*) suggested that there would be considerable health benefits from food and agriculture strategies aimed at reducing greenhouse gas emissions (Friel et al., 2009). Margaret Chan, Director General of the World Health Organization (WHO), commenting on the article, stated that 'reduced consumption of animal products in developed countries would bring public health benefits' (Chan, 2009).

However, the WHO has yet to say this in its official reports. The definitive WHO statement on diet and health is still *Diet, Nutrition and the Prevention of Chronic Diseases* published in 2003 (WHO, 2003) with recent updates for guidelines on salt and carbohydrates (WHO, 2015) and new guidelines for fats, including saturated fat and trans-fats to be published later in 2017. *Diet, Nutrition and the Prevention of Chronic Diseases* merely notes that: 'Excessive consumption of animal products in some countries and social classes can lead to excessive intakes of fat'.

In the UK the most authoritative expert body on nutrition is the Government's Scientific Advisory Committee on Nutrition (SACN). SACN has not, to date, advised a reduction in average meat and/or dairy consumption in the UK. The closest it has got is to say: 'Lower consumption of red and processed meat would probably reduce the risk of colorectal cancer. Although the evidence is not conclusive, as a precaution, it may be advisable for intakes of red and processed meat not to increase above the current average (70g/day) and for high consumers of red and processed meat (100g/day or more) to reduce their intakes' (SACN, 2009). Moreover SACN have never argued that we need to cut down on MDPs themselves to reduce the risk of CVD. They have merely indicated a need to cut down on MDPs high in fat, particularly saturated fat and also salt (Department of Health, 1994).

However Public Health England – responsible for turning SACN's dietary recommendations for the UK population into advice for the general public – has recently revised the UK Government's official food-based dietary guidelines – the 'Eatwell Guide' (Public Health England, 2016), originally developed in the 1990s and then called the 'National Food Guide' (Hunt et al., 1995). The Eatwell Guide is a pie chart where the size of the segments represents the amount of foods that consumers should eat from each of five food groups: 'fruit and vegetables', 'potatoes, bread, rice, pasta and other starchy carbohydrates', 'beans, pulses, fish, eggs, meat and other proteins', 'dairy and alternatives', and 'oils and spreads' with another group – 'fatty and sugary foods' – placed outside the pie.

The Eatwell Guide indicates – perhaps unsurprisingly – that we need to eat more 'fruit and vegetables' and 'potatoes, bread, rice, pasta and other starchy carbohydrates' and less 'fatty and sugary foods'. But perhaps more surprisingly the new Eatwell Guide also indicates that reductions in the consumption of foods in the 'beans, pulses, fish, eggs, meat and other proteins' category by 24 per cent, and of foods in the 'dairy and alternatives' category by 29 per cent will also be necessary if all SACN's dietary recommendations (including new guidelines on sugar and fibre) are to be met (Scarborough et al., in preparation).

The analyses, involving optimization modelling, that we have done to support the development of the Eatwell Guide also suggest necessary changes in the consumption of particular MDPs including a reduction in red and processed meat consumption by 79 per cent but an increase in consumption of beans, pulses and other legumes by 86 per cent, a large reduction in consumption of cheese by 85 per cent but only a small reduction in milk consumption of 10 per cent (Scarborough et al., in preparation).

Conclusion

How then might we decide: 'How much meat and milk is optimal for health?' and 'What type of MDPs are optimal for health?' These are different, separate, but of course interrelated questions.

How much meat and milk is optimal for health?

Our discussion in this chapter about the positive and negative aspects of MDP consumption suggests that the costs and benefits to health from MDP consumption can be balanced against each other, and a consensus can therefore be achieved as to the exact level of meat and dairy consumption that should be recommended in order to gain optimal benefits with acceptable risk levels. In reality, this balancing of the positive and negative aspects is complicated. There are two main reasons for this.

First, human beings need to eat and drink to live, and MDPs represent only a proportion of the total number of foods and drinks that are available to meet energy and nutritional needs. The consumption of MDPs cannot be considered a closed system in which a change in consumption levels will have negligible impacts on other behaviours – rather, if consumption of MDPs is reduced, then consumption of other foods must increase and vice versa. Such displacement effects are not well understood but are likely to have a profound impact on the health effects of reducing or increasing MDP consumption. For example, successful vegans generally tend to have lower adverse health outcomes compared to the general population, which suggests that it is possible for some people to remove all MDPs from the diet and obtain the nutrients commonly found in MDPs from plant-based sources. However, not all people who remove MDPs from their diets, or to whom MDPs are unavailable, are successful at this replacement. There is another important aspect of this displacement effect: it may obscure some of the mechanisms for the relationship between MDP consumption and health. Adverse health outcomes associated with high MDP intake may in part be due to a related low intake of fruits and vegetables, for example. Adjustment for this potential confounding in observational studies is hindered by the difficulty of accurately measuring dietary intakes.

The second reason for the difficulty in balancing the positive and negative aspects of MDP consumption is that the positive health aspects tend to be about averting poor quality of life in the immediate term whereas the negative aspects tend to be about increased risk of mortality in the long term, and these two metrics are notoriously difficult to combine and compare. Methods have been developed that combine years of life lost due to early death and years of life lost in ill health within a single index (e.g. the disability adjusted life years lost (DALY)). But DALYs (and similar indices) have yet to be widely used to compare the positive and negative aspects of MDP consumption.

This all being said, it does seem likely that the negative consequences of eating large amounts of meat (and to a lesser extent dairy) in countries like the UK outweigh the positive benefits.

What type of meat and dairy products are optimal for health?

On the face of it this seems a simpler question. It seems clear that if we are to eat MDPs, then on a routine basis we should eat those products that are lower in saturated fat and salt, e.g. fresh meat rather than processed meat, semi-skimmed and skimmed milks rather than whole milk, etc. Furthermore, on the basis that it seems that red and processed meats eaten in excess, rather than white and unprocessed meats, increase the risk of disease, we might consider eating less of the former type of product and more of the latter (particularly if we are high meat consumers). It may also be worth paying some attention to new ideas about how grass-fed animals produce healthier MDPs than intensively reared animals.

How much and what type of meat and dairy products are optimal for our health and that of the planet?

But finally these questions: 'How much meat and dairy is optimal for health?' and 'What type of meat and dairy products are optimal for health?' need to be set in the context of the even more important question: 'How much and what type of MDP is optimal for our health *but also that of the planet*?' This is one of the most important questions for our time. It is clear that greenhouse gas emissions are strongly correlated with the production and thereby consumption of MDPs (see Garnett's chapter in this book). We have estimated that vegan diets in the UK have half the carbon footprint of meat-based diets and also (importantly) that diets with high levels of meat consumption (>100g/d) are the cause of over 50 per cent more greenhouse gas emissions than diets with low levels of meat consumption (<50g/d) (Scarborough et al., 2014). Globally, our recent analysis suggests that '[t]ransitioning toward more plant-based diets that are in line with standard dietary guidelines could reduce global mortality by 6–10% and food-related greenhouse gas emissions by 29–70% compared with a reference scenario in 2050'. However it is also clear that significant changes in the global food system will be necessary for this to happen and that this will be a challenge to us all (Springmann et al., 2016).

References

Aburto, N.J., Ziolkovska, A., Hooper, L., Elliott, P., Cappuccio, F.P., and Meerpohl, J.J. (2013) 'Effect of lower sodium intake on health: Systematic review and meta-analyses', *BMJ*, vol 346, pp1326.

Alexander, D.D., Bylsma, L.C., Vargas, A.J., Cohen, S.S., Doucette, A., Mohamed, M., Irvin, S.R., Miller, P.E., Watson, H., and Fryzek, J.P. (2016) 'Dairy consumption and CVD: A systematic review and meta-analysis', *British Journal of Nutrition*, vol 115, no 4, pp737–750.

Bouvard, V., Loomis, D., Guyton, K.Z., Grosse, Y., El Ghissassi, F., Benbrahim-Tallaa, L., Guha, N., Mattock, H., and Straif, K. (2015) 'Carcinogenicity of consumption of red and processed meat', *The Lancet Oncology*, vol 16, pp1599–1600.

Cannon, G. (2003) The Fate of Nations: Food and Nutrition Policy in the New World, The Caroline Walker Trust, London.

Chan, M. (2009) 'Cutting carbon, improving health', *The Lancet*, vol 374, no 9705, pp1870–1871.

Department for Environment, Food and Rural Affairs (2016) 'Family food statistics' available from www.gov.uk/government/statistical-data-sets/family-food-datasets, last accessed 1 June 2016.

Department of Health (1991) *Dietary Reference Values for Food Energy and Nutrients for the United Kingdom*, Report on Health and Social Subjects 41, HMSO, London.

Department of Health (1994) *Nutritional Aspects of Cardiovascular Disease*, Report on Health and Social Subjects 46, HMSO, London.

Fiddes, N. (1991) *Meat: A Natural Symbol*, Routledge, London.

Friel, S., Dangour, A., Garnett, T., Lock, K., Chalabi, Z., Roberts, I., Butler, A., Butler, C., Waage, J., McMichael A.J., and Haines, A. (2009) 'Public health benefits of strategies to reduce greenhouse-gas emissions: Food and agriculture', *Lancet*, vol 374, no 9706, pp145–152.

Givens, D.I. (2005) 'The role of animal nutrition in improving the nutritive value of animal derived foods in relation to chronic disease', *Proceedings of the Nutrition Society*, vol 64, pp395–402.

Gonzalez Fischer, C., and Garnett, T. (2016) *Plates, Pyramids and Planets: Developments in National Healthy and Sustainable Dietary Guidelines: A State of Play Assessment*, FAO and the University of Oxford, Oxford.

Hooper, L., Martin, N., Abdelhamid, A., and Davey Smith, G. (2015) 'Reduction in saturated fat intake for cardiovascular disease.' *Cochrane Database of Systematic Reviews* 2015, no 6, Art. No.: CD011737.

Hunt, P., Rayner, M., and Gatenby, S.J. (1995) 'A national food guide for the UK? Background and development', *Journal of Human Nutrition and Dietetics*, vol 8, pp315–322.

Institute for Health Metrics and Evaluation (IHME) (2015) 'GBD compare'. Seattle, WA: IHME, University of Washington, available from http://vizhub.healthdata.org/gbd-compare, last accessed 1 June 2016.

Kaluza, J., Wolk, A., and Larsson, S.C. (2012) 'Red meat consumption and risk of stroke. A meta-analysis of prospective studies', *Stroke*, vol 43, no 10, pp2556–2560.

Key, T.J., Fraser, G.E., Thorogood, M., Appleby, P.N., Beral, V., Reeves, G., Burr, M.I., Chang-Claude, J., Frentzel-Beyme, R., Kuzma, J.W., Mann, J., and McPherson, K. (1999) 'Mortality in vegetarians and nonvegetarians: Detailed findings from a collaborative analysis of 5 prospective studies', *American Journal of Clinical Nutrition*, vol 70, pp516S–524S.

Laatikainen, T., Critchley, J., Vartianen, E., Saloma, V., Ketonen, M., and Capwell, S. (2005) 'Explaining the decline in coronary heart disease mortality in Finland between 1982 and 1997', *American Journal of Epidemiology*, vol 162, pp764–773.

Larsson, S., and Orsini, N. (2014) 'Red meat and processed meat consumption and all-cause mortality: A meta-analysis', *American Journal of Epidemiology*, vol 179, pp282–289.

McKee, F. (1997) 'The popularisation of milk as beverage during the 1930s', in Smith, D.E. (ed.) *Nutrition in Britain*, Routledge, London, pp123–139.

Mann, J. (2009) 'Vegetarian diets: Health benefits are not necessarily unique but there may be ecological advantages', *BMJ*, vol 339, pp525–526.

Micha, R., Michas, G. and Mozaffarian, D. (2012). 'Unprocessed red and processed meats and risk of coronary artery disease and type 2 diabetes: An updated review of the evidence. *Current Atherosclerosis Reports*, vol 14, no 6, pp515–524.

Millward, D.J., and Garnett, T. (2010) 'Food and the planet: Nutritional dilemmas of greenhouse gas emission reductions through reduced intakes of meat and dairy foods', *Proceedings of the Nutrition Society*, vol 69, pp103–118, Cambridge University Press, doi: 10.1017/S0029665109991868

Mozaffarian, D., Katan, M.B., Ascherio, A., Stampfer, M.J., and Willett, C. (2006) 'Trans fatty acid and cardiovascular disease', *New England Journal of Medicine*, vol 354, pp1601–1613.

NatCen Social Research, MRC Human Nutrition Research and University College London Medical School (2015) *National Diet and Nutrition Survey Years 1–4, 2008/09–2011/12*. Public Health England and Food Standards Agency, London.

National Food Administration and Swedish Environmental Protection Agency (2009) The National Food Administration's Environmentally Effective Food Choices: Proposal Notified to the EU, NFA, Stockholm.

Public Health England (2016) 'The eatwell guide' available from www.gov.uk/government/publications/the-eatwell-guide, last accessed 1 June 2016.

SACN (2009) *Iron and Health*, SACN, London.

Scarborough, P., Appleby, P.N., Mizdrak, A., Briggs, A.D.M., Travis, R.C., Bradbury, K.E., and Key, T.J. (2014). 'Dietary greenhouse gas emissions of meat-eaters, fish-eaters, vegetarians and vegans in the UK', *Climatic Change*, vol 125, no 2, pp179–192.

Scarborough, P., Kaur, A., Cobiac, L., Owens, P., Parlesak, A., Sweeney, K., and Rayner, M. (2016). 'The Eatwell Guide: modelling the dietary and cost implications of incorporating new sugar and fibre guidelines', *BMJ Open*, vol 6, no 12, p.e013182. doi:10.1136/bmjopen-2016-013182.

Scarborough, P., Nnoaham, K., Clarke, D., Capewell, S., and Rayner, M. (2012) 'Modelling the impact of a healthy diet on cardiovascular disease and cancer mortality', *Journal of Epidemiology and Community Health*, vol 66, no 5, pp420–426.

Skeaff, C.M., and Miller, J. (2009) 'Dietary fat and coronary heart diseases: Summary of evidence from prospective cohort and randomised controlled trials', *Annals of Nutrition and Metabolism*, vol 55, pp173–201.

Souza, R.J.de, Mente, A., Maroleanu, A., Cozma A.I., Ha, V., Kishibe, T., Uleryk, E., Budylowski, P., Schünemann, H., Beyene, J., and Anand, S.S. (2015) 'Intake of saturated and trans unsaturated fatty acids and risk of all cause mortality, cardiovascular disease, and type 2 diabetes: Systematic review and meta-analysis of observational studies', *BMJ*, vol 35, pp3978.

Springmann, M., Godfray, H.C., Rayner, M., and Scarborough, P. (2016) 'Analysis and valuation of the health and climate change cobenefits of dietary change', *Proceedings of the National Academy of Sciences of the United States of America*, vol 113, pp4146–4151.

Townsend, N., Bhatnagar P., Wilkins, E., Wickramasinghe, K., and Rayner, M. (2015) *Cardiovascular Disease Statistics 2015*, British Heart Foundation, London.

Von Liebig, J. (1846) *Animal Chemistry*, Scholarly Publishing Office, University of Michigan Library; 3 Revised edition (13 September 2006), available from http://tinyurl.com/397tgua, last accessed 25 May 2010.

Von Liebig, J. (1847) *Researches on the Chemistry of Food*, Taylor and Walton, London, available from http://tinyurl.com/37ev953, last accessed 24 May 2010.

WCRF/AICR (1997) *Food, Nutrition, Physical Activity and the Prevention of Cancer: A Global Perspective*, World Cancer Research Fund/American Institute for Cancer Research, Washington DC.

WCRF/AICR (2007) *Food, Nutrition, Physical Activity and the Prevention of Cancer: A Global Perspective*, World Cancer Research Fund/American Institute for Cancer Research, Washington, DC.

WHO (2003) *Diet, Nutrition and the Prevention of Chronic Diseases*, WHO Technical Report Series, No 916, WHO, Geneva.

WHO (2007) *Protein and Amino Acid Requirements in Human Nutrition*, Report of a Joint WHO/FAO/UNU Expert Consultation, WHO Technical Report Series, No 724, WHO, Geneva.

WHO (2015) 'Healthy diet' available from www.who.int/mediacentre/factsheets/fs394/en, last accessed 1 June 2016.

PART IV

Politics, philosophy and economics

15

DEVELOPING ETHICAL, SUSTAINABLE AND COMPASSIONATE FOOD POLICIES

Kate Rawles

Introduction

The anthropologist nervously stroked her antennae. The renewal – or not – of her research grant most likely depended on what she said next.

'And the update on Earth food production systems?'

The request came from the chief Martian Institute Research Coordinator himself. This was it.

'Well', she began, 'we have observed very different patterns of food consumption emerging over the last hundred or so Earth years. Some sectors of Earth human population are especially intriguing, and it is these sectors I believe warrant further study'.

'Go on', the chief said.

The anthropologist flicked through her files.

'We have observed', she said, hesitantly, 'a very substantial rise in the consumption of "meat" – flesh from deceased animals – across a range of human populations, largely facilitated by changes in farming technology. What many of these Earth beings have now realized, however', she said, warming to her theme, 'is that this rise in meat consumption, initially thought to be beneficial, is generating multiple interlocking problems. These include human health issues, such as ischaemic heart disease, obesity and possibly cancers as well as aggravated incidence of zoonotic diseases, such as swine flu. In addition, meat production as practiced in the societies under observation is highly water intensive and, typically, extremely inefficient in relation to land use, thus exacerbating pressure on critical resources at a time when both human populations and resource scarcity are increasing. The systems in question are also extremely negative in relation to the welfare of the beings who are "produced". And, perhaps most significantly, recent research by Earth scientists themselves has revealed that the production of meat, especially from ruminants, is one of the largest single contributors to anthropogenic climate change. This climate change is on a trajectory predicted to cause the extinction of about one half of Earth's current suite of species and widespread resource conflict, death and displacement of the human species, by the end of the Earth century. Many negative impacts will of course occur well in advance of that and a significant number are already underway. In our view, as well as that of Earth scientists, it is not clear that Earth's human societies can survive this degree of climate change. They certainly cannot in their current form'.

'Fascinating, indeed', the chief MIRC acknowledged. 'Presumably your research interest lies in assessing the efficacy of the humans' strategies for radically restructuring their current food systems and reversing their adverse consequences?'

'No', the anthropologist replied. 'That is precisely the point. It lies in our discovery – quite unique in my cosmic career – that this species appears intent on acting against its own interests. All these problems could be greatly reduced, if not resolved, by eating non-animal derivatives – without loss of nutritional content. Yet, despite humanity's rapidly burgeoning knowledge and understanding of these issues, and notwithstanding their reasonably well-developed analytical brains (by outer arm Milky Way standards at least) and even an average compassion rating (ironically especially well developed in relation to large animals with eyes), dominant sectors of these societies are not only maintaining but even increasing their own meat consumption, as well as exporting it to previously low-meat consumption sectors of the Earth community as a desirable norm'.

'Cosmos above!' the chief MIRC said, visibly astonished. 'What is the likelihood of this policy – if it can be called a policy – being reversed?'

'In our view, that greatly depends on the frequency with which the occasional and highly fortuitous Earth economic "credit crunches" recur, allowing a rare window of opportunity for intervention in the typically rather blind allegiance to a largely market-led system by principled, compassionate, farsighted, scientifically informed ethicists creating and taking up positions of influence within a greatly strengthened International Food Policy decision making board'.

'Unlikely, in other words', said the chief MIRC. 'I see. Grant application request extended – we can clearly learn more about the features of fatally flawed decision-making processes from this research. Meanwhile, memo to security: advise in the strongest terms that we continue to reprogram all satellite imagery in order to foil attempts by Earth scientists to find our community here on Mars. Record of peaceful interactions by Earth beings with benign cultures, particularly under times of resource stress, is exceedingly poor. Next applicant!'

★★★

The first step in developing ethical, sustainable and compassionate food policies is to acknowledge that we need them. In the 2006 Stern Report, Sir (now Lord) Nicholas Stern famously described anthropogenic climate change as the greatest market failure ever witnessed. Climate change, he argued, can be seen as the disastrous but unintended outcome of millions of consumer choices made in a relatively unregulated market shaped largely by short-term economic priorities – in the wider context, as analysts like Naomi Klein have since added, of a pro-consumption, pro-growth, aggressively neoliberal socio-economic worldview. Stern is not a critic of pro-growth world views, but he does argue strongly, along with Klein and others, that tackling climate change will require systematic and rigorous intervention in market-led systems, in the light of a very different set of priorities.

Stern might have made similar points about high levels of meat consumption had he been studying it and had he had the good fortune to view the issue with the clarity and lack of bias of a detached Martian observer, as opposed to the somewhat distorted perspective occasionally associated with the vested interests of, for example, a meat eater resident on Earth. The outcome of millions of consumer choices, made in a socio-economic context in which, for various reasons and in various ways, meat eating is encouraged, advertised and advocated, has led to a situation in which meat production and consumption in its current form is a major contributor to a suite of serious problems, as sketched at the beginning of this chapter and explored throughout this book. Nobody has deliberately set out to create this system, but this is the system we have. The idea that ethical, sane approaches to food production will spontaneously emerge from it – from the 'free' market – with a bit of consumer education and product labelling is, unfortunately, delusional. If we are to reorient food production along sane, sustainable, compassionate and ethical lines then we need to intervene. In what follows, I will sketch out the principles and values that should, arguably, guide this intervention.

The triple crunch context

The 2008–2013 recession, and the 'credit crunch' that initiated it, dominated the news for years, and took centre stage in political activity from local to global. As the main focus of several G20 summits, world leaders grappled with the implications of global recession, not least in relation to what rising unemployment, rising inequity and a slowdown in economic growth actually mean in terms of human lives and human suffering. But a number of analysts argued compellingly that the credit crunch would prove as nothing compared to the impacts of climate change or the so-called 'nature crunch' more generally.

When Stern published the climate change report mentioned earlier, he essentially overturned the last argument against robust action on climate change that had any shred of credibility. He did this by demonstrating that the economic costs of letting climate change rip and mopping up the damage would vastly outweigh the costs of taking action now to try to mitigate its worst effects. Since then, the scientific evidence on which those conclusions were based has been revealed as optimistic – including by Stern himself. The predictions in terms of average global temperature rise, and the likely impacts of this on social, financial, ecological and climactic systems, have systematically worsened. The good news is that we now have global consensus on anthropogenic climate change as a serious threat that must be tackled; and an historic agreement at the 2015 Paris climate negotiations that average global temperature increase be kept at most to 2 degrees above pre-industrial levels and, ideally, 1.5 degrees.[1] Even assuming the agreed emissions reductions are enacted, though, the current deal would still commit us to between 2.7 and 3 degrees of warming. The commitment to reconvene every five years and negotiate a 'ratcheting up' of emissions reduction gives hope that the 2 degrees target can still be met. But there is no doubt that even 2 degrees will bring extremely serious consequences, including the loss of a number of small island states and exacerbation of the climate change impacts we've already experienced, such as extreme weather events and consequent disruption to lives and livelihoods. In terms of species extinction, droughts, floods, desertification, impacts on agriculture, sea level rise, impacts on fresh water, spread of disease, displacement of people, resource conflict and human security generally, we really don't want to contemplate 3 degrees.

Climate change, for all its seriousness, is not the only critical environmental issue we face. Human encroachment on habitat, not least for agriculture, is contributing to 'the sixth great extinction', with the United Nations, amongst others, stating that our mid- to long-term survival is now genuinely in doubt because of the impact of the way we acquire our resources on biodiversity and ecological systems. Rockstrom and his team have endeavored to calculate the implications of this impact on what he calls 'the safe operating space for humanity' across a range of environmental issues, several of which we've already breached. And this in turn has already seriously compromised the aims of reducing malnutrition and other aspects of absolute poverty as set out, for example, in the Millennium Development Goals (now the Sustainable Development Goals). The credit crunch is indeed nothing to the nature crunch, even if our politicians and the media might have it the other way around.

In short, considering the increases in human poverty and inequality that these combined economic and environmental issues are delivering right now; a cluster of research concluding that inequality *per se* (i.e. independently of the absolute position of the worst off) has significant negative impacts on human health and well-being; the predicted impacts of climate change and other anthropogenic environmental issues on human and other-than-human lives and well-being; and the ongoing fragility and volatility of the global economy, it makes sense to talk about a triple crunch: economic, environmental and social. And this emphasizes, yet again, that the need for humans to get their collective act together in relation to sustainable development – often characterized in terms of the sustainability triangle, with economy, environment and society as its three points (see later in the chapter) – is absolutely compelling.

Why animals?

Implementing actions and policies to deal with climate change and other urgent environmental issues is – at least in theory! – relatively easy to justify. Preserving our own habitat is clearly in our own interests, even if it has taken us a while to figure this out (and not that this conclusion has exactly been dominating mainstream political activity). But why should we be concerned about compassion and ethics in relation to animals? On the face of it, whether or not farm animals, for example, live out their lives in poor conditions, does not appear to affect our own human lives very much at all. The animal welfare agenda attempts to implement the ethical obligations that we have towards *other* sentient beings; to make compassion for other animals systematic and practical. This has positive implications for how many millions of real animals live and die but may appear irrelevant to human interests. Add the concern about climate change, and the priority this issue is at last beginning to receive, as well as the consistently prioritized economic growth agenda, and it is easy to see how concern with animal welfare is often marginalized. It is not unusual to hear the argument that animal welfare is something we must trade off against more urgent concerns: a luxury that, in the current economic and environmental context, we have to relinquish as simply unaffordable.

In the rest of this chapter, I will argue that this is deeply mistaken. High standards of animal welfare are, or should be, a core value of food animal production and one that – alongside environmental, climate and human health and well-being concerns – should guide the ethically appropriate recrafting of our food policies. They are also a critical, if often neglected, dimension of sustainable development more generally. Indeed, far from being a luxury, I will argue that dealing with poor animal welfare, or at least the mindset that legitimizes it, is a necessity. For it is precisely this mindset that has given us the nature crunch and the credit crunch. And, to paraphrase that much used Einstein quote, 'You can't solve a problem with the same kind of thinking that caused it'.

Animal welfare should be a core value – two arguments

I will sketch two arguments, the first to do with sustainable development and the second to do with problematic mindsets.

Animal welfare and sustainable development

To paraphrase something that Roland Bonney (a Director of the Food Animal Initiative, Oxford) once said: sustainable development is about being able to do tomorrow what you can do today. Fine as far it goes, as he pointed out. But today's societies, complete with gross inequity and unacceptable levels of poverty – a little under one in five people across the world currently lack clean drinking water and basic nourishment – could certainly be around tomorrow. And this clearly shows that sustainable development is not just about 'carrying on'. It is about carrying on in a way that manifests our core values as civilized societies. Or, remembering Gandhi's famous quip, 'what do I think about Western civilization? I think it would be a good idea', sustainable development is *ethically aspirational*. It is about the values we *want* societies to manifest, the values we consider critical if we are to continue our residence on Earth in civilized, humane and meaningful ways.

The core values of sustainable development are often represented as points on a triangle – or legs on a three-legged stool (see Figure 15.1).

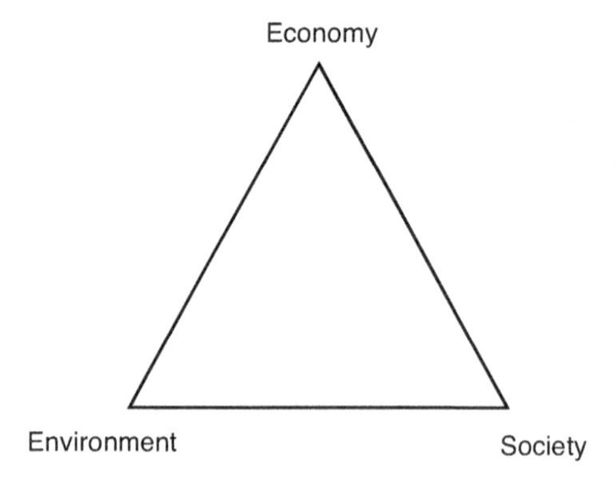

FIGURE 15.1 The sustainable development triangle

What is striking from the perspective of this chapter is, as I have argued elsewhere, that on this model, concern with animal welfare doesn't really fit anywhere. Economic development is (or is supposed to be) in the interests of meeting human needs and improving human quality of life. The 'society' end of the triangle represents values to do with equity, within and between generations, as well as the opportunity for meaningful participation in social and political institutions – again between humans. And 'environment' is concerned with protecting resources for people or, on less anthropocentric interpretations, coexisting with other species and ecosystems, valued in their own right as well as in relation to their undeniable usefulness to ourselves. On either interpretation, the environmental focus is on 'ecological collectives' of various kinds. But the concern with animal welfare is a concern with animals as individuals rather than as species or part of ecosystems; and it is a concern with animals that are typically domesticated or tamed rather than wild. Animal welfare does not naturally fit any point of the sustainable development triangle, and, although this may be changing, it has often been excluded from mainstream sustainable development rhetoric, concerns and policies.

We've already argued that sustainable development is ethically aspirational. Indeed, with its focus on dealing with poverty and intergenerational equity, sustainable development has ethics at its very core. But there is a whole flock of arguments to the effect that restricting ethics exclusively to inter-human concerns makes no rational sense, ranging from Peter Singer's condemnation of 'speciesism' to Mary Midgley's 'animals are part of our community' approach.[2] I can't review these here but suffice it to say that, if sustainable development is ethically aspirational (and, if it isn't, it is of highly dubious value) then the humane treatment of the animals we use for our own purposes and that we are responsible for in relation to farming, pet-keeping and so on must surely be included. What counts as 'humane' is then another debate, of course. But if there is a non-speciesist argument to the effect that

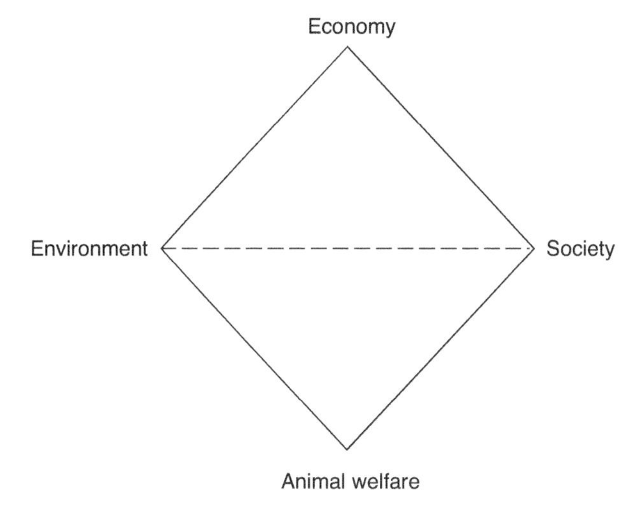

FIGURE 15.2 The sustainable development diamond

humane treatment of animals in our care is irrelevant, I'd be really interested to read it. Meanwhile, I argue that we should adapt the sustainable development triangle to a diamond, with animal welfare as the fourth point (see Figure 15.2). Without it, a key ethical commitment, and one that affects billions of sentient beings, can simply be overlooked.[3]

Of course, there is a further ethical issue here about the legitimacy of both domestication and animal-based agriculture. Tom Regan (1985), for example, maintains that campaigning for improved farm animal welfare is as ethically misguided as working to improve the well-being of slaves.[4] In both cases, he believes, the institution should be abolished. Doing justice to this argument is beyond the scope of this chapter and the abolition of domestication in general and farmed animals in particular is clearly a long way off. Moreover, even if Regan were right that this should be our ultimate aim, it certainly wouldn't follow that poor animal welfare in existing (pre-abolition) farms would be acceptable in the interim.

Instrumental thinking underpins the triple crunches – and the dismissal of animal welfare as a luxury

Various philosophers and other commentators have discussed 'instrumental rationality' as part of the mindset that has its roots in Enlightenment thinking and that has proved to be, to say the least, a double-edged sword. On the plus side, it has allowed us to develop fantastically efficient systems and greatly increased production, in agriculture amongst other contexts. But the negatives are stacking up to the point of being overwhelming.

Instrumental rationality or 'means/end' thinking focuses on one particular value, or suite of values, most commonly economic growth and/or profit, often in the short term. It then looks at the world, and everything in it, entirely from this perspective. Thus the environment is viewed as a set of resources to be managed for human gain rather than as a complex, living system on which we utterly depend and of which we are a part; people are viewed as workers or resources of other kinds, or irrelevant; farm animals are viewed as cogs in a machine designed with the aim of turning animal fodder into human food as efficiently as possible. In other words, a whole host of beings are considered, well, instrumentally – as a means to the end of economic growth, often in ways that are typically detrimental to their own well-being. From this perspective, more or less anything becomes acceptable in the efficient pursuit of profit or economic growth (to stay with that example), and other values – such as environmental protection, social welfare or animal welfare – are *all* overridden as luxuries we can't afford.

A current example of concern about this kind of means/end thinking is the fear expressed by numerous NGOs, campaign bodies and other commentators that the proposed Transatlantic Trade and Investment Partnership (TTIP) will, via the slashing of regulatory barriers to trade, render it increasingly difficult for states to legislate on environmental and social issues, with dire results. It is a supreme example of the neoliberal model of unfettered global markets in action and a classic example of instrumental rationality. The justification usually offered in its defence – until recently almost unchallengeable without being labelled a lunatic – is that only with increasingly unfettered markets can we achieve continuous economic growth, and only with continuing economic growth can we tackle poverty (despite the mass of evidence that, decades of growth notwithstanding, the poorest have remained poor) or, even more bizarrely, that only with economic growth can we afford to fix the environment.

This kind of thinking has its place. As indicated above, it has facilitated, for example, increased productivity across a range of contexts. But when it becomes dominant, in the way that it has in modern industrialized societies, the result is a focus on one set of values that are too limited and that are pursued at the expense of myriad other values of critical importance. This kind of means/end, instrumental thinking has delivered us economic systems that have become increasingly divorced from 'real wealth' as well as from the values such as trust, openness, honesty, accountability and caring that turn out to be crucial to the sustainable functioning of the economic system itself. This kind of thinking has overridden the need to look after the ecological systems we are part of to the extent that climate change and biodiversity loss now threaten our own survival as a species – let alone that of millions of the other species we coexist with. It has led us to ignore the inconvenient truth that our current model of indefinite resource-based growth is totally at odds with the reality of living on a planet that has ecological limits – limits to space, to resources, to the capacity to absorb pollution. And it has given us the kind of intensive systems that systematically deny animals basic welfare as outlined, for example, in the Five Freedoms (see later in the chapter).

If we are to deal with the nature crunch, the credit crunch, the poverty crunch and the welfare crunch – if we are to move towards sustainable development in any meaningful sense of that term – we absolutely have to challenge this kind of thinking, not legitimize it in yet another guise. The view that animal welfare is a luxury we can't afford and should be overridden to achieve economic and environmental priorities is precisely a case in point: a clear example of means/end, instrumental thinking, with appalling practical consequences for the billions of animals that go through our farming systems every year. Instead of seeking to ease our economic and environmental problems by compromising on animal welfare – a bit like responding to the knowledge that a loud noise is making us deaf by turning the sound up – we need to tackle the problematic thinking that underpins all of these problems, in the full understanding that they are not separate, but profoundly interconnected, issues.

A wiser worldview

What, then, is the way forward? First, we need to insist that our food production systems be shaped by other values beyond efficiency in profit production. The way we produce our food is not just another industry. Food production is critical to our health and well-being, and the systems we put in place to produce our food have immense impacts upon the health and well-being of the animals involved, as well as on the wider environment – on other living beings, species, ecological systems. Human health, environmental well-being, good animal welfare – these are all important values that our systems for providing us with food need to embody and reflect, not displace in the name of efficiency. Food production should not be – *cannot* be if we are to continue our tenancy on planet Earth – just a question of efficiency. It plays a critical role in sustainable development and it urgently needs to be reoriented along explicitly ethical lines.

The second point, as Stern, Klein and others have argued in the climate change context, is that we can't expect ethical and sustainable food production systems to be delivered by the market. The market cannot deliver unaided in this way, for reasons we've outlined above. We need to intervene; to intentionally reorient our food production systems in relation to a much richer and more appropriate set of values than it currently serves, in the context of a saner, wiser worldview.

What would such a worldview entail? We can develop this by looking briefly at the problematic one in a little more detail. Scratch the surface of modern industrialized societies and, alongside the predominance of means/end thinking, you find a whole set of attitudes, beliefs and assumptions that add up to an implicit worldview. Once this worldview is made explicit, our stunningly unsustainable approach to meeting our needs suddenly appears much less surprising. Indeed it is hard to see how societies with this kind of conceptual underpinning could be anything *other* than unsustainable.

In the current context, four interconnected aspects of this worldview merit particular comment. First, as already argued, this is a worldview that typically understands the Earth and everything in it as a vast repository of resources for the sole benefit of humans. In relation to the other-than-human world, instrumental thinking is supreme. Second, these resources have often been assumed to be infinite. Take these together and, in Ray Anderson's (2007) words, you get a picture of the world 'as a sort of gigantic production system, capable of producing ever-increasing outputs'. Third comes the particularly bizarre phenomenon I've referred to as the 'allotment mindset'. This is the belief that humans are somehow *outside* ecological systems. Ecological systems – the 'environment' in general – are out there, like a vast allotment, and we stride out and take from them when we need to. But we are not really *in* them. An extraordinary techno-optimism often accompanies this belief, to the effect that, even if Earth's resources turn out not to be infinite after all, we don't need to worry because we will find ways of manufacturing our own resources. So long, Earth, and thanks for all the fish – but now we can make our own. Fourth, and clearly rooted in the previous aspects of the modern, industrial worldview, is the view that not only is increasing consumption of resources (by increasing numbers of people) unproblematic; it is to be encouraged. If we accept this worldview, then growth of consumption leads to growth of economy and economic growth is good. Indeed it is, as we have seen, our overriding aim and number one value. It is certainly not a problem. Economic growth, premised on continuously increased consumption, can and should continue indefinitely; it is the best and only way of ensuring high standards of living for all.

The outline characteristics of a saner, wiser worldview, and the ethics that would follow from it, will by now be obvious. For a start, we need to challenge our own out-of-control human-centrism. Of course the environment is a resource for humans and, like all species, we have to relate to it partly in this way. But it is not only a resource. The vast complex of astonishing diversity, energy and sheer will to live that is 'the environment' has value far beyond its usefulness to us. Basking sharks and blue tits, savannah and rainforests, clouds, stars and streams – as well as cats, dogs, cattle and pigs – have value beyond the extent to which one species amongst millions happens to need them. To deny this is to take an astonishingly arrogant stance, positioning humans as the only species of true worth and the rest of relevance only in relation to ourselves. This is a pre-Copernican view of ethics: the values equivalent of believing that the sun spins around the Earth.

In addition, we need to acknowledge and fully understand that we are part of ecological systems, not apart from them. We are not on the outside looking in. Our experience of life may distance us from the reality that all our basic needs are sourced in planet Earth and its ecological and physical systems. But however many layers of technical brilliance intervene between natural resources and our end products, we cannot detach ourselves from our ultimate dependence on Earth ecology. For all our technology, we remain earthbound creatures, relying on ecological systems for our basic needs, including food, as the reports of the Millennium Ecosystem Assessment, the UN, WWF and others have all made shockingly clear. Finally, and crucially, we have to acknowledge that Earth's biophysical systems have limits. We cannot, as modern societies have assumed we can – and astonishingly some forms of farming have to be included here – simply ignore biophysical realities and endlessly extract resources at one end and produce pollution at the other without consequence. We need to reorient the way we live and meet our needs so that we can live within biophysical limits, not endeavour to ignore them.

This is where many part company with Stern. His analysis of the climate change problem is compelling but he only has part of the solution. Stern believes we can simply (well, not simply, but we can) decouple the economy from carbon and continue to grow. Continue with the same mindset, the same instrumentalizing view of the Earth and other living things (including people); the same commitment to growth that, even if it acknowledges limits to Earth's capacity to absorb carbon, fails to acknowledge there are limits to space; to the Earth's capacity to absorb other forms of pollution; to ecological systems' ability to continue to function even as we decimate the species that make them up. In sum, not only is the challenge of decoupling the economy from carbon actually, in the context of increasing consumption and increasing human population, immense beyond Stern's recognition as Monbiot and others point out; the Earth has other limits too. We cannot grow indefinitely on a finite planet. It is already the case that, as World Wildlife Fund (WWF) has so powerfully expressed it, if everyone on Earth lived the lifestyle of an average Western European, we would need three planet Earths. Yet this is the lifestyle whose consumer-oriented material values underpin what is meant by 'development', 'success' and 'progress' and are exported around the world as something to be emulated. As a recent Chatham House report (amongst others) states, the production of meat in industrialized countries and the predicted global rise in meat consumption is in itself one of the biggest impediments to climate change safety we face: a seriously neglected issue at the 2015 Paris climate negotiations. Meat production in turn needs to be understood as embedded in agricultural systems that are profoundly unsustainable, that are themselves embedded in industrialized cultures whose concepts of progress and success are profoundly unsustainable and that have set human societies on a trajectory that is, literally, self-destructive.

Crucially, then, we need a worldview that supports a different set of values. Values that emphasize quality of life rather than a materialistic high standard of living, and values that acknowledge the worth of people, animals and environment in their own right, not just as a set of resources to service out of control industrialized growth economies. We need to get a grip of our runaway market-led system that exemplifies instrumental, means/end thinking, that is embedded in a deeply flawed worldview and that has delivered us the range of interconnected problems sketched above. We need to reshape the current system, along firmly ethical, values-led lines, in the context of a wiser, saner worldview as sketched in this section – fully realizing our own interdependence with other living things, understanding ourselves as part of a wider ecological and community (and one that includes our domesticated animals) rather than as detached managers of a set of resources and aspiring towards a very different conception of quality of life than the current materialistically conceived understanding of a what 'high' standard of living entails.[5]

An outline ethical framework

To translate this wiser, saner, compassionate worldview into actionable ethical policies, I suggest we need a quadruple bottom line approach – in keeping with the sustainability diamond.

The quadruple bottom line would make positive recommendations and some core prohibitions. Policies would be judged against their positive and negative contributions to:

- Environmental values – with a range of indicators here in relation to biodiversity, ecosystem integrity, climate change, other forms of pollution reduction and so on.
- Social values – with a focus on reducing inequality across current generations; increasing participation; and developing less materialistic, conceptions of quality of life (which could also be more fulfilling).
- Economic values – with a refocusing on the core aim of meeting human needs both now and in the future (and a big issue here in relation to distinguishing real needs from wants or luxuries).
- Animal welfare values – articulated, for example, in relation to the Five Freedoms or similar.

This approach would recognize these as discrete if interconnected values, rather than attempt to reduce them to one core value, and it would pursue them all. It would *prohibit* policies, actions and activities if they violated core principles in any area, for example, if they caused serious environmental degradation, or violated human rights or significantly increased inequity or entailed bad animal welfare. It would *recommend* policies to the extent that they contribute positively.

Clearly, there will sometimes need to be trade-offs, but this would be done on a case-by-case approach, and trade-offs would not be acceptable in relation to core prohibitions. So, for example, violating human rights in the interests of economic development or environmental protection would not be permitted, nor would seriously degrading the environment in the interests of economic development and so on. If any one value *were* to take priority it would need to be environmental – as, beyond a rapidly approaching point, environmental degradation will render all other values unachievable.

Interestingly, core prohibitions in relation to the environment are in fact quite hard to establish in more than general terms. Clearly, the degradation of ecological systems, the loss of biodiversity and various kinds of pollution will all need to be included; but identifying what actually counts as 'degradation' rather than change in a constantly changing system and at what point biodiversity loss and pollution become unacceptable is more challenging than it first appears. Nevertheless, it is not impossible. Polly Higgins, e.g., has worked on this in the context of establishing what constitutes 'ecocide'. And other areas are much more straightforward. Establishing what counts as the core prohibitions in relation to animal welfare would, for example, be relatively easy. Arguably, they have already been identified as something very like the Five Freedoms, the Farm Animal Welfare Council's version of these being:

1 Freedom from Hunger and Thirst: by ready access to fresh water and a diet to maintain full health and vigour.
2 Freedom from Discomfort: by providing an appropriate environment including shelter and a comfortable resting area.
3 Freedom from Pain, Injury or Disease: by prevention or rapid diagnosis and treatment.
4 Freedom to Express Normal Behaviour: by providing sufficient space, proper facilities and company of the animal's own kind.
5 Freedom from Fear and Distress: by ensuring conditions and treatment which avoid mental suffering.

Source: Farm Animal Welfare Council (2009).

The fourth of these is especially significant. Marthe Kiley-Worthington's (1993) version of this – ensuring that the animal has the opportunity to express all the behaviour in their natural repertoire, provided this does not cause prolonged or acute suffering to others – is particularly useful, offering real insight into how to develop appropriate husbandry systems. Either version, of course, has profound implications for current food production systems. The majority of intensive systems, for example, clearly fail to provide animals these opportunities and many violate other freedoms as well.

This is in no sense meant to be a completed approach and clearly there is much to be filled in. Meanwhile, there are two key points that sound rather abstract but whose practical implications are in fact hard to overstate. The first is the means/end point. The diamond values counter this. They are firmly rooted in an acknowledgement that other living things – people, animals, the environment – have intrinsic value. Other living things and systems are ends as well as means and should not be treated merely instrumentally. Second, and following from this, the framework proposed above is of a deontological variety rather than a utilitarian one. Within utilitarianism, an approach that underpins all forms of cost-benefit analysis and the justification of deregulated market systems, trade-offs are always possible, and as witnessed in the reality of environmental collapse, structural inequity, persistent poverty and systematically poor animal welfare – all a result of trade-offs in pursuit of narrowly conceived economic goals.

Practical implications

What would all this mean in practice? Restructuring food production systems in the light of the diamond values would mean systems that were fair to people – producers and consumers across the world – and good for human health and well-being. These would be systems in which people had a say and which we could all help to shape. They would provide high-quality, affordable, accessible food for all, in a way that did not leave an impossibly degraded environment for the future and, indeed, could readily coexist and even support a huge range of wild species. Farming would work within local ecosystems rather than seek to displace them and it would be rooted in a view of ourselves as members of a vast, complex ecological community. A pragmatic sensitivity towards others in the light of our mutual interdependence and a deep respect for others in their own right is implied by the community metaphor. And this, of course, would apply to the domestic animals in these communities, who would be treated in ways that respected them as animals, instead of as the unfeeling components of machines.

All of this would be an immense challenge, of course. The evidence from so many different angles – human health, environment, animal welfare, food security – overwhelmingly suggests that this would have to mean much less (if any) meat and dairy consumption, with far fewer animals living lives of a much, much higher quality, in environments of a much, much higher quality. But it is not impossible. As Colin Tudge (2007), Vandana Shiva and others argue, the main tenets of this have effectively been in place in varieties of traditional agriculture practised across the world for thousands of years. This is not about going back, though. It is about shaking off our brief, temporary obsession with a narrowly conceived set of economic values and moving towards a saner future. Farming systems based on respect for other forms of life – including the animals within them – should be pursued because this is the right ethics, and also because we need to think like this if we are to continue our tenancy on our one and only planet. High standards of animal welfare are an absolutely necessary part of this. They are, or should be, a core aim of sustainable development, which itself should be an overriding priority, given our current multiple crises. The mindset that acknowledges the importance of animal welfare as well as the other 'diamond' values is part of the solution in all these cases. And if you ain't part of the solution . . .

Optimistic postscript

'What in cosmos happened to you, then? Your career looked so promising. And now . . .'

The anthropologist shrugged.

'It was so unexpected. So utterly unlikely. But they did it. They turned it around. The Earth humans took control. Against all the odds they started to act rationally in relation to the information about the problems their food production systems were causing; and they began to respond compassionately and wisely – in their own limited ways – in relation to their impacts on other beings. Before I could say "galactic worm-hole", most humans were eating primarily vegetarian food, of a very high quality. Their health gains were massive, of course, and their media was temporarily dominated by meal-makeovers with vegetarian chefs as the new screen idols – completely displacing footballers, and even that inane vehicle worshipper,

Clarkson whatshisname. Malnutrition was practically abolished from the planet, and, at the same time, because of the farming methods they adopted, biodiversity increased and the integrity of some extremely compromised ecological systems was largely restored. And of course, because of the reduction in carbon emissions and the increase in natural biomass, this all had the effect of reducing the extent of climate change and, in turn, conflict over other resources, like water'.

'And what happened to "meat"?'

'It was still eaten, but only occasionally. It came to be considered a real luxury, to be savoured on special occasions. And the animals concerned were kept in immeasurably better conditions. So-called "intensive farms" – more like factories than farms – became a thing of the past, as did animals kept in painful, cramped conditions, performing stereotypical behaviours and transported long distances in appalling conditions while still alive to be killed in substandard abattoirs. All gone. A much smaller number of animals living extensive, high-quality lives and slaughtered locally and humanely were all that remained. Which made human agriculture vastly more efficient of course. Hence the ability to feed their population and coexist with other species. Wonderful from an Earth perspective. But it completely finished me as a researcher. Examples of sane, wise, rational, compassionate thinking, albeit rare on Earth, are commonplace in the rest of the cosmos. I never got another grant after that'.

'So what are you doing now? You don't look as distressed as you might'.

'Well, oddly enough, it's all worked out rather positively. I realized academia could be a bit of a, well, to use an Earth expression, "rat-race". All that pressure to publish. And I rather took to some of the Earth conclusions about quality of life being about quality of time. I'm working half-time now, on my own book. It's loosely based on my previous research, but it's written for a wider audience. Travel. Pictures. Anecdotes. Even a few Earth recipes'.

Notes

1 Discussion of the emissions associated with livestock and the predicted rise in meat consumption was largely omitted from the Paris talks. See e.g. Kristie Middleton (2015) "The livestock sector is already responsible for 7.1 gigatons of CO_2 equivalent a year of greenhouse gas (GHG) emissions – just under 15 percent of the global total, and equivalent to tailpipe emissions from all the world's vehicles." Chatham House Report quoted in: www.triplepundit.com/2015/12/chicken-room-paris-climate-talks/.

2 See, for example, key works by these authors: Singer, P. (1975) *Animal Liberation*, Pimlico, London; Midgley, M. (1983) *Animals and Why They Matter: A Journey Around the Species Barrier*, University of Georgia Press, Athens, GA.

3 Roland Bonney has argued that an alternative and better approach is via the 'Three E's' – environment, economy and ethics, with good animal welfare included, alongside decent treatment of people, under 'ethics'. His argument is that this makes it more likely that animal welfare will be included as, once 'ethics' is admitted as a valid component of sustainable development, it is very hard to argue that animal welfare is not a relevant aspect of ethics. The 'diamond' approach in his view still leaves animal welfare vulnerable – it is easy enough to lop off or ignore the extra arm.

4 See, for example, Regan, T. (2004) *Empty Cages: Facing the Challenge of Animal Rights*, Rowman and Littlefield, Lanham, MA, and www.tomregan-animalrights.com/home.html.

5 The community metaphor was powerfully articulated by Aldo Leopold (1949) in the 1950s and has since been reworked by e.g. Baird Callicott (1989) and Robert Macfarlane (2016).

Further reading

Eshel, G. and Martin, P.; (2006) 'Diet, energy and global warming', *Earth Interactions*, vol 10.

Global Humanitarian Forum; (2009) 'The anatomy of a silent crisis' www.ghf-ge.org/humanimpact-report.pdf last accessed 16/12/15.

Lymbery, P. and Oakeshott, I.; (2014) *Farmageddon: The True Cost of Cheap Meat*, Bloomsbury, London, New Delhi, New York, Sydney.

McMichael, A. J., Powles, J. W., Butler, C. D. and Uauy, R.; (2007) 'Food, livestock production, energy, climate change, and health', *Lancet*, vol 370, pp1253–1263.

Monbiot, G.; (2008) 'This stock collapse is petty when compared to the nature crunch', *The Guardian* www.theguardian.com/commentisfree/2008/oct/14/climatechange-market turmoil last accessed 17/12/15.

Monbiot, G.; (2015a) 'There's a population crisis all right: But probably not the one you think' www.theguardian.com/commentisfree/2015/nov/19/population-crisis-farm-animals-laying-waste-to-planet last accessed 16/12/15.

Monbiot, G.; (2015b) 'Consume more, conserve more: Sorry but we just can't do both' www.theguardian.com/commentisfree/2015/nov/24/consume-conserve-economic-growth sustainability last accessed 16/12/15.Rawles, K.; (2006) 'Sustainable development and animal welfare: The neglected dimension', in Turner, J. and D'Silva, J. (eds) *Animals, Ethics and Trade*, Earthscan, London, pp208–216.

Rawles, K.; (2008) 'Environmental ethics and animal welfare: Reforging a necessary alliance', in Dawkins, M. S. and Bonney, R. (eds) *The Future of Animal Farming: Renewing the Ancient Contract*, Blackwell Publishing, Malden, Oxford, Victoria.

Stehfest, E., Bouwman, L., van Vuuren, D. P., den Elzen, M. G. J., Eickhout, B. and Kabat, P.; (2009) 'Climate benefits of changing diet', *Climatic Change*, vol 95, nos 1–2, pp83–102.

Stern, N.; (2009) A Blueprint for a Safer Planet: How to Manage Climate Change and Create a New Era of Progress and Prosperity, The Bodley Head, London.

United Nations Environment Programme; (2007) *Global Environment Outlook GEO4 Environment for Development*, Progress Press Ltd, Malta, www.unep.org/geo/geo4.asp last accessed 16/12/15.

United Nations Environment Programme; (2012) 'Global environment outlook GEO5 environment for the future we want' www.unep.org/geo/geo5.asp accessed 16/12/15 last accessed 17/12/15.

Wilkinson, R. and Pickett, K.; (2009) *The Spirit Level: Why More Equal Societies Almost Always Do Better*, Allen Lane, London.

Williams, L.; (2015) 'What is TTIP? and six reasons why the answer should scare you', *The Independent* www.independent.co.uk/voices/comment/what-is-ttip-and-six-reasons-why-theanswer-should-scare-you-9779688.html last accessed 16/12/15.

References

Anderson, R.; (2007) 'Mid-course correction', *Resurgence*, no 242.

Bonney, R.; (2008) 'Ethics in action: Farming, the environment and animal welfare', presentation at 'Reconnections', Forum for the Future, Yewfield, Cumbria.

Bonney, R.; (2009) 'How do livestock producers balance the demands for food production and environmental responsibility with animal welfare?' presentation at 'Animal welfare, sustainable farming and food security', AWSELVA conference at the Food Animal Initiative, Wytham, Oxford, UK.

Callicott, J. B.; (1989) *In Defence of the Land Ethic: Essays in Environmental Ethics*, SUNY Press, Albany, New York.

Chatham House; (2015) 'Changing climate, changing diets: Pathways to lower meat consumption' www.chathamhouse.org/publication/changing-climate-changingdiets?dm_i=1TYD,3U28I,CERIHT,DTI0E,1#sthash.qzXClZOf.dpuf last accessed 16/12/15.

Farm Animal Welfare Council; (2009) 'Five freedoms' http://webarchive.nationalarchives.gov.uk/20121007104210/http:/www.fawc.org.uk/freedoms.htm last accessed 16/12/15.

Kiley-Worthington, M.; (1993) *Eco-Agriculture: Food First Farming – Theory and Practice*, Souvenir Press, London.

Leopold, A.; (1949) *A Sand County Almanac*, reprinted Oxford University Press (1968), Oxford.

Macfarlane, R.; (2006) 'Turning points', in Buckland et al. (eds) *Burning Ice; Art and Climate Change*, Cape Farewell, London, UK.

Middleton, K.; (2015) 'The chicken in the room at the Paris climate change talks', *Triple Pundit* 10th December www.triplepundit.com/2015/12/chicken-room-paris-climate-talks/ last accessed 17/12/15.

Regan, T.; (1985) 'The case for animal rights', in Singer, P. (ed.) *In Defence of Animals*, Blackwell Publishers, Oxford.

Stern, N.; (2006) *The Economics of Climate Change: The Stern Review*, Cambridge University Press, Cambridge.

Tudge, C.; (2007) *Feeding People Is Easy*, Pari Publishing, Italy.

United Nations; (2015) 'Sustainable development goals' https://sustainabledevelopment.un.org/?menu=1300 last accessed 16/12/15.

WWF; (2014, 2012, 2010) 'Living planet reports' http://wwf.panda.org/about_our_earth/all_publications/living_planet_report/ last accessed 16/12/15

16

THE POLITICS AND ECONOMICS OF FARM ANIMAL WELFARE AND SUSTAINABLE AGRICULTURE

Peter Stevenson

Introduction

Since the 1980s the welfare of farm animals has been a subject of growing importance. Progress has been driven by both governments and commercial bodies: this has involved legislation and codes and also the setting of standards by producers' own organisations and food businesses including retailers, foodservice operators and food manufacturers.

Despite this, industrial livestock production – with its inherently low welfare standards – remains the norm in developed countries and has taken root in much of the developing world. There is increasing recognition that if we are to attain high welfare standards, fundamental restructuring of our food and farming system is necessary.

Two very different models of future agriculture are currently vying for primacy. Some espouse further industrialisation. Others argue that agriculture must nurture the natural resources on which it depends: arable land and water should be used sparingly, pollution of air and water should be avoided and degraded soils and biodiversity restored. This model recognises that each animal is an individual and that good welfare entails not just the prevention of negative states but enabling animals to enjoy positive, even pleasurable experiences.

Progress to date

The EU has banned the three most egregious aspects of factory farming: veal crates (Council Directive, 2008/119/EC), sow stalls (though these are still permitted for the first four weeks after service) (Council Directive, 2008/120/EC) and barren battery cages (Council Directive, 1999/74/EC).

The move away from sow stalls (also known as 'gestation crates') is gaining momentum in a range of countries. In addition to the EU ban, sow stalls have been prohibited in nine US states (HSUS, 2012) and in New Zealand (Ministry for Primary Industries, 2010). The Code of Practice for Canada calls for a phase-out by 2024 (National Farm Animal Care Council, 2014). The Australian pork industry has committed to voluntarily phasing out sow stalls by 2017 (Australian Pork, no date). All major pork processors in Brazil have announced they will phase out the use of sow stalls (Perrett, 2015; Pacelle, 2014; Globo Rural, 2015). The South African Pork Producers organisation has committed to a final phase out date of 2020 (South African Pork Producers' Organisation, 2013).

In 2007, Smithfield Foods, the world's largest pig producer, committed to phase out gestation crates by 2017 (although sows are housed individually until confirmed pregnant) (Smithfield, 2016). Smithfield is also asking its US contract farmers to convert to group housing by 2022 (Gyton, 2015).

Similarly, battery cages for laying hens are increasingly being rejected. In addition to the EU ban, five US states ban or restrict the use of battery cages (Farm Sanctuary, 2016) and well over 100 US retailers and other food businesses are committed to going cage free; these include McDonald's and Walmart. The Retail Council of Canada is committed to being cage-free by 2025 (CNW, 2016).

Twenty years ago the impetus for change came from legislation, but now we are seeing voluntary industry initiatives and moves by retailers and other food businesses also playing a part and in some countries such as the US being at the forefront of change.

EU progress is faltering

Progress in the EU in the 2010s has been disappointing. Enforcement of EU welfare legislation is poor particularly as regards transport,[1] the ban on routine tail docking of pigs (European Parliament, 2014) and the requirement that pigs must be given effective enrichment materials. A few examples of the reluctance of the European Commission and most Member States to tackle welfare problems are set out in this chapter.

The EU has a large live animal export trade (mainly cattle and sheep) to the Middle East, Turkey and North Africa. Animal welfare organisations have regularly informed the Commission and the exporting Member States of frequent breaches of EU welfare legislation (Council Regulation, 1/2005) in the course of these journeys. They have also been told that slaughter practices in the destination countries are almost always in breach of the OIE international standards on welfare at slaughter (OIE, 2015b) resulting in extreme suffering for EU animals. The Commission and the exporting Member States have taken no effective steps to address these problems. Indeed, both the Commission and the Agriculture Council have welcomed the increase in live exports (European Commission, 2015b, 2016; Council of the European Union, 2016). For the EU the profits that pour in from this harsh trade outweigh any qualms about the concomitant suffering and illegality.

The Commission has been alerted to the fact that many chickens – possibly one billion per year – are stunned with ineffective electrical parameters (Compassion in

World Farming, 2014 and 2015). Birds that are ineffectively stunned may suffer an electric shock and be immobilised while remaining fully conscious when the neck is cut. The Commission has refused to address this problem.

The EU dairy sector is rapidly industrialising as farmers move from pasture-based systems to 'zero-grazing' in which cows are housed all year round and are pushed to ever higher milk yields. The European Food Safety Authority has warned that these practices are highly detrimental to dairy cow health and welfare (EFSA, 2009). However, the Commission and Member States fail to act to reverse these damaging trends.

The Treaty on the Functioning of the EU recognises animals as 'sentient beings' and requires the EU and the Member States, in formulating and implementing policy on agriculture, transport, fisheries and technological development, to "pay full regard to the welfare requirements of animals" (TFEU, 2007). However, this requirement is largely ignored by the Commission and the Member States.[2] This rather reduces this Treaty provision to the status of legislative window dressing, designed to look pleasing but lacking in substance.

There are a number of reasons for the EU's faltering progress. Enlargement of the EU has resulted in Member States that accord low priority to welfare having a large majority.

The Court of Justice of the EU has ruled that, with only a few exceptions, non-governmental organisations (NGOs) have not got the legal standing to challenge the legality of Commission acts or omissions at the Court. This has bred a certain disdain in the Commission as they know that animal welfare NGOs cannot take them to the Court for their failure to respect the Treaty obligation to "pay full regard to the welfare requirements of animals".

A further impediment is the fear that in raising its welfare standards the EU will leave its farmers vulnerable to lower welfare imports. The Commission and Member States frequently cite the rules of the World Trade Organisation (WTO) as preventing restrictions on imports on welfare grounds, thereby making it unfair to EU farmers to raise EU welfare requirements above global levels.

The WTO rules do indeed place important constraints on member countries' actions. However, the WTO is also often used as a respectable excuse for inaction. In fact WTO case law over recent years indicates that trade measures aimed at the protection of animals can in certain circumstances be justified provided that there is no element of discrimination against imports (WTO, 2011; WTO, 2012; WTO, 2013; WTO, 2014).[3] The EU and other WTO members could arguably be more confident in recognising that, subject to certain provisos, they may set high standards of animal welfare and require imports to be derived from animals reared to standards that are comparable in effectiveness to their own (WTO, 2001).

The EU places great weight on the need for consumers to drive the market; the Commission stresses the importance of empowering consumers (European Commission, 2012a). Despite this the Commission and most Member States are determined to keep consumers in the dark and firmly oppose proposals that meat and milk should be labelled as to farming method (even though eggs and egg packs have to be so labelled). There is a real fear that if consumers knew how most animals are farmed they would reject these products.

The politics of sustainable food and farming

Some see the challenge of feeding the growing world population – which is expected to reach 9.6 billion by 2050 – primarily in quantitative terms. They argue that major increases in food production are needed and that accordingly further industrialisation of agriculture is necessary. In the EU this view tends to dominate both in the Commission and the Member States.

Others point out that we already produce enough food to feed 13–14 billion people but that over half of this is wasted – for example by being thrown out by retailers and consumers, used as biofuels or fed to animals which convert it very inefficiently into meat and milk (Cassidy *et al.*, 2013). They argue that we do not need to produce large amounts of additional food but rather that we need to use what we produce more wisely (Lundqvist *et al.*, 2008; De Schutter, 2014). They point out that further industrialisation will undermine the key natural resources – soil, water, biodiversity – on which the ability of future generations to feed themselves depends. The case against industrialisation has been powerfully expressed by the UN Special Rapporteur on the right to food, Hilal Elver (United Nations, 2015), who writes:

> [T]he view has emerged that humankind will not be able to feed itself unless current industrial modes of agriculture are expanded and intensified. This approach is wrong and counterproductive and will only serve to exacerbate the problems experienced by the current mode of agriculture. . . . [T]here is a need to encourage a major shift from current industrial agriculture to transformative activities such as conservation agriculture (agroecology).

Industrial livestock production is increasingly recognised as playing a leading part in many of the problems that beset today's food and farming system. Industrial production is dependent on feeding human-edible cereals to farm animals. In the EU 56% of cereal production is used to feed animals (European Commission, 2016). Globally the figure is 36%, while in the US 67% of crop calories are used as animal feed (Cassidy *et al.*, 2013).

Studies show that for every 100 calories fed to animals in the form of human-edible crops, we receive on average just 17–30 calories as meat and milk (Lundqvist *et al.*, 2008; Nellemann *et al.*, 2009). One paper indicates that the efficiency rates may be even lower for some animal products (Cassidy *et al.*, 2013).

The Royal Institute of International Affairs states that the feeding of cereals to animals is "staggeringly inefficient" (Bailey *et al.*, 2014). The International Institute for Environment and Development stresses that using arable land to produce crops for animal feed rather than to grow food for direct human consumption is "a colossally inefficient" use of resources (IIED, 2015).

The sheer scale of the losses entailed in feeding cereals to animals means that this practice is increasingly being recognised as undermining food security. The UN Food and Agriculture Organisation (FAO) warns that further use of cereals as animal feed could threaten food security by reducing the grain available for human consumption (FAO, 2013).

Industrial livestock's huge need for grain has fuelled the intensification of crop production which, with its monocultures and agrochemicals, leads to soil degradation (Edmondson *et al.*, 2014), biodiversity loss (European Commission, 2011), nitrogen pollution (Sutton *et al.*, 2011) and overuse of water (Mekonnen and Hoekstra, 2012).

Industrial production relies on routine preventive use of antibiotics to ward off the diseases that would otherwise be inevitable when large numbers of animals are kept in crowded conditions (Review on AMR, 2015; WHO, 2016). This contributes to the development of antibiotic-resistant bacteria; these can then infect people and be resistant to some of the antibiotics used to treat serious human disease (European Medicines Agency, 2006).

Industrial production has also facilitated the high levels of consumption of red and processed meat that typify the Western diet and which contribute to obesity, diabetes, heart diseases and certain cancers (European Commission, 2012b; Anand *et al.*, 2015; Bouvard *et al.*, 2015).

Despite the strong evidence that the current food and farming system undermines food security and natural resources, contributes to climate change and is damaging to public health, antibiotics and animal welfare, the European Commission and most Member States remain firmly committed to a productivist approach and to the industrial model of agriculture.

This problem is compounded by the tendency of governments to deal with the different aspects of food and farming in silos thereby failing to provide a cohesive plan that integrates objectives on food security, health, the environment, farmers' livelihoods and animal welfare. Their policies also rarely consider both production and consumption. They tend to focus on production and assume that consumption patterns are a largely unchangeable given.

The European Commission's narrow perspective was seen when in 2015 it abandoned its proposed Communication on sustainable food in part due to fears that it might prove to be a modest first step in the eventual unravelling of the EU's industrial model of agriculture.

The EU's failure to take a cohesive approach to food and farming is highlighted in its position on climate change. Studies indicate that on a business-as-usual basis our diets alone – and in particular our high levels of meat and dairy consumption – will by 2050 take us over the Paris Climate Agreement's target of limiting global temperature rises to well below 2°C (Bajželj *et al.*, 2014; Bailey *et al.*, 2014). However, the Commission and the Member States refuse to include food consumption in their plans for implementing the Paris Agreement despite clear warnings from the science that failure to do so will make it almost impossible to avoid a dangerous level of climate change.

The ability of governments worldwide to take an approach that encompasses all dimensions of food and farming will be tested by the need to implement the 2030 Sustainable Development Goals (SDGs). There is a danger that they will focus on Goal 2.4 which calls for increased food production and advocate industrial agriculture to achieve this Goal.

Further industrialisation, however, will make it impossible to achieve food security and sustainable agriculture, both of which are key facets of Goal 2. In addition, industrial farming will undermine the following Goals and targets: reverse land degradation and improve soil quality (Goals 2.4 & 15); use water sparingly (6.3 & 6.4); reduce nutrient pollution (3.9, 6.3, 14.1 & 15); halt biodiversity loss (15); halt deforestation (15.2); and implement agricultural practices that strengthen capacity for adaptation to climate change, extreme weather, drought, flooding and other disasters (2.4).[4]

The SDGs stress that their interlinkages and integrated nature are of crucial importance in ensuring that the purpose of the 2030 Agenda is realised. However, will governments be able to resist opting for the simplistic solution of industrialisation while ignoring its detrimental impact on many of the Goals relating to the environment and health?

Agribusiness has massive influence in much of the world. In Brussels it has 'captured' DG Agriculture of the Commission and the Agriculture Committee of the European Parliament. Both bodies perceive their primary role to be the protection of agribusiness and the furtherance of its interests. They fail to recognise that food and farming policy has to serve a wide range of legitimate concerns.[5] Of course, farmers must have decent livelihoods, but dietary health, the environment and animal welfare should not be seen as subservient to this.

Corporations that provide inputs to farming (fertilisers, pesticides, commercial seeds, livestock genetics and pharmaceuticals) and that trade in agricultural commodities such as grain are perhaps the most powerful players within agribusiness. They have a huge interest in the maintenance and further expansion of industrial agriculture. Demand for their products would be much reduced if farming were to move away from the industrial model that dominates in the West and that is increasingly becoming embedded in the developing world.

The weight of these interests can be seen from the fact that the EU fertiliser industry has an annual turnover of €13.2 billion (Fertilisers Europe, 2015). Fifty-one per cent of EU fertilisers are used for the production of wheat and coarse grains (Fertilisers Europe, 2015); 56% of these crops are used as animal feed (European Commission, 2015a). Another 23% of EU fertilisers are used for grassland and forage crops. Ten per cent is used for oilseeds; oilseed meal is used extensively in animal feeds (Fediol, no date). The EU pesticide sector has an annual turnover of €7.7 billion (ECPA, 2013).

The global muscle of these sectors flows from their sheer size. Table 16.1 sets out the annual turnover of key agri-input sectors.

Within the EU the Common Agricultural Policy (CAP), despite its environmental elements, has driven – and continues to support – a primarily industrial

TABLE 16.1 Value of global sales of key agri-input sectors, 2011

Sector	*Value of sales in US$ of top 10 companies in each sector*
Commercial seeds	25.9 billion
Pesticides	41.6 billion
Fertilisers	65.7 billion
Animal pharmaceuticals	21.9 billion*

*Livestock-related products make up 60% of the total animal health market

Source: (ETC Group, 2013)

model of agriculture. The CAP appears to take the environment seriously. The larger part of the CAP budget – 77% – provides direct payments for farmers; 30% of these payments are conditional on compliance with certain greening requirements. However, research indicates that these greening payments are not being used well and are likely to provide little counterbalance to the dominant industrial thrust of EU agriculture (Institute for Agroecology and Biodiversity, 2015; Hart, 2015).

The smaller part of the CAP budget – 23% – supports rural development (European Commission, 2013). Part of this funding is used for agri-environment schemes. However, it is also used to foster competitiveness and innovation, both of which have to date tended to steer agriculture in an industrial direction. In the 2014–2020 period 23% of rural development funding has been ear-marked for physical investments (European Parliament, 2016). Experience indicates that some of this money is likely to be used to 'modernise' farms in ways that are detrimental to animal welfare (Bergschmidt and Schrader, 2009; Hogan, 2015a, 2015b). In contrast, just 1.4% of the rural development budget has been allocated to animal welfare (European Commission, no date).

An example of the CAP's tendency to foster industrial agriculture is provided by the damaging symbiotic relationship between the EU's arable sector and its pig and poultry sectors. Commission data show that 56% of EU cereals are used as animal feed (European Commission, 2015a); most of this is used in the intensive pig and poultry industries and in the intensive part of the dairy and beef sectors (Westhoek *et al.*, 2014).

If EU animal production were to move away from the use of cereals as feed, the EU cereal sector would experience the loss of much of its principal market. Thus the EU cereal sector as currently formulated is highly dependent on demand from industrial livestock production while the latter's survival hinges on the supply of plentiful cheap subsidised cereals. So we have the anomaly of a subsidised intensive crop sector that erodes soil quality and biodiversity, which would not have to be intensive but for the fact that it needs to feed industrial animal production, which in turn contributes to unhealthy diets. This is a vicious circle of mutually reinforcing damage.

The emergence of global animal welfare standards

Since the turn of the century progress has been made in the development of global animal welfare standards and recommendations. The OIE (World Organisation for Animal Health) has adopted standards on the welfare of animals (including farmed fish) during transport and slaughter and also on the on-farm welfare of beef cattle, dairy cows and broiler chickens (OIE, 2015a, 2015b). The OIE intends to produce standards regarding the on-farm welfare of all the main farmed species.

The UN Food and Agriculture Organisation has been involved in animal welfare–related activities for many years and has developed the *Gateway to Farm Animal Welfare*, an informative web-based platform (UN FAO, no date).

The International Finance Corporation (IFC) is part of the World Bank Group. The IFC is the largest multilateral financial institution investing in private enterprises in emerging markets. It has published a strong and helpful Good Practice Note entitled *Improving Animal Welfare in Livestock Operations* (IFC, 2014).

The role of international lending and investment institutions has generally been damaging as they have financed industrial livestock operations with low welfare standards (HSI *et al.*, 2013). However, international finance institutions are now beginning to recognise the need to take animal welfare into account. For example, the European Bank for Reconstruction and Development (EBRD) states that it will only finance livestock operations that conform to EU animal welfare standards (EBRD, 2014). Rabobank has adopted a *Sustainable Policy Framework* which includes a helpful section on animal welfare though regrettably it does not eschew the most egregious farming systems such as battery cages and sow stalls (Rabobank, 2016). Despite this encouraging progress, international finance institutions such as IFC and EBRD continue to finance large-scale industrial livestock operations (HSI, 2016).

Economics

There is a widespread assumption that moving to high welfare systems and outcomes for farm animals invariably entails a substantial increase in production costs. However, analysis of industry data shows that in certain cases, such as changing from battery to free-range eggs or from sow stalls to group housing, higher welfare farming adds little to the costs of production.[6]

Moreover, high welfare farming practices can achieve economic benefits as compared with intensive production. In better welfare systems, animals tend to be healthier. This can lead to savings in terms of reduced expenditure on veterinary medicines and lower mortality rates. The provision of straw and/or additional space for finishing pigs can result in better feed conversion ratios and improved growth rates (Beattie *et al.*, 2000). Similarly, compared with high-yielding dairy cows, lower-yielding but healthier cows with better fertility and longevity can deliver higher net margins due to lower heifer replacement costs and higher sale prices for the calves and cull cows (Darwent, 2009).

A study of chickens reared to *Freedom Food* and UK *Red Tractor* (standard intensive) standards shows that measurably better welfare outcomes were achieved by the *Freedom Food* birds (RSPCA, 2006). The *Freedom Food* chickens had lower levels of hock burn, foot pad burn, mortality and transport deaths. The study shows that the higher welfare of the *Freedom Food* birds translates into improved economic performance.

Industrial farming is justified by the assertion that it gives us cheap food. But the low cost of animal products is achieved only by an economic sleight of hand. We have devised a distorting economics which takes account of some costs such as housing and feeding animals but ignores others including the detrimental impact of industrial agriculture on human health, natural resources and animal welfare. Farming's damaging impacts are referred to as 'negative externalities'. The costs of industrial farming's negative externalities are immense and have been detailed in the report *Cheap Food Costs Dear* (Compassion in World Farming, 2016).

Economists argue that these negative externalities should be internalised i.e. incorporated into the prices paid by farmers and consumers. If they are not internalised, the costs associated with them are borne by third parties or society as a whole, for example taxpayers funding the costs of treating diet-related disease. In some cases the costs are borne by no one and key resources such as soil and biodiversity are allowed to deteriorate, undermining the ability of future generations to feed themselves.

The Foresight report stressed: "There needs to be much greater realisation that market failures exist in the food system that, if not corrected, will lead to irreversible environmental damage and long term threats to the viability of the food system. Moves to internalise the costs of these negative environmental externalities are critical to provide incentives for their reduction" (Foresight, 2011). A report by the UN Food and Agriculture Organisation states: "In many countries there is a worrying disconnect between the retail price of food and the true cost of its production. As a consequence, food produced at great environmental cost in the form of greenhouse gas emissions, water pollution, air pollution, and habitat destruction, can appear to be cheaper than more sustainably produced alternatives" (FAO, 2015).

The consequence of unhealthy food being cheaper in the West than healthy food is that poorer members of society find themselves having to rely on poor-quality food. Olivier De Schutter, former UN Special Rapporteur on the right to food, stresses that "any society where a healthy diet is more expensive than an unhealthy diet is a society that must mend its price system" (De Schutter, 2011). This applies equally to a society where environmentally damaging, low-animal-welfare food is cheaper than food that respects natural resources and animals' well-being.

A wide range of mechanisms will be needed to mend our price system. These include much better public information about the consequences of today's farming, mandatory labelling as to farming method and supportive public procurement. Fiscal measures will be of particular importance. The CAP must be reformed. The distinction between Pillars 1 and 2 must be removed. All its funds should be used to support positive externalities e.g. as payments for environmental services and high standards of animal welfare that the market cannot, or can only partially, deliver.

Taxation should entail two intertwined approaches. Taxes can be levied equal to a particular negative externality; this will very precisely internalise them. Taxes should also be used to positively lower the cost of quality food and farming for both farmers and consumers. Farmers adopting high standards could be given generous capital allowances and/or an extra tranche of tax-free income.

The cost of high-quality food could be reduced for consumers in two ways. Income generated by taxes levied to internalise negative externalities could be used to subsidise quality food such as meat raised to high welfare standards, fruit and vegetables. In countries, where VAT is charged on food, a low or zero rate should be placed on healthy food that respects the environment and animal welfare.

Notes

1 Reports by the European Commission's Food and Veterinary Office and by animal welfare organisations reveal regular breaches of Council Regulation (EC) No 1/2005 on the protection of animals during transport.
2 For a full account of this see Stevenson P., 2014. Animal welfare article of the Treaty on the Functioning of the European Union is undermined by absence of access to justice. www.ciwf.org/accesstojustice
3 For a full account of this see Stevenson P., 2015. The impact of the World Trade Organisation rules on animal welfare. www.ciwf.org.uk/research/animal-welfare/
4 For a fuller discussion of this see Compassion in World Farming, 2016. Implementing the Paris Climate Agreement and the 2030 Sustainable Development Goals. www.ciwf.org/ParisandSDGs
5 The undue influence currently given to industry is highlighted by the Decision of the European Ombudsman in her inquiry concerning the composition of the Civil Dialogue Groups (CDGs) brought together by the Commission's DG Agriculture. The CDGs provide a forum for dialogue with representative associations and civil society on matters relating to the CAP; they also provide advice and expertise to DG Agriculture on all CAP matters.
6 For a full account of this see Stevenson P., 2011. Reviewing the costs: The economics of moving to higher welfare farming and Stevenson P., 2014. Economic implications of moving to improved standards of animal welfare, both via www.ciwf.org.uk/research/policy-economics/.

References

Anand, S.S., Hawkes, C., De Souza, R.J., Mente, A., Dehghan, M., Nugent, R., Zulyniak, M.A., Weis, T., Bernstein, A.M., Krauss, R.M. and Kromhout, D., 2015. Food consumption and its impact on cardiovascular disease: Importance of solutions focused on the globalized food system: A report from the workshop convened by the world heart federation. *Journal of the American College of Cardiology*, *66*(14), pp. 1590–1614.

Australian Pork, no date. Industry focus: Housing. http://australianpork.com.au/industry-focus/animal-welfare/housing/ Accessed 25 March 2016.

Bailey, R., Froggatt, A. and Wellesley, L., 2014. Livestock: Climate change's forgotten sector. *Chatham House*. www.chathamhouse.org/publication/livestock-climate-change-forgotten-sector-global-public-opinion-meat-and-dairy Accessed 20 June 2016.

Bajželj, B., Richards, K.S., Allwood, J.M., Smith, P., Dennis, J.S., Curmi, E. and Gilligan, C.A., 2014. Importance of food-demand management for climate mitigation. *Nature Climate Change*, *4*(10), pp. 924–929. www.nature.com/doifinder/10.1038/nclimate2353

Beattie, V.E., O'Connell, NE., Moss, B.W., 2000. Influence of environmental enrichment on the behaviour, performance and meat quality of domestic pigs. *Livestock Production Science*, 65: 71–79.

Bergschmidt, A. and Schrader, L., 2009. Application of an animal welfare assessment system for policy evaluation: Does the farm investment scheme improve animal welfare in subsidised new stables. *Landbauforschung – vTI Agriculture and Forestry Research*, *2*(59), p. 95. http://literatur.vti.bund.de/digbib_extern/bitv/dk041902.pdf

Bouvard, V., Loomis, D., Guyton, K.Z., Grosse, Y., Ghissassi, F.E., Benbrahim-Tallaa, L., Guha, N., Mattock, H., Straif, K. and Monograph Working Group, 2015. Carcinogenicity of consumption of red and processed meat. *The Lancet Oncology*, *16*(16), p. 1599.

Cassidy, E.S., West, P.C., Gerber, J.S. and Foley, J.A., 2013. Redefining agricultural yields: From tonnes to people nourished per hectare. *Environmental Research Letters*, *8*(3), p. 034015.

CNW, 2016. Retail Council of Canada grocery members voluntarily commit to source cage-free eggs by the end of 2025. www.newswire.ca/news-releases/retail-council-of-canada-grocery-members-voluntarily-commit-to-source-cage-free-eggs-by-the-end-of-2025–572574901.html Accessed 9 June 2016.

Compassion in World Farming, 2014 and 2015. Letters from compassion in world farming to the European Commission dated 17 October 2014, 9 December 2014 and 16 March 2015.

Compassion in World Farming, 2016. Cheap food costs dear. www.ciwf.org.uk/media/7426410/cheap-food-costs-dear.pdf Accessed 23 April 2016

Council Directive, 1999/74/EC. Laying down minimum standards for the protection of laying hens. http://eur-lex.europa.eu/legal-content/EN/TXT/PDF/?uri=CELEX:31999L0074&rid=2 Accessed 27 March 2016.

Council Directive, 2008/119/EC. Laying down minimum standards for the protection of calves. http://eur-lex.europa.eu/legal-content/EN/TXT/PDF/?uri=CELEX:32008L0119&qid=1459116293547&from=EN Accessed 27 March 2016.Council Directive, 2008/120/EC. Laying down minimum standards for the protection of pigs. http://eur-lex.europa.eu/legal-content/EN/TXT/PDF/?uri=CELEX:32008L0120&rid=2 Accessed 27 March 2016.

Council of the European Union, 2016. Note from the Presidency to the Council, 10 February 2016. International agricultural trade issues. http://data.consilium.europa.eu/doc/document/ST-5888-2016-INIT/en/pdf

Council Regulation, 1/2005 of 22 December 2004. On the protection of animals during transport and related operations. http://eur-lex.europa.eu/legal-content/en/ALL/?uri=CELEX:32005R0001 Accessed 20 June 2016.

Darwent, N., 2009. Understanding the economics of robust dairy breeds. Attitudes to male dairy calves are becoming more black and white. www.ciwf.org.uk/includes/documents/cm_docs/2009/c/calf_forum_report.pdf

De Schutter, O., 2011. Report of the Special Rapporteur on the right to food, A/HRC/19/59. www.ohchr.org/Documents/HRBodies/HRCouncil/RegularSession/Session19/A-HRC-19-59_en.pdf

De Schutter, O., 2014. Nous pourrions nourrir deux fois la population mondiale, et pourtant. . .*Le point.fr*. www.lepoint.fr/environnement/nous-pourrions-nourrir-deux-fois-la-population-mondiale-et-pourtant-09-09–2014–1861529_1927.php Accessed 3 April 2016.

EBRD, 2014. Paragraph 28 of performance requirement 6 of the EBRD Environmental and Social Policy 2014. www.ebrd.com/downloads/research/policies/esp-final.pdf Accessed 11 April 2016.

ECPA, 2013. *European Crop Protection Association Annual Review 2011–12*. Brussels: ECPA

Edmondson, J.L., Davies, Z.G., Gaston, K.J. and Leake, J.R., 2014. Urban cultivation in allotments maintains soil qualities adversely affected by conventional agriculture. *Journal of Applied Ecology*, *51*(4), pp. 880–889.

EFSA, 2009. Scientific opinion on the overall effects of farming systems on dairy cow welfare and disease. *The EFSA Journal*, *1143*, pp. 1–38. www.efsa.europa.eu/sites/default/files/scientific_output/files/main_documents/1143.pdf

ETC Group, 2013. Putting the Cartel before the Horse. . .and Farm, Seeds, Soil, Peasants, etc. *ETC Group Communique*, 111, pp. 1–39.

European Commission, 2011. Analysis associated with the Roadmap to a Resource Efficient Europe Part II, SEC (2011) 1067 final. Commission staff working paper. http://ec.europa.eu/environment/resource_efficiency/pdf/working_paper_part2.pdf

European Commission, 2012a. Communication on the European Union Strategy for the Protection and Welfare of Animals 2012–2015. http://ec.europa.eu/food/animals/docs/aw_eu_strategy_19012012_en.pdf

European Commission, 2012b. Consultation paper: Options for resource efficiency indicators. http://ec.europa.eu/environment/consultations/pdf/consultation_resource.pdf

European Commission, 2013. Overview of CAP reform 2014–2020. http://ec.europa.eu/agriculture/policy-perspectives/policy-briefs/05_en.pdf Accessed 12 April 2016.

European Commission, 2015a. EU market: Cereals supply & demand. http://ec.europa.eu/agriculture/cereals/balance-sheets/cereals/overview_en.pdf Accessed 20 June 2016.

European Commission, 2015b. Short-term outlook for EU arable crops, dairy and meat markets in 2015 and 2016. http://ec.europa.eu/agriculture/markets-and-prices/short-term-outlook/index_en.htm

European Commission, 2016. Short-term outlook for EU arable crops, dairy and meat markets in 2016 and 2017. http://ec.europa.eu/agriculture/markets-and-prices/short-term-outlook/index_en.htm

European Commission, no date. Rural development programmes 2014–2020. http://ec.europa.eu/agriculture/rural-development-2014-2020/country-files/common/rdp-list_en.pdf Accessed 12 April 2016.

European Medicines Agency, 2006. Reflection paper on the use of fluoroquinolones in food-producing animals in the European Union: Development of resistance and impact on human and animal health. www.ema.europa.eu/docs/en_GB/document_library/Other/2009/10/WC500005155.pdf

European Parliament, 2016. Fact Sheet: Second pillar of the CAP: Rural development policy. www.europarl.europa.eu/atyourservice/en/displayFtu.html?ftuId=FTU_5.2.6.html Accessed 12 April 2016.

European Parliament Directorate-General for Internal Policies, 2014. Routine tail docking of pigs. Study for the PETI Committee. http://www.europarl.europa.eu/RegData/etudes/STUD/2014/509997/IPOL_STU(2014)509997_EN.pdf Accessed 26 April 2017.

FAO, 2013. Tackling climate change through livestock. www.fao.org/3/i3437e.pdf

FAO, 2015. Natural capital impacts in agriculture. www.fao.org/fileadmin/templates/nr/sustainability_pathways/docs/Natural_Capital_Impacts_in_Agriculture_final.pdf Accessed 23 April 2016.

Farm Sanctuary, 2016. State legislation. www.farmsanctuary.org/get-involved/federal-legislation/state-legislation/ Accessed 25 April 2016.

Fediol, undated. Feed. www.fediol.be/web/feed/1011306087/list1187970125/f1.html

Fertilizers Europe, 2015. Industry facts and figures 2015. http://tinyurl.com/feff2015

Foresight, 2011. The future of food and farming: Final project report. The Government Office for Science, London.

Globo Rural, 2015. Aurora diz que vai eliminar gaiolas de gestação de suínos, 29 December. http://revistagloborural.globo.com/Noticias/Criacao/Suinos/noticia/2015/12/aurora-diz-que-vai-eliminar-gaiolas-de-gestacao-de-suinos.html Accessed 22 January 2016.

Gyton, G., 2015. Smithfield Foods announces progress on sow housing. *Global Meat News*, January. www.globalmeatnews.com/Industry-Markets/Smithfield-Foods-announces-progress-on-sow-housing Accessed 6 December 2015.

Hart, K., 2015. Green direct payments: Implementation choices of nine Member States and their environmental implications. www.eeb.org/index.cfm?LinkServID=0DFEF8B2-5056-B741-DB05EBEF517EDCCB Accessed 12 April 2016.

Hogan, P., 2015a. Modern farm facility part-funded by #EU_RDP in Arges County Romania. https://twitter.com/PhilHoganEU/status/576035320761839617 Accessed 12 March 2015.

Hogan, P., 2015b. Weekly update. https://ec.europa.eu/commission/2014-2019/hogan/blog/my-weekly-update-13_en Accessed 17 March 2015.

HSI, 2016. International finance institutions, export credit agencies and farm animal welfare, February 2016. Humane society international. www.hsi.org/assets/pdfs/ifi-report.pdf Accessed 10 June 2016.

HSI, Compassion in World Farming and Four Paws International, 2013. Finance institutions, export credit agencies and farm animal welfare. www.hsi.org/assets/pdfs/hsi_ifi_report_june_2013.pdf Accessed 11 April 2016.

HSUS, 2012. Rhode Island enacts legislation to prohibit extreme confinement crates for pigs and calves and the routine docking of cows' tails. Humane Society of the United States. www.humanesociety.org/news/press_releases/2012/06/rhode_island_gestation_crates_ban_062112.html?credit=web_id311355019 Accessed 21 January 2016.

IFC, 2014. Good practice note: Improving animal welfare in livestock operations. International Finance Corporation. www.ifc.org/wps/wcm/connect/67013c8046c48b889c6cbd9916182e35/IFC+Good+Practice+Note+Animal+Welfare+2014.pdf?MOD=AJPERES Accessed 11 April 2016.

IIED, 2015. Sustainable intensification revisited. Briefing, March 2015. http://pubs.iied.org/17283IIED.html

Institute for Agroecology and Biodiversity, 2015. Landscape infrastructure and sustainable agriculture. www.eeb.org/index.cfm?LinkServID=0E2EEC07-5056-B741-DBA777455AA46334 Accessed 12 April 2016.

Lundqvist, J., de Fraiture, C. and Molden, D., 2008. Saving water: From field to fork: Curbing losses and wastage in the Food chain. SIWI policy brief. https://center.sustainability.duke.edu/sites/default/files/documents/from_field_to_fork_0.pdf Accessed 3 April 2016.

Mekonnen, M.M. and Hoekstra, A.Y., 2012. A global assessment of the water footprint of farm animal products. *Ecosystems*, *15*(3), pp. 401–415.

Ministry for Primary Industries, National Animal Welfare Advisory Committee, 2010. Pigs code of welfare, p. 21. www.mpi.govt.nz/protection-and-response/animal-welfare/codes-of-welfare/ Accessed 25 March 2016.

National Farm Animal Care Council, 2014. *Code of Practice for the Care and Handling of Pigs*, p. 11. www.nfacc.ca/pdfs/codes/pig_code_of_practice.pdf Accessed 25 March 2016.

Nellemann, C., MacDevette, M., Manders, T., Eickhout, B., Svihus, B., Prins, A. G. and Kaltenborn, B. P. (Eds), 2009. The environmental food crisis: The environment's role in averting future food crises. A UNEP rapid response assessment. United Nations Environment Programme, GRID-Arendal. www.unep.org/pdf/foodcrisis_lores.pdf

OIE (World Organisation for Animal Health), 2015a. Aquatic Animal Health Code, section 7. www.oie.int/index.php?id=171&L=0&htmfile=titre_1.7.htm

OIE (World Organisation for Animal Health), 2015b. Terrestrial Animal Health Code, section 7. www.oie.int/index.php?id=169&L=0&htmfile=titre_1.7.htm

Pacelle, W. 2014. Brazil adds its might to the move to end gestation crates. *Huffington Post*. www.huffingtonpost.com/wayne-pacelle/brazil-adds-its-might-to_b_6221032.html Accessed 11 January 2016.

Perrett, M., 2015. End of gestation crates for JBS SA. www.globalmeatnews.com/Industry-Markets/End-of-gestation-crates-for-JBS-SA Accessed 10 June 2016.

Rabobank, 2016. Sustainable policy framework. www.rabobank.com/en/images/sustainability-policy-framework.pdf Accessed 11 April 2016.

Review on AMR, 2015. Antimicrobials in agriculture and the environment: Reducing unnecessary use and waste. Review on antimicrobial resistance. http://amrreview.org/sites/default/files/Antimicrobials%20in%20agriculture%20and%20the%20environment%20-%20Reducing%20unnecessary%20use%20and%20waste.pdf Accessed 3 April 2016.

RSPCA, 2006. Everyone's a winner. How rearing chickens to higher welfare standards can benefit the chicken, producer, retailer and consumer. http://tinyurl.com/RSPCA2006

Smithfield, 2016. Smithfield Foods reports significant progress toward conversion to group housing systems for pregnant sows. Press release, 4 January. www.smithfieldfoods.com/newsroom/press-releases-and-news/smithfield-foods-reports-significant-progress-toward-conversion-to-group-housing-systems-for-pregnant-sows Accessed 22 February 2016.

South African Pork Producers' Organization, 2013. South African Pork Producers' Organisation making strides to loose housing for sows. Organisation says not enough credit is given for developments so far to reach targets by 2020. Press release, 18 March. www.sapork.biz/news-2/ Accessed 22 February 2016.

Sutton, M.A., Howard, C.M., Erisman, J.W., Billen, G., Bleeker, A., Grennfelt, P., van Grinsven, H. and Grizzetti, B., (Eds), 2011. *The European Nitrogen Assessment*. Cambridge: Cambridge University Press.

TFEU, 2007. Treaty on the Functioning of the European Union, article 13. http://eur-lex.europa.eu/legal-content/EN/ALL/?uri=OJ:C:2010:083:TOC

UN FAO, undated. Food and Agriculture Organisation. Gateway to farm animal welfare. www.fao.org/ag/againfo/themes/animal-welfare/aw-abthegat/aw-whaistgate/en/ Accessed 11 April 2016.

United Nations, 2015. Interim report of the Special Rapporteur on the right to food. www.ohchr.org/Documents/Issues/Food/A-70-287.pdf. Accessed 9 June 2016.

Westhoek, H., Lesschen, J.P., Rood, T., Wagner, S., De Marco, A., Murphy-Bokern, D., Leip, A., van Grinsven, H., Sutton, M. and Oenema, O., 2014. Food choices, health and environment: Effects of cutting Europe's meat and dairy intake. *Global Environmental Change*, *26*(May 2014), pp. 196–205. Supplementary material, table S3.

WHO, 2016. WHO Director-General addresses ministerial conference on antimicrobial resistance. www.who.int/dg/speeches/2016/antimicrobial-resistance-conference/en/ Accessed 3 April 2016.

WTO, 2001. Report of the Appellate Body in US-*Shrimp*, WT/DS 58/AB/RW. 22 October 2001, paragraph 144.

WTO, 2011. Panel Report, *United States – Measures Concerning the Importation, Marketing and Sale of Tuna and Tuna Products*, WT/DS381/R, adopted 15 September 2011, as modified by Appellate Body Report WT/DS381/AB/R.

WTO, 2012. Appellate Body Report, United States – Measures Concerning the Importation, Marketing and Sale of Tuna and Tuna Products, WT/DS381/AB/R, adopted 13 June 2012.

WTO, 2013. Panel Reports, European Communities – Measures Prohibiting the Importation and Marketing of Seal Products, WT/DS400/R/WT/DS401/R/.

WTO, 2014. Appellate Body Report, European Communities – Measures Prohibiting the Importation and Marketing of Seal Products, WT/DS400/AB/R and WT/DS401/AB/R, adopted 22 May 2014.

17

RELIGION, CULTURE AND DIET

Martin Palmer

As the world begins seriously to take stock of the true cost of our food consumption – especially meat – the need to find powerful forces within ourselves and our cultures to help us change becomes more urgent. One of the most powerful but often most neglected is the power of religious tradition. In every faith there are millennia-old traditions of simplicity, fasting and appropriate foods. Long dismissed as simply old-fashioned, superstitious or irrelevant, they are being rediscovered by the faiths and recognized by environmentalists as profoundly wise. For within these traditions lie the experience and wisdom of generations of humanity and, as far as the faiths are concerned, the wisdom of the Divine as to how we should live as part of this complex, beautiful world of creation. This wisdom relates not just to good ecology, or even good spirituality. It is also the wisdom of how to live and eat well and keep well.

In the early 1990s research undertaken by the Greek medical authorities into the reasons for heart attacks cast light on an unexpected insight. They discovered that heart attacks happened far less frequently to Greek men and women over 50 years old than to similarly aged people living in other European countries (Chliaoutaki, 2002; Sarri et al., 2003, 2004). After investigating and discarding various possible reasons for this they arrived at the conclusion that this was to do with the fasting laws of Greek Orthodox Christianity. It was shown that observing these laws and traditions ensured a far greater possibility of a long and healthy life than those who did not follow the laws and traditions.

The tradition in Orthodoxy was to fast one day a week every week, twice a week in certain periods and then three days a week during special seasons such as Lent and Advent. Fasting involved no meat, no oil, no cheese or milk products and no wine. This means that for example during Lent – preceding Easter – the diet is effectively vegan with no oil except on Sundays and no wine.

In 2007, similar medical research into monks on Mount Athos in Greece found that these men were far less likely to suffer heart attacks or certain kinds of cancer than other European men and concluded that this was largely because of the religious fasting laws.

Fasting, abstinence and the following of specific diets is an important feature of many faiths and could be one of the most powerful sources possible for redirecting lifestyles. The revival of interest in religion and in the religious life worldwide is of such a scale as to bring new energy to old traditions, which have now been found to be of extraordinary relevance to a world that thought they were just old superstitions or practices. Not only have these practices been found to be beneficial medically – see later in the chapter for further specific examples – but they are being built into the long-term plans that almost every major religious tradition is now developing worldwide to respond to the environmental crises that press upon us.

In 2009, the United Nations Development Programme (UNDP) in partnership with the Alliance of Religions and Conservation (ARC) launched an ambitious project. They asked dozens of major religious traditions – such as the Daoists of China, the Shinto of Japan, Mongolian Buddhist, East African Protestants and so forth – to create long-term plans to help protect our living planet. Since then over seventy such long-term plans have been launched and a second round for many of these traditions was launched in Bristol, UK at a joint UN/ARC meeting relating such plans to the new Sustainable Development Goals (SDGs). In all of these lifestyle changes was one of the three main foci for the commitments of the faiths to respond to environmental challenges. For example, Judaism, Islam, Hinduism and Sikhism each decided to start faith-based labelling systems for the faithful to promote organic, free-range, more environmentally friendly production – e.g. Forest Stewardship Council (FSC) products; Marine Stewardship Council (MSC) fish supplies; and energy-efficient products, while every major faith committed to purchasing ethically.

The Daoists of China in 2013 reinstated two vegetarian fast days into the lunar month, reviving an ancient tradition. This is now being taken up also by Chinese Buddhists, and as China is the fastest rising country for meat consumption, this could make a significant difference in the long run.

The reason this was possible and will be effective is that such traditions of conscious decision making about what to eat and how that food should be considered lies deep in every faith tradition and far back in time. In the case of Judaism and Islam this was building upon traditions of prohibition – kosher and halal – but with a twist. Kosher and halal are essentially about what not to eat. The new programmes are about what you should eat – organic, free range, fair trade, etc. In the case of Hinduism and Sikhism the plans take basic notions of compassion and respect and highlight new areas of concern for those faith traditions.

For some faiths that have launched their long-term plans, there are no such ancient traditions of kosher, halal or Hindu vegetarianism. Instead these faiths – Christianity, Shinto and Buddhism – sought to explore monastic or priestly traditions of simple living that embody many insights about healthy and thoughtful eating – as has been highlighted by the Christian Orthodox examples mentioned previously.

Also arising from this joint UN/ARC initiative has come a whole programme called Faith in Food which in 2014 published a book of that name (Weldon and Campbell, 2014) that explores six faith traditions in terms of what they believe, what they practice, what they eat and how they treat the growing of food or the rearing of livestock. It is one of the most comprehensive – and attractive – of such resources.

There is therefore a vast and powerful series of forces, models and lifestyles to be explored within each faith and to do this we need to understand how these work and what their cultural roots and significance are.

There are many stories told within the myths and legends (myths here meaning truth-bearing) from diverse traditions that emphasize the need to have a diet directed by spiritual concerns. For example this is captured in the shift in diet recorded in the bible with regards to Adam and Eve and then a few generations later, Noah and his family. In the *Genesis* story of God creating a man and woman on the last day of Creation (*Genesis*, Chapter 1:29), the man and woman are told that they can only eat vegetables and fruit. This is seen, in biblical terms, as being the natural and right food for human beings, prior to the coming of sin.

However, after the disaster of the moral decline of human beings that later results in the sending of the flood by God to purge and purify the world, God allows human beings to eat meat for the first time, albeit with the beginnings of the strict kosher laws that were to come to define Judaism later (*Genesis*, Chapter 9:2–3). The traditional interpretation of this new dietary permission is that God recognized that humanity was no longer capable of living the life he had hoped they would, and that he also recognized the fallen nature of humanity, with meat eating as a concession to this imperfect life that now existed. A corollary of this is that in Paradise, we will return to being vegetarians (if indeed we eat at all). Based on this tradition, Hazon, the world's largest Jewish social and environmental network, works with thousands of synagogues and Jewish organizations on community-supported farming projects. Underlying this is a discussion about whether we now need to return to that primal diet – whether in other words we can now become responsible again in our relationships with God and with the rest of creation. One of the Jewish community's commitments is to reduce communal meat consumption by 50 per cent by 2015 (Jewish Seven Year Plan, 2009). This has not been achieved but neither has it been discarded. Hazon's focus on ethical or faith-consistent food is a central plank of their entire work and the numbers involved – even if not yet reaching 50 per cent – is growing rapidly.

We thus find in one of the most influential stories in the world – a story that has shaped Judaism, Christianity, Islam and the Baha'i faiths representing some 50 per cent of all human beings and which gives many people a sense of their origin and meaning – that the issue of appropriate food, diet and abstinence is a central theme. It is a powerful indicator of how diet has always been a key issue for faiths and cultures.

Earliest references to dietary laws

The earliest detailed references we have to dietary and fasting laws occur in the Hebrew bible, especially in the Torah (the Five Books of Moses) dating from before 1000 BC, as well as in the Laws of Manu from Hinduism also known as Ma¯nava-Dharmas´a¯stra, which were recorded in around 200 BC but are traced back to oral traditions before 1000 BC. From Greek and Latin sources including Porphyry of Tyre's third-century book *De Abstinentia* we learn of reports about the dietary laws of Egyptian priests at that time. He quoted the philosopher Xenocrates, asserting that three of his laws still remain in Eleusis, which are these: 'Honour your parents; Sacrifice to the Gods from the fruits of the earth; Injure not animals.'

The laws from the Torah and from the Law of Manu probably both date from the middle of the second millennium BC in their earliest forms. The Jewish laws are still observed to this day by Orthodox Jews, while many of the contemporary dietary traditions and laws of Hinduism, Jainism and Buddhism have their roots in the Laws of Manu.

From the Torah, and in particular the Book of Leviticus, comes the prohibition on pork, camel, the hare and rock-badger as well as less likely food stuff such as lizards, weasels, mice and the chameleon. There is considerable debate as to why these laws came into being and what they mean. The Jewish Encyclopedia lists four main reasons:

- Hygiene: meat rots quickly in hot climates and pork in particular rots very swiftly, and eating rotten meat can cause considerable illness and even death.
- Ethnic identity: the Jews set themselves apart from others by these practices and made it easier to retain their identity amongst stronger nations.
- Symbolic: the animals named are each linked to a vice so that avoidance of eating them means you avoid the vice.
- These were totem animals for neighbouring tribes and thus were taboo.

Whatever the reason, the health benefits of the Jewish diet are now a consideration, though their significance does not appear to be as strong as the fasting traditions of other faiths.

The Hindu laws in the Laws of Manu, especially in Chapter 5, are as detailed as those in the Torah of Judaism. The classic statement on why adherence to a strict diet is essential is spelt out in the opening verses:

> The sages, having heard the duties of a Snataka thus declared, spoke to the great-souled Bhrigu, who sprang from fire: 'How can Death have power over Brahmanas who know the sacred science, the Vedas and who fulfil their duties as they have been explained by Thee O Lord?' Righteous Bhrigu, the son of Manu answered the sages: 'Hear in punishment of what faults Death seeks to shorten the lives of Brahmanas. Through neglect of the Veda-study, through deviation from the rule of conduct, through remissness in the fulfilment of

> duties, *and through faults committed by eating forbidden food*, Death becomes eager to shorten the lives of Brahmanas.
>
> *[author's emphasis] (Manu, n.d./1886)*

It is clear from this early text that diet was viewed as on a par with spiritual exercises and wisdom and that it can cause the same spiritual and actual death as ignorance or wilful disobedience of the will of the gods.

The Daoist dietary laws

The long list of forbidden animals, birds and fish as well as such root plants as garlic and onions in the Laws of Manu is very close to elements of Judaism and also bears a remarkable similarity to the Daoist dietary laws. These date from around the fourth to sixth centuries AD and are concerned with the maintenance of the *qi* – the life energy that animates the body. In Daoist thought (which itself is based upon philosophical notions of the body and soul dating from the sixth to third centuries BC) when we are born we have within our bodies all the *qi* we can ever have. The moment we start to breathe out we begin to lose this *qi*. Hence the dietary laws prohibit any foods that cause wind or indigestion as this means the wasteful loss of *qi* and thus an earlier death. This, coupled with almost exclusively vegetarian food, has led to many Daoists living long lives of remarkable healthiness, much commented upon by writers down the centuries. However, to the best of my knowledge there have been no scientific studies to compare with the work on Orthodox Christian monks and Greek Orthodox lay people.

When the Daoists launched their long-term plans and commitments in 2009 they drew upon this notion of *qi* and also on the Daoist philosophy of yin and yang. The relevance of this to contemporary environmental and welfare issues was powerfully captured by Olav Kjorven, Assistant Secretary General of UNDP, when he addressed the heads of all the Daoist temples in China in 2008 as they prepared their long-term commitment to protect the living planet:

> Over the past couple of days I've had a chance to learn a bit from your tradition although I have to humbly say that I'm only scratching the surface. I have visited the White Cloud Temple in Beijing and yesterday I went to Mao Shan Temple here in this area. And I have learned that in your tradition as well, our duty as humanity is to restore balance, and to care for and respect nature – and that human wellbeing fundamentally depends on maintaining this balance.
>
> Let me quote from one of your holy books: Chapter 42 of the *Dao De Jing*.
> 'The Tao gives birth to the origin;
> The origin gives birth to the two – yin and yang.
> The two gives birth to the three – heaven, earth and humanity.
> The three gives birth to all creation, all of nature.'

> This is very important teaching for our world today. I'm sure that many of you have heard of the common challenge we are facing around the world: that of climate change.
>
> Because of the way we utilize energy and organize our economies around the world we are in danger of severely disrupting the balance of the climate, which conditions everything around us.
>
> But what is climate change in its most simplistic scientific sense? It is all about the balance of carbon – a very important component in our natural system which makes life possible as we know it. It is about the balance of the carbon that exists in the air, in the clouds, in the atmosphere that surrounds us on the one hand and the carbon in the earth on the other, including in living things. And what we have been busily doing as humanity – particularly in the rich countries, but also increasingly in other countries around the world including China – is to disrupt that balance and move a lot of carbon out of the earth and into the clouds. This is familiar to you, I think because if this is anything at all it is the disruption of the balance between the yin and the yang.
>
> And I think that your tradition as Daoists in China – your expression of the yin and the yang and how it relates to our existence as human beings – expresses better than any other religious tradition that I know of the challenge that we are facing when it comes to environmental degradation and climate change.

Given the role of meat production and animal by-products the yin/yang imagery speaks not just to the general issues but also to our lifestyle choices. This has been picked up in the rediscovery of the two days a lunar month fasting or vegetarian tradition.

What becomes clear already from the three cases cited above is that dietary laws and fasting are intimately interwoven with spiritual practices. Echoes of this can still be discerned in Europe today when the Christian fasting period of Lent – the seven weeks before Easter – are still used by many who often have little or no formal contact with organized religion, as an excuse that society validates, to commence a diet. The strength of communal acceptance of a time of restraint, fasting or dieting still has a role and place even in countries where the observance of religion has waned.

The fast of Ramadan in Islam is perhaps the best-known example of a fasting tradition that has maintained its power to today. The 30 days of the month of Ramadan are devoted to fasting from sunrise to sunset. This combined with the total ban on alcohol and the halal rules on what may be eaten and what may not has created a diet and way of life that is considered very healthy. The scientific fascination with the Islamic dietary laws and especially the Ramadan fast has led to many studies of its nutritional and medical significance.

Islamic dietary laws

Fundamentally, diet is seen to be a key element of Islamic well-being. Interestingly, traditionally, the first thing that an apprentice physician would learn was how to cook – both for himself and others.

Islamic laws – Unani – being the laws associated with healthy living – provide two major openings into the lifestyles of the Muslim world that need to be more properly considered than has been the case thus far by animal welfare groups and environmental organizations:

- Because of core beliefs, Unani very strongly supports the move towards better understanding and care for food nurturing and growing because these are seen as both a gift from God but also as our responsibility because we have been appointed as khalifas – vice-regents upon Earth – and have the moral and spiritual responsibility to ensure the world functions well at all levels. A problem has been that Islam has never been properly asked to take part and indeed misunderstanding of halal has often created barriers of mistrust.
- Kindness to the food you eat: there is a Hadith (account of the words of Muhammad) that suggests that the family or community wanting to eat a chicken must let it live with them, to be taken care of, for three days. Re-emphasizing such a ruling, again, would be excellent for the free-range movement.
- Apart from the well-known Islamic concepts of halal, allowed/permissible, and haram, forbidden, is the concept of tayyib. The Qur'an is explicit: 'O mankind, eat from whatever is on earth [that is] lawful (halal) and good (tayyib) and do not follow the footsteps of Satan' (Qur'an 2:168). Given teachings elsewhere in the Qur'an about respecting the family and community nature of all creatures, good in this context has to be seen as part of Islamic compassion for the family feelings of all creatures. What therefore good (tayyib) cannot be is cruel or destructive to the natural, God-given nature of animals living in family and community relationships. Nor can it be good to cause any such creatures undue pain or distress. This increasingly Muslims are coming to agree means a ban on factory farming. With the new fatwas (official Islamic ban) against the illegal wildlife trade perhaps it is time also for a fatwa against factory farming.

In Islam itself, fasting and the dietary laws are seen as essentially spiritual. Indeed, the institution of fasting in Islam comes second only to that of prayer. In the Qur'an, those who fast are called *saih* meaning spiritual travellers – see Surah 9:112 and Surah 66:5. Fasting is seen as preparing oneself for the spiritual struggle to remain faithful to the Will of God. In one of the Hadiths (sayings of Muhammad) he said, 'Fasting is a shield.'

Once again the question of the ban on certain foods, especially pork, raises questions of whether we have here a sanctification of sensible hygiene laws. Islam is quite clear that it has inherited its basic dietary laws from those traditions that came before it – Judaism and Christianity in particular. The Qur'an makes this quite clear in Surah 2:183: 'O you who believe, fasting is prescribed for you as it was for those before you, so that you may guard against evil.'

The evil is overindulgence and lack of restraint and self-possession. These are exactly the tools that we need, the entry points into cultures that we seek if we are to be serious about lifestyle choices.

One could ask: how does a culture prescribe good dietary and ecological practices? The best way is to build them into annual rituals and rites sanctioned by faith and maintained by social pressure. The question that is open to so many answers is which came first. Did religion always equate food, restraint and taboos with spirituality and by accident discover the health benefits that we now also see as being environmental benefits; or did religion encode discoveries about a healthy diet and appropriate foods into a set of rituals that were designed as much for physical well-being as for spiritual development?

Either way, it is clear that modern scientific research is finding in these ancient traditions models for healthy sustainable living, which fascinate the scientific community. Perhaps it is time that the environmental and animal welfare organizations paid academic attention to the ecological implications of such diets, cultures and faiths, as the traditions outlined above offer unique structural and psychological entry points for engagement with people and their lifestyles.

There is no other form of social pressure that can so well enable, enforce or assist the following of a specific diet and fasting regime. In studying the health traditions of the faiths, this significant contribution to generations of well-being should be given a special place and consideration.

References

Chliaoutaki, M. (2002) 'Greek Christian Orthodox ecclesiastical lifestyle: Could it become a pattern of health-related behavior?', *Preventative Medicine*, vol 34, pp428–435.

Jewish Seven Year Plan for Climate Change (2009) http://jewishclimatecampaign.org/aboutThisCampaign.php, last accessed 25 May 2010.

Manu (n.d.) 'The Laws of Manu', translated by G. Buhler, edited by Max Muller (1886), *Sacred Books of the East*, vol 25, Oxford University Press, Oxford, pp169–170.

Sarri, K. O., Linardakis, M. K., Bervanaki, F. N., Tzanakis, N. E. and Kafatos, A. G. (2004) 'Greek Orthodox fasting rituals: A hidden characteristic of the Mediterranean diet of Crete', *British Journal of Nutrition*, vol 92, pp277–284.

Sarri, K. O., Tzanakis, N. E., Linardakis, M. K., Mamalakis, G. D. and Kafatos, A. G. (2003) 'Effects of Greek Orthodox Christian church fasting on serum lipids and obesity', *BMC Public Health*, vol 3, p16.

Weldon, S. and Campbell, S. (2014) *Faith in Food: Changing the World One Meal at a Time*, Bene Factum Publishing, UK.

PART V

Devising farming and food policies for a sustainable future

18

POLICY STRATEGIES FOR REDUCING THE CLIMATE IMPACT OF FOOD AND AGRICULTURE

Stefan Wirsenius, Fredrik Hedenus and David Bryngelsson

In this chapter we argue that in order to substantially reduce greenhouse gas (GHG) emissions from food production and to preserve natural and agricultural biodiversity, policies that separately address the demand and the supply sides of the food system will be required. Taxes on animal food, and other policies that shift consumption patterns towards less GHG-intensive and land-demanding food, will be crucial for reducing agricultural GHG emissions as well as for mitigating biodiversity losses related to the expansion of agriculture into natural ecosystems. Demand-moderating policies are vital because of the overall low potential for reducing agricultural GHG emissions by technological means, and because of the inherently large land requirements of ruminant meat (beef and lamb) production. However, demand-side policies alone are far from enough. Comprehensive supply-side policies will also be required, especially for containing agricultural land expansion in order to protect biodiversity in tropical regions. Supply-side policies, such as direct subsidies, will also be fundamental for preserving agricultural-related biodiversity in Europe and other regions holding biodiversity-rich permanent pastures. The latter holds for Europe even if no policies that moderate the demand for ruminant meat are put in place, since the low-intensive land use characteristic of these areas in either case is not economically viable in the long run. Furthermore, the biodiversity-rich areas represent a minor share of the total agricultural land in Europe. Therefore, the goal to preserve agricultural biodiversity in Europe should not be taken as a counter-argument against reducing global ruminant meat production by the implementation of demand-moderating policies.

Major sustainability issues of food and agriculture systems: climate and biodiversity

This chapter deals with the arguably two most severe effects on the Earth systems caused by food production – climatic change and loss of natural ecosystems and their biodiversity. In this section, we briefly describe some of the basics related to these issues.

The food and agriculture systems' role in climatic change has increasingly been put on the political and scientific agenda. Even though carbon dioxide from the energy and transport systems is the largest contributor to climate change, carbon dioxide from agricultural land expansion and methane and nitrous oxide from agriculture represent roughly 20% of global GHG emissions (based on IPCC, 2014, and other sources given for Figure 18.1).

At the global level, GHG emissions from food and agriculture are dominated by soil/vegetation carbon losses from conversion of forests and other land to agricultural land, nitrous oxide from nitrogen-fertilized agricultural soils, and methane from the feed digestion in ruminants ('enteric fermentation'); see Figure 18.1. Emissions from energy use (on farms) and fertilizer production make up roughly 10% of global agricultural emissions, and are small compared to those of methane and nitrous oxide. In the EU, soil and vegetation carbon losses from agricultural land are negligible (or possibly even negative), and methane and nitrous oxide by far make up the great majority of agricultural GHG emissions.

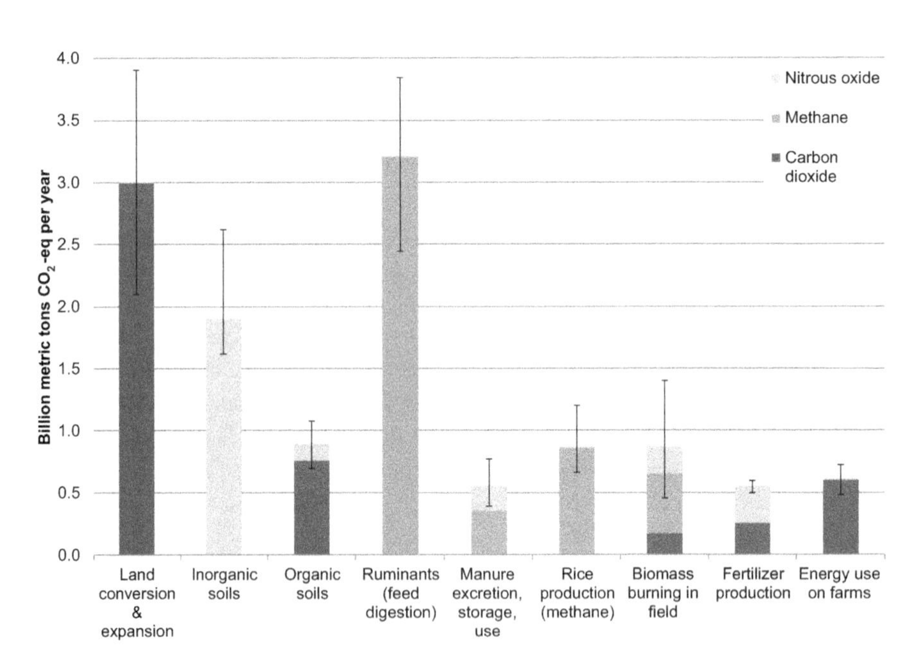

FIGURE 18.1 Current (around 2005) global greenhouse gas emissions from agriculture, with error bars indicating variation across sources.

Sources: Author compilation from FAOSTAT (2015), Humpenöder et al. (2015), JRC-IES (2015), Hedenus et al. (2014), IPCC (2014), Gerber et al. (2013), Herrero et al. (2013), MacLeod et al. (2013), Opio et al. (2013), Valin et al. (2013), Bodirsky et al. (2012), EPA (2012), Popp et al. (2010), Lal (2004), Koungshaug (1998). Note: For consistency, numbers in sources were here recalculated into CO_2 equivalents using the most recent GWP_{100} factors as compiled by the IPCC (Myhre et al., 2013).

Avoiding dangerous climate change involves reducing the global greenhouse gas emissions by at least 50% by 2050, or even more if the climate turns out to be more sensitive to increased levels of greenhouse gases. To make this deep cut in emissions, a number of studies have shown that costs would be considerably less if not only carbon dioxide emissions were reduced but also those of other greenhouse gases, particularly methane and nitrous oxide (Reilly et al., 1999; Manne and Richels, 2001; Weyant et al., 2006). A wider inclusion of methane and nitrous oxide in climate policies would have implications particularly for agriculture, since that sector is responsible for about 60% of the emissions of these gases. In their review of policies to reduce agricultural GHG emissions, Povellato et al. (2007) concluded that the agricultural sector potentially offers GHG abatement at relatively low costs. But they also noted that in reality the potential efficiency gains from introducing price-based instruments in agricultural production may be offset by high transaction and monitoring costs.

Of relevance for policies aiming at achieving deep emissions cuts is that there are very large differences between the GHG emissions from different kinds of food, also within the group of meats and other protein-rich food. This is illustrated in Figure 18.2, which shows characteristic greenhouse gas emission intensities of major types of protein-rich food.

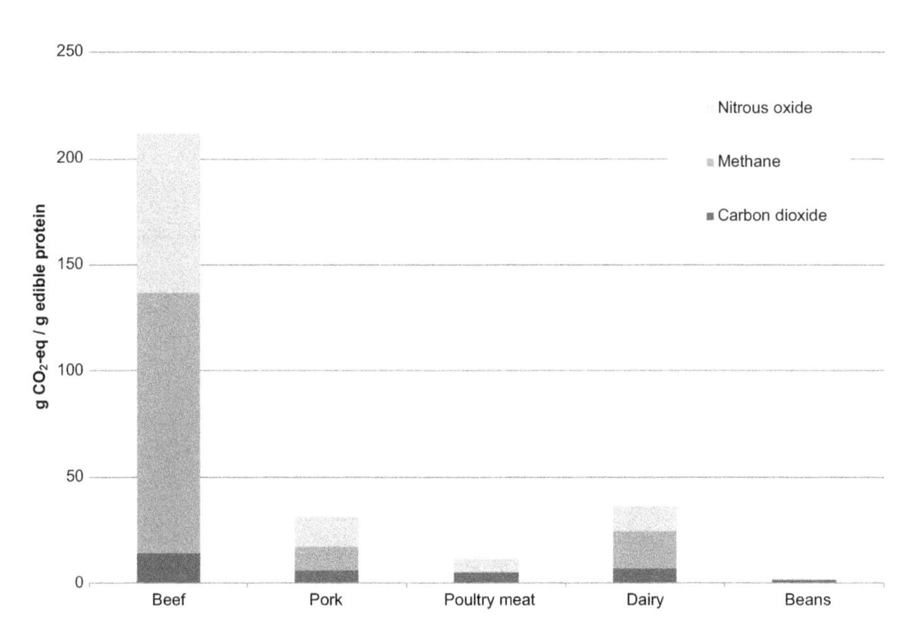

FIGURE 18.2 Current greenhouse gas emissions per unit of food produced (in protein terms) by major animal food types and beans. Data for animal food refer to average conditions in Sweden; EU average emission levels are somewhat higher overall, but the pattern is essentially the same. Note: Soil and vegetation carbon balances are not included; beef refers to suckler beef (non-dairy) production.

Source: Bryngelsson et al. (2016).

There are a number of reasons for these large differences between different food types. The main factor is the magnitude of use of land and biomass per unit of food produced – the more land and biomass that are used, the higher the GHG emissions are, since emissions are correlated with land area and turnover of crops and feedstuff. Overall, land and biomass use per unit of food is substantially higher for animal than vegetable food due to the inevitable losses in the conversion of crops and grass into animal tissue. Within the meat group, land and biomass use per food unit is several times higher for beef and lamb (ruminants) meat than for pork and poultry (monogastrics); see Figure 18.3. In addition to these differences in feed required per food unit, due to the nature of the digestive system of ruminants, significant amounts of methane are produced during feed digestion (of the order of 5–9% of feed energy intake), which adds to the emission gap between beef and lamb versus pork and poultry.

The differences in land and feed requirements are mainly due to ruminants having much lower reproduction rates (i.e. offspring produced per female parent per year) than pigs and poultry – in the EU, breeding cows typically give birth to one calf per year, whereas sows have about 15–20 piglets and breeding hens up to 150 chicks annually. Feed eaten by reproducing adult females essentially represents a loss from a meat production perspective, since virtually all the feed energy is converted to body heat lost to the surroundings, and only a tiny fraction (less than 1%) is

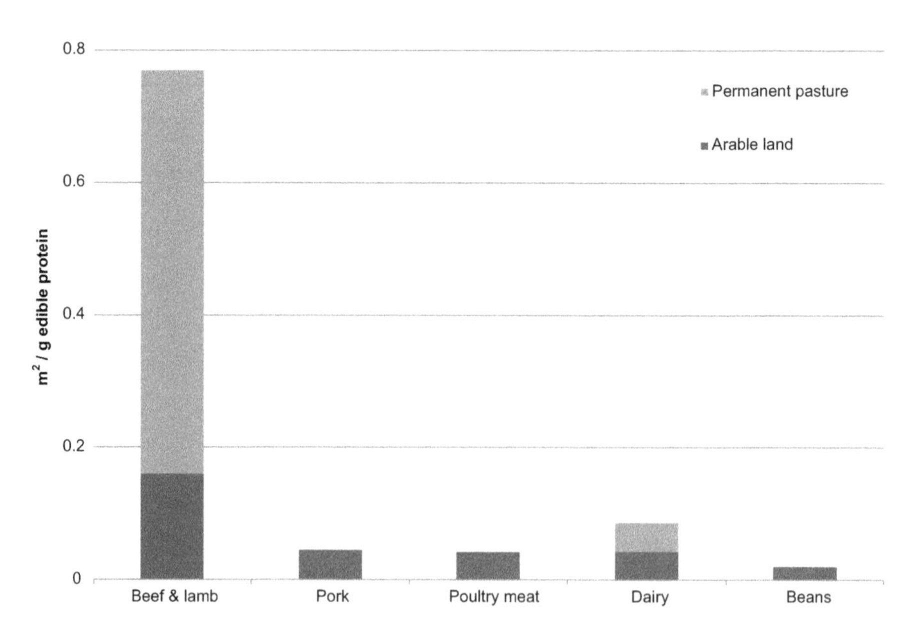

FIGURE 18.3 Current land use per unit of food produced in the EU (in protein terms) by major animal food types and beans. Note: Beef refers to suckler beef (non-dairy) production.

Source: Wirsenius et al. (2011).

converted into offspring reared for slaughter. Therefore, the lower the reproduction rate, the larger is the share of total feed use that does not result in produce, i.e. meat. This means that the total feed (i.e. feed eaten by adult females plus that eaten by offspring reared for slaughter) required for producing one unit of meat is higher.

The carbon dioxide emissions due to transportation of food often gain large attention in media and among NGOs. However, the total energy-related carbon dioxide emissions are small, as seen in Figure 18.2, and transportation is only a small fraction of these emissions. Thus, in the context of GHG mitigation in food systems, freight-related emissions are insignificant, with the notable exception of food items transported via aviation.

It should be noted that the numbers in Figure 18.2 do not include carbon dioxide emissions related to land use change, i.e. conversion of forests and other natural habitats to agricultural land, nor does it include the opposite process, which is sequestration of carbon in soils and vegetation. As shown in Figure 18.1, carbon emissions from land use and land use change are substantial, accounting for about 30% of global agricultural GHG emissions. To what extent different food types contribute to these emissions is not very well known, due to methodological obstacles and data limitations. Yet it is clear that ruminant production accounts for a large share, since conversion of natural habitats into pastures is a major land use change process, particularly in the tropics (Steinfeld et al., 2006).

In addition to releasing large amounts of carbon dioxide into the atmosphere, conversion of forests, natural grasslands and other natural habitats into cropland and pastures also leads to loss of biodiversity. Destruction, fragmentation and degradation of natural habitats in the tropics and sub-tropics are considered the major threats to global biodiversity, and agricultural expansion, especially in the form of pastures, is a major driver of these habitat changes. Although managed pastures represent a more spatially diffuse and less intensive form of land use than cropping, globally it is considered a major driver of deforestation and encroachment into natural grasslands and woodlands (Asner et al., 2004).

Although ruminant production overall constitutes a substantial menace to global biodiversity, in some regions the opposite can be the case. In many parts of Europe, grazing cattle and sheep are fundamental for conserving agricultural land that holds high biodiversity, landscape and cultural values. These 'high nature value farmland' areas comprise hot spots of grazing-dependent biodiversity and are usually characterized by extensive farming practices. The majority of the areas consist of semi-natural grasslands, and are estimated to comprise 15–25% of EU agricultural land area (EEA, 2004).

As agricultural expansion in the tropics contributes to large GHG emissions and biodiversity loss, a relevant question is whether these negative effects could be attributed only to the food produced on recently exploited land (most often ruminant meat), or all food produced in the entire region or country, or to all food produced in the world. We argue that to significant extent they should be attributed to food products with high land requirements regardless of location of production. As demand for land increases anywhere in the world, this translates into increased global food prices, which leads to three things. Food is grown more intensively, demand for food is somewhat reduced and new land is converted into agricultural land. Which of these knock-on effects is most prominent varies between regions, but to some extent increased demand for land in Europe does lead to increased pressure on tropical forests, as has been illustrated by Searchinger et al. (2008) in the case of increased demand for US cropland for biofuels. This phenomenon will also prevail in the long run as i) food and feed markets are largely global, with relatively low transportation costs for several major commodities (cereals, oil crops, meat), and ii) there are strong supply-side constraints due to finite land area and biophysical limitations in yields.

Scarce agricultural land resources become an even larger challenge as the world calls for large-scale climate mitigation. If stringent policies aimed at achieving deep cuts in carbon dioxide emissions from the energy system are implemented, by substantially increasing the cost of emitting carbon dioxide through, e.g. taxes or emissions cap and trade schemes, demand for biomass for energy purposes is likely to increase considerably. As a high enough price on carbon dioxide makes fossil fuels costlier than bioenergy, the demand for biomass and thereby agricultural land will increase. Estimates indicate that a stringent climate policy may increase grain prices by between 50% and 200% by 2050 (Johansson and Azar, 2007; Wise et al., 2009). The magnitude of the food price increase as well as the technical potential of bioenergy is dependent on the area efficiency in the agricultural as well as the bioenergy system.

It can be concluded that increasing the land use efficiency of food production across the board, not only in tropical regions, is crucial for preserving biodiversity in the tropics and for mitigating land use change–related GHG emissions. In the longer run, increased area efficiency in food production is also central for allowing bioenergy to expand and thereby reducing carbon dioxide emissions from the energy system in a more cost-efficient way.

Options for mitigating the climate impact from food systems

Overall, options for reducing GHG emissions from food production may be divided into either technological, or structural/behavioural, where the latter includes changes in human diets, which switches the supply structure towards less emission-intensive food types.

The technology group includes a wide array of options, from measures that increase productivity and efficiency (e.g. in land and nitrogen use), to specific mitigation technology options, such as low-emitting manure storage techniques. In many world regions, there is great scope for increasing crop and livestock productivity and thereby reducing the amount of greenhouse gases emitted per unit of food produced (Tilman et al., 2011; Valin et al., 2013; Wirsenius et al., 2010). In most of the EU, however, agricultural productivity is already relatively high and the remaining potential is unlikely to contribute substantially to reducing agricultural emissions. In contrast, specific technology options could offer substantial reductions, at least for some sources, such as manure management (Montes et al., 2013). However, many other, potentially significant, options, such as nitrification inhibitors that reduce nitrous oxide emissions from soils (Akiyama et al., 2010), and fat additives that reduce methane from ruminants (Grainger and Beauchemin, 2011), are still only at the experimental or pilot-scale level, and do not yet have any proven long-term records of sustained emission reductions. Hence, for these large sources, nitrous oxide from soils and methane from ruminants (cf. Figure 18.1), specific mitigation technologies offer only relatively limited and, more importantly, uncertain reduction potentials.

Only a handful of studies have systematically explored the mitigation potential from major technology options combined. Bryngelsson et al. (2016) estimated the potential in year 2050 for methane and nitrous oxide reductions in Swedish agriculture related to both improved productivity and efficiency, and the implementation of a range of specific mitigation technologies. The productivity and efficiency analysis in Bryngelsson et al. focused mainly on increasing livestock systems' feed and nitrogen efficiency, whereas the specific technology options included feed additives (that reduce methane from feed digestion), low-emitting manure storage and application technologies, nitrification inhibitors (that reduce nitrous oxide from soils) and end-of-pipe cleaning in fertilizer production. Figure 18.4 shows the combined

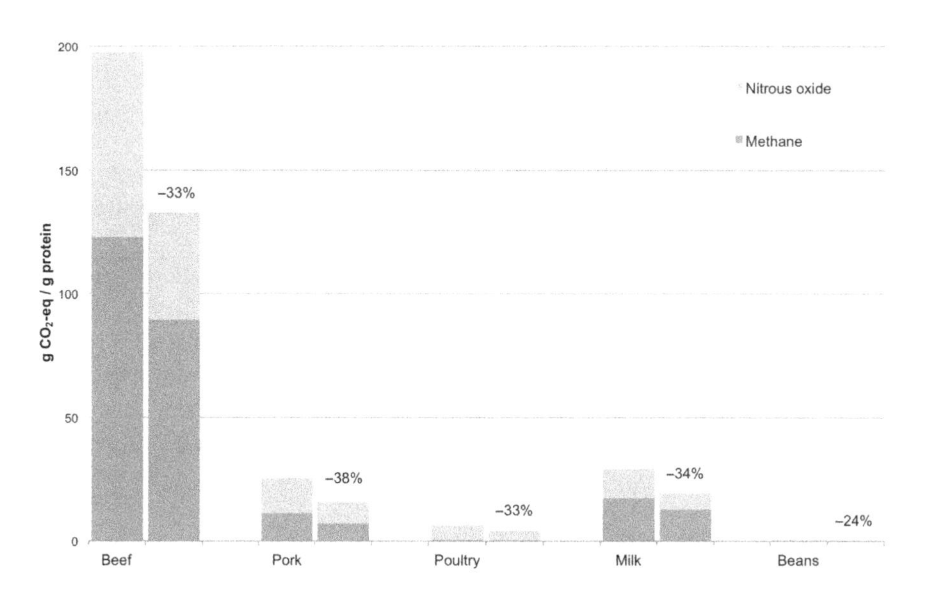

FIGURE 18.4 Methane and nitrous oxide reduction potentials in 2050 from implementation of a wide range of technology options (bars to the right; current emissions shown by bars to the left). Potentials here refer specifically to Swedish systems, but numbers are likely to be similar for systems in the EU overall.

Note: Beef refers to suckler beef (non-dairy) production; emission levels for beans are negligible (cf. Figure 15.2).

Source: Bryngelsson et al. (2016).

potential from these options for meat and other protein-rich food types; overall the potentials hover around 30%.

These rather limited technological potentials are related to the fact that these methane and nitrous oxide emissions occur due to intrinsic characteristics of the systems. The digestive system of ruminants inevitably involves production of methane at significant levels that cannot be drastically reduced without fundamentally manipulating the digestive process. Similarly, nitrous oxide production is an inherent part of the nitrogen cycle, and a high nitrogen turnover per land area – which is required for medium to high crop yields – inevitably entails production and release of significant amounts of nitrous oxide.

The technological potentials reported above do not include carbon sequestration in soils. The potential to actively increase the sequestration rate by specific changes in land use is highly uncertain, and the long-term mitigation effect is inherently unstable since sequestered carbon at any time may be released back to the atmosphere if land use practices are changed. Furthermore, using land for bioenergy instead of ruminant production will in many cases offer much higher, and definite, GHG mitigation per area unit. For instance, if European grassland were used for production of biomass that substituted for coal in power plants, avoided GHG emissions would amount to some 3 ton C per ha per year (Wirsenius et al., 2011), which is several times higher than plausible long-term soil carbon sequestration rates. This means that even if carbon sequestration rates in grasslands could be maintained at high levels, the combined GHG mitigation effect in the beef and energy systems would still be higher if beef were produced more area efficiently (i.e. using a smaller pasture area), assuming that bioenergy were produced on the land made available. Even though this is an efficient measure to mitigate carbon emissions, it may imply negative effects on biodiversity – clearly so in the case where unfertilized, native permanent pastures are replaced by intensive bioenergy plantations.

A crucial consequence of the limited technological GHG mitigation potentials is that the large emission gaps between different types of food remain about the same as in the case without mitigation, as is illustrated in Figure 18.4. This means that the potential to reduce GHG emissions by structural changes in human diets is large, even if technology options are implemented. For instance, if pork or poultry are substituted for beef, GHG emissions are reduced by about 90% and 95%, respectively. If beans containing an equal amount of protein are substituted for cattle meat, emissions are cut by more than 99%.

The GHG mitigation potentials of changes in diets from ruminant meat towards less GHG-intensive food are even larger if also taking into account land use change–related emissions, and production of bioenergy on land made available. As mentioned in the previous section, land use change–related carbon dioxide emissions from beef production in the tropics may be several times larger than all other GHG emissions from the production. Since some (~5–10%) of the beef consumed in the EU is imported from the tropics, and since there exist knock-on effects between regional beef markets, it is reasonable to assume that reduced beef consumption in the EU also leads to reduced land use change–related emissions in the tropics. Also, due to the large differences in land requirements between ruminant meat and virtually all other types of food (see Figure 18.3), changing the diet away from beef reduces land use substantially, not only of permanent pastures but also that of cropland. If the land made available is used for bioenergy in order to replace fossil fuels, additional reductions in GHG emissions can be achieved. The magnitude of the mitigation effect from bioenergy varies substantially, depending on the crops used and which kind of fossil-based energy use is replaced (see further next section).

We may thus conclude that changed consumption patterns hold far greater GHG mitigation potentials than does the adoption of improved technology and practices, for the food system. In this respect, the food system differs fundamentally from the other major contributors to human GHG emissions, the energy and transport systems. In the energy and transport systems, new technology, such as wind and solar power, carbon capture and storage in fossil-based power production, plug-in hybrid or electric vehicles, biofuels, etc, has the potential to make these systems almost carbon-neutral, which means that reduction of energy use by changed consumption patterns and lifestyles, although desirable, will not play the same key role as in the food system. For this reason, quite different policy options should be considered for promoting a sustainable food system as compared to sustainable energy and transport systems.

Policy strategies

Broadly speaking, environmental policy instruments can be divided into command-and-control instruments (e.g. performance standards, stipulated technology) and price-based approaches (e.g. taxes, tradable emission permits, subsidies). Within the domain of price-based instruments, there is also the choice between taxes on the emissions as such and taxes on the outputs (i.e. the produce), or inputs (energy, feedstock, etc.), that are related to, but normally not perfectly correlated with, the emissions. Taxes on emissions are generally preferable because they directly address the discrepancy between private and social cost – however, in some cases they may be less practical and cost-effective than taxes on outputs or inputs. The latter is the case when the costs of monitoring emissions are high, the technological options for reducing emissions are limited or when the potential for reducing emissions by substitution in output or input is high (Schmutzler and Goulder, 1997).

In this section, we argue that these conditions are fulfilled for GHG emissions from food production and that, therefore, GHG weighted consumption taxes should be imposed on animal food with the purpose to stimulate substitution towards less emission-intensive diets. This policy strategy to promote low-emission food consumption should be complemented with measures that stimulate the exploitation of the low-cost technical reduction potentials and subsidies to support grazing on biodiversity-rich permanent pastures.

Taxes on emissions have in several cases, such as carbon dioxide from fossil fuels and sulphur, proven to be cost-effective policy tools for reducing emissions. However, a prerequisite for a cost-effective application of emission taxes is that emissions can be accurately monitored. In the cases of carbon dioxide and sulphur from fossil fuels, monitoring is possible at relatively low cost. For methane and nitrous oxide emissions from farm operations, however, monitoring costs would most likely be prohibitively expensive. Emissions of methane from enteric fermentation in the digestive tract of ruminants are correlated with feed intake but can differ considerably between individual animals, even when feed composition and other factors are similar. For instance, for cattle consuming the same feed, emissions can vary by up to a factor of two (Lassey, 2007). Therefore, to accurately monitor methane from enteric fermentation, emissions from a significant sample of animals at the farm would have to be measured regularly. Nitrous oxide emissions from agricultural soils are correlated with nitrogen fertilizer input, but variation is much larger than in the case of enteric methane, with fluctuations of several orders of magnitudes over short time scales (Bouwman and Boumans, 2002). An accurate monitoring of nitrous oxide emissions would require virtually continuous measurement for a great fraction of the fields at a farm. Obviously, for both methane and nitrous oxide the costs of such extensive emission monitoring schemes would be extremely high.

Furthermore, the effectiveness of emission taxes is lower if the technological options for reducing emissions are limited, and as was shown in previous section, for GHG emissions from food production, the technical potentials are overall minor (Figure 18.4). In contrast, the potential for reducing emissions by substitution between food products of similar characteristics (e.g. between different types of meat) is very large, as also was shown in previous section.

We conclude, therefore, that output taxes on emission-intensive food products are likely to be a far more effective policy instrument than emission taxes for mitigating agricultural GHG emissions. An effective scheme for such output taxes could be one where the tax is imposed at the consumption level, with the tax differentiated by the GHG emission levels per unit of food. The differentiation by GHG emissions means that taxes are weighted according to the average production emission intensities for the food categories. This means that the tax on ruminant meat should be around 20 times higher than on chicken (compare data in Figure 18.2). In principle, all categories of food should be subject to a GHG weighted consumption tax. However, for practical reasons, it is reasonable to exempt vegetable food, since their much lower GHG emissions per food unit mean that the administrative costs of vegetable food taxation compared to the achieved emission reduction would be much higher than for animal food.

Assuming that such a tax scheme was introduced in the EU, significant reductions in GHG emissions would be obtained due to the tax-induced changes in food consumption. For a tax level of €60 per ton CO_2-eq, which is not an unlikely level of future carbon costs assuming a stringent climate policy in the EU, total net reduction of agricultural emissions (excluding land use change–related emissions) would be about 33 million ton CO_2-eq; see Figure 18.5 (Wirsenius et al., 2011). This corresponds to about a 7% reduction of current GHG emissions in EU agriculture. This relatively modest mitigation effect from imposing emission costs at the consumer level has been observed in other, more recent studies. Edjabou and Smed

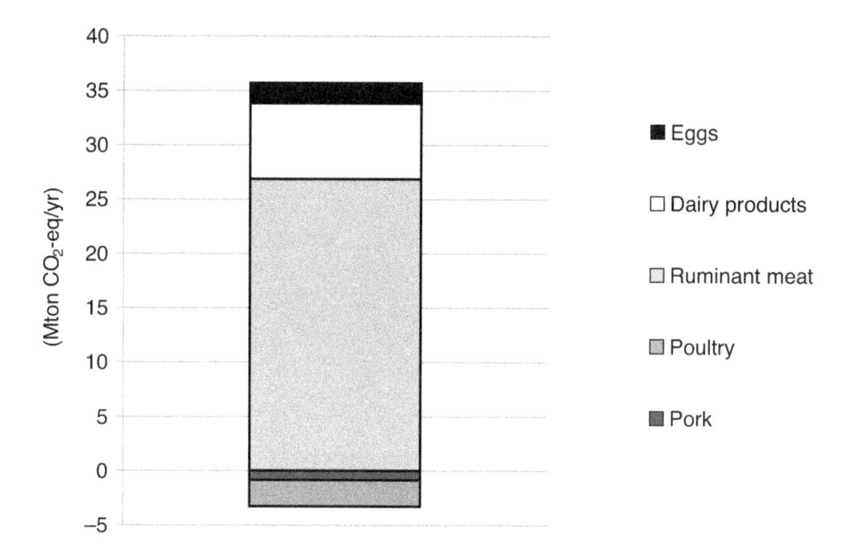

FIGURE 18.5 Reductions in GHG emissions from animal food production in the EU for GHG weighted consumption taxes on animal food equivalent to €60 per ton CO_2-eq.

Source: Wirsenius et al. (2011).

(2013) estimated the mitigation effect of tax levels corresponding to €35 and €100 per ton CO_2-eq on Danish food consumption at about 6% and 15%, respectively. Notably, the tax schemes were found to have lower mitigation effect in additional scenario variants where the increased tax burden on high-emission foods was compensated by reduced value added tax (VAT) on low-emission foods. In a study with a broader environmental scope that included also nitrogen and phosphorus pollutants, Säll and Gren (2015) estimated the GHG mitigation effect at 12% assuming an implementation of an environmental tax on Swedish meat and dairy consumption corresponding to about €110 per ton CO_2-eq.

GHG weighted consumption taxes on animal food would only be considered in a world aiming at strongly mitigating climate change. In such a case, bioenergy would turn out as a profitable source of energy, since prices of fossil fuels would increase (either through a carbon tax or a cap and trade system). Therefore it is reasonable to assume that land made available due to the tax-induced changes in food consumption (see Figure 18.6) would be used for bioenergy (or afforestation that sequesters carbon) rather than remaining unused. In that case much larger emission reductions could be achieved. If the land made available were used for production of lignocellulosic crops that replace coal in electricity production, GHG emissions would be reduced by some additional 200 million ton CO_2-eq, or around seven times higher emissions reductions compared to those that stem from reduced animal food production only (Wirsenius et al., 2011). In addition to these reductions, land use change–related carbon emissions in beef-exporting regions (e.g. Brazil) would

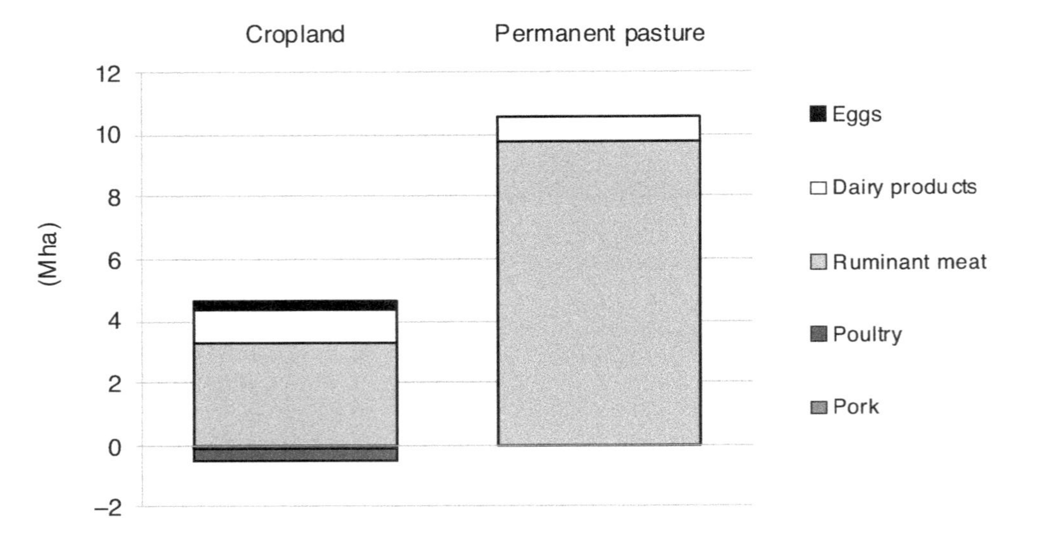

FIGURE 18.6 Reductions in land use for animal food production in the EU for GHG weighted consumption taxes on animal food equivalent to €60 per ton CO_2-eq.

Source: Wirsenius et al. (2011).

also be reduced to some extent, since a decreased beef consumption in the EU would reduce non-EU regional beef supply through global market mechanisms.

An advantage of a consumption tax instead of an emission tax is that it would not entail substantial distortionary effects between domestic production and imports. Emission taxes imposed on production in the EU would create a cost disadvantage for EU producers in relation to producers outside the EU, which would lead to higher import ratio in EU food supply. Although the GHG emission from EU food production would decrease due to lower production in the EU, global emissions would not decrease to the same extent but would rather be moved to other parts of the world (so-called 'carbon leakage'). In contrast, a tax levied at the consumption level is not likely to cause emission leakage, since the tax most likely would affect EU and non-EU producers equally.

A major disadvantage of a GHG weighted consumption tax scheme is that it does not provide incentives for the producers to reduce emissions by using improved technology and practices. Therefore, a consumption tax scheme should be supplemented by policies that promote or prescribe adoption of mitigation technologies. For example, for manure storage systems, the implementation of specific mitigation options (e.g. gas-proof sealing or anaerobic digesters) could be stipulated or subsidized. In this way, most of the low-cost technical mitigation potential could potentially be captured.

Choosing policy strategies for containing biodiversity-threatening agricultural expansion, especially deforestation, in the tropics is a complex topic, and it is beyond the scope of this chapter to deal with it thoroughly. Policies that moderate demand for ruminant meat – such as the scheme of GHG weighted taxes on animal food discussed earlier – would mitigate the expansion pressure. However, in many areas, such as parts of the Amazon, agricultural expansion for beef and crop production is profitable under current circumstances (Margulis, 2003), which means that expansion will persist, albeit perhaps more slowly, even if there is a drop in global demand. In many of the affected areas, lack of proper land titles is also a major factor that encourages speculative and short-sighted land use – for instance in the Brazilian Amazon only about 15% of privately owned land is backed by a secure title deed (IMAZON, 2009). Introduction of policy elements such as improved land regularization and changed economic incentives also needs to be accompanied by enhanced capacity of enforcement of legislation and surveillance of illegal clearing.

The conclusion that reduced ruminant meat production is a central policy objective for mitigating GHG emissions from the food and energy systems, as well as for protecting tropical biodiversity, raises the issue of conservation of grazing-dependent biodiversity on cultural permanent pastures in Europe and elsewhere. On the face of it, these two goals – reducing ruminant meat production and conserving pasture biodiversity – may seem to be in tension. However, in a global perspective the size of these hot spots of biodiversity-rich permanent pastures is small and does not play a major role in world ruminant supply. This means that the biodiversity-rich pastures may be maintained also in the case of lower ruminant meat and milk production. In the case of Europe, ruminant demand at current, or even higher, levels will not prevent these areas from being abandoned, due to unfavourable economic conditions and depopulation (EEA, 2004). Therefore, to protect biodiversity-rich pastures in the EU from being abandoned, by far the most effective policy strategy is to provide specific subsidies that enhance their economic viability – rather than keeping total ruminant production at a higher level.

In the analysis in Wirsenius et al. (2011), the assumed GHG weighted consumption tax led to increased consumption in poultry and pork. This result is quite sensitive to assumptions on cross-price elasticities, and available data on cross-price elasticities are sparse. Still, it is not unreasonable to assume that a GHG weighted consumption tax would increase poultry consumption. From an animal welfare perspective this would be an unwarranted effect, since the animal welfare problems in broiler chicken industry are well known (Butterworth, 2010). For instance, the birds are selected to grow very fast, which partly contributes to the relatively low GHG emissions from the production. However, the fast growth also leaves up to a quarter of the birds lame during the last week of their lives. Thus, a more holistic approach to a climate-friendly diet would be to substitute vegetables and pulses for meat, in particular beef and lamb. In that way, a diet to reduce greenhouse gases would not result in additional numbers of chickens suffering from lameness, skin damages, respiratory dieses, etc., that are prevalent in the current broiler industry.

In the chapter we have shown that the special features of the agricultural system call for an unorthodox policy mix. We suggest policies that aim at altering the diet towards less GHG-intensive food types. Just as policies have long aimed at increasing the energy efficiency in cars by fuel taxes, it is time to also address the GHG efficiency in our diets. After all, the food system today is a larger climate problem than the transport system. However, these policies, we have shown, must also be complemented by policies that ensure a more environmentally friendly production, by introducing measures to mitigate GHG emissions by technical means and subsidies to ensure continuous grazing of biodiversity-rich permanent pastures in Europe.

References

Akiyama, H., Yan, X. and Yagi, K., (2010) 'Evaluation of effectiveness of enhanced-efficiency fertilizers as mitigation options for N2O and NO emissions from agricultural soils: Meta analysis', *Global Change Biology*, vol 16, pp 1837–1846.

Asner, G. P., Elmore, A. J., Olander, L. P., Martin, R. E. and Harris, T. (2004) 'Grazing systems, ecosystem responses, and global change', *Annual Review of Environment and Resources*, vol 29, no 1, pp. 261–299.

Bodirsky, B. L., Popp, A., Weindl, I., Dietrich, J. P., Rolinski, S., Scheiffele, L., Schmitz, C. and Lotze-Campen, H.. (2012) 'N2O emissions from the global agricultural nitrogen cycle: Current state and future scenarios', *Biogeosciences*, vol 9, pp 4169–4197.

Bouwman, A. F. and Boumans, L. J. M. (2002) 'Emissions of N2O and NO from fertilized fields: Summary of available measurement data', *Global Biogeochemical Cycles*, vol 16, no 4, p 1058.

Bryngelsson, D., Wirsenius, S., Hedenus, F. and Sonesson, U. (2016) 'How can the EU climate targets be met? A combined analysis of technological and demand-side changes in food and agriculture', *Food Policy*, vol 59, pp 152–164.

Butterworth, A. (2010) 'Cheap as chicken', In: Webster, J. and D'Silva, J. (eds.) *The crisis in meat and dairy consumption: Developing a sustainable and greener future*, Earthscan, London, pp 133–148.

Edjabou, L. D. and Smed, S. (2013) 'The effect of using consumption taxes on foods to promote climate friendly diets: The case of Denmark', *Food Policy*, vol 39, pp 84–96.

EEA (2004) *High nature value farmland: Characteristics, trends and policy challenges*, European Environment Agency (EEA), Copenhagen, Denmark.

EPA (2012) *Global anthropogenic non-CO2 greenhouse gas emissions: 1990–2030*, U.S. Environmental Protection Agency, Washington, DC.

FAOSTAT (2015) FAO statistics. http://faostat3.fao.org/

Gerber, P. J., Steinfeld, H., Henderson, B., et al. (2013) *Tackling climate change through livestock: A global assessment of emissions and mitigation opportunities*, FAO, Rome, Italy.

Grainger, C. and Beauchemin, K. A. (2011) 'Can enteric methane emissions from ruminants be lowered without lowering their production?' *Animal Feed Science and Technology*, vol 166–167, pp 308–320.

Hedenus, F., Wirsenius, S. and Johansson, D. J. A. (2014) 'The importance of reduced meat and dairy consumption for meeting stringent climate change targets', *Climatic Change*, vol 124, pp 79–91.

Herrero, M., Havlík, P., Valin, H., et al. (2013) 'Biomass use, production, feed efficiencies, and greenhouse gas emissions from global livestock systems', *Proceedings of the National Academy of Science*, vol 110, no 52, pp 20888–20893.

Humpenöder, F., Popp, A., Stevanovic, M., et al. (2015) 'Land-use and carbon cycle responses to moderate climate change: Implications for land-based mitigation?' *Environmental Science Technology*, vol 49, no 11, pp 6731–6739.

IMAZON (2009) *The risks and the principles for landholding regularization in the Amazon*, Instituto do Homem e Meio Ambiente da Amazônia (IMAZON), www.imazon.org.br

IPCC (2014) Climate change 2014: Synthesis report: Contribution of Working Groups I, II and III to the Fifth Assessment Report of the Intergovernmental Panel on Climate Change [Core Writing Team, R. K. Pachauri and L. A. Meyer (eds.)], IPCC, Geneva, Switzerland.

Johansson, D. J. A. and Azar, C. (2007) 'A scenario based analysis of land competition between food and bioenergy production in the US', *Climatic Change*, vol 82, pp 267–291.

JRC-IES (2015) EDGAR: Emission database for global atmospheric research. http://edgar.jrc.ec.europa.eu/

Koungshaug, G. (1998) 'Energy consumption and greenhouse gas emissions in fertilizer production', IFA Technical Conference, 28 Sept–1 Oct 1998, Marrakech, Morocco.

Lal, R. (2004) 'Carbon emission from farm operations', *Environment International*, vol 30, no 7, pp 981–990.

Lassey, K. R. (2007) 'Livestock methane emission: From the individual grazing animal through national inventories to the global methane cycle', *Agricultural and Forest Meteorology*, vol 142, no 2–4, pp 120–132.

MacLeod, M., Gerber, P., Mottet, A., et al. (2013) *Greenhouse gas emissions from pig and chicken supply chains*, FAO, Rome, Italy.

Manne, A. S. and Richels, R. G. (2001) 'An alternative approach to establishing trade-offs among greenhouse gases', *Nature*, vol 410, pp 675–677.

Margulis, S. (2003) *Causes of deforestation of the Brazilian Amazon*, World Bank Working Paper No. 22, The World Bank, Washington, DC, USA.

Montes, F., Meinen, R., Dell, C., et al. (2013) 'Special topics: Mitigation of methane and nitrous oxide emissions from animal operations, II: A review of manure management mitigation options', *Journal of Animal Science*, vol 91, pp 5070–5094.

Myhre, G., Shindell, D., Bréon, F.-M., et al. (2013) 'Anthropogenic and natural radiative forcing', In: Stocker, T. F., Qin, D., Plattner, G.-K., et al. (eds) *Climate change 2013: Physical science basis: Contribution of working group I to fifth Assessment Report of the intergovernmental panel on climate chang*, Cambridge University Press, Cambridge, UK, pp 659–740.

Opio, C., Gerber, P., Mottet, A., et al. (2013) *Greenhouse gas emissions from ruminant supply chains*, FAO, Rome, Italy.

Popp, A., Lotze-Campen, H. and Bodirsky, B. (2010) 'Food consumption, diet shifts and associated non-CO2 greenhouse gases from agricultural production', *Global Environmental Change*, vol 20, pp 451–462.

Povellato, A., Bosello, F. and Giupponi, C. (2007) 'Cost-effectiveness of greenhouse gases mitigation measures in the European agro-forestry sector: A literature survey', *Environmental Science & Policy*, vol 10, pp 474–490.

Reilly, J., Prinn, R., Harnisch, J., et al. (1999) 'Multi-gas assessment of the Kyoto Protocol', *Nature*, vol 401, pp 549–555.

Säll, S. and Gren, I. M. (2015) 'Effects of an environmental tax on meat and dairy consumption in Sweden', *Food Policy*, vol 55, pp 41–53.

Schmutzler, A. and Goulder, L. H. (1997) 'The choice between emission taxes and output taxes under imperfect monitoring', *Journal of Environmental Economics and Management*, vol 32, no 1, pp 51–64.

Searchinger, T., Heimlich, R., Houghton, R. A., et al. (2008) 'Use of US croplands for biofuels increases greenhouse gases through emissions from land-use change', *Science*, vol 319, pp 1238–1240.

Steinfeld, H., Gerber, P., Wassenaar, T., Castel, V., Rosales, M. and de Haan, C. (2006) *Livestock's long shadow: Environmental issues and options*, Food and Agriculture Organization of the United Nations (FAO), Rome, Italy.

Tilman, D., Balzer, C., Hill, J. and Befort, B. L. (2011) 'Global food demand and the sustainable intensification of agriculture', *Proceedings of the National Academy of Science U. S. A.*, vol 108, pp 20260–20264.

Valin, H., Havlík, P., Mosnier, A., et al. (2013) 'Agricultural productivity and greenhouse gas emissions: Trade-offs or synergies between mitigation and food security?' *Environmental Research Letters*, vol 8, p 035019.

Weyant, J. P., De la Chesnaye, F. C. and Blanford, G. J. (2006) 'Overview of EMF-21: Multigas mitigation and climate policy', *Energy Journal*, vol 27, Sp. Iss. 3, pp. 1–32.

Wirsenius, S., Azar, C. and Berndes, G. (2010) 'How much land is needed for global food production under scenarios of dietary changes and livestock productivity increases in 2030?' *Agricultural Systems*, vol 103, pp 621–638.

Wirsenius, S., Hedenus, F. and Mohlin, K. (2011) 'Greenhouse gas taxes on animal food products: Rationale, tax scheme and climate mitigation effects', *Climatic Change*, vol 108, pp 159–184.

Wise, M., Calvin, K., Thomson, A., et al. (2009) 'Implications of limiting CO_2 concentrations for land use and energy', *Science*, vol 324, p 1183.

19

MEAT AND POLICY

Charting a course through the complexity[1]

Tim Lang

Meat is a 'hot' policy issue for the food industry, governments and consumers. Half a century ago, to question unrestricted meat consumption would have been to stand in the way of what was deemed to be culinary progress and the expansion of personal choice. The Western world judged vegetarians as rather weird or eccentric or worse, certainly not progress. Progress was not what ancient culinary cultures such as vegetarian India or carnivorous China had developed, namely low- or no-meat plant-based diets, but was firmly in the 'meat at the centre of the plate' school of thought, and the more meat the better! Policy makers worldwide in post–World War II reconstruction were generally committed to increasing meat production and servicing rising demand, and an intensification of modes of production was unleashed (Brandt, 1945; Nierenberg, 2005). Even in India, the cattle population was expanded for milk, if not meat. That policy support for meat (and dairy, the flipside of the policy coin) delivered the astonishing growth in meat production and consumption, evidenced in this book and elsewhere (Steinfeld et al., 2006). This chapter addresses the challenge to policy makers now that meat's policy status is so in doubt and indeed in some quarters is almost inverted. Far from being a good thing, data suggest the need to curtail and almost certainly either reverse or radically transform its production and consumption. Whichever route is followed, past policy is certainly looking increasingly ragged. The chapter concludes with an overview of the policy options. Although the battles over meat's role in public health and environment are ever clearer, I argue that the cultural battle over the place of meat in culinary and consumer culture is going to be critical. This is a battle for hearts and minds, not just mouths. This is about reconfiguring food progress.

Policy arguments for and against meat

In the last two decades, there has been a veritable explosion of analyses and data about meat production, which has emerged as central to a number of key public and planetary health challenges. These range from climate change to water use (Gerber et al., 2013; Hoekstra, 2010; Bailey et al., 2014); from land use to culinary culture (Holm and Møhl, 2004; Elferink and Nonhebel, 2007); from economic development to social inequalities (Larsen, 2012; Bailey et al., 2014); from heart disease to cancers (IARC, 2015; Bouvard et al., 2015; Sinha et al., 2009; Aune et al., 2013; Chan et al., 2011); and to sources of communicable disease such as *salmonella, campylobacter,* and *e coli.* Because the biodiversity on which humanity depends looks to be currently part threatened by meat consumption, we now find conservation bodies increasingly worried about the seemingly inexorable rise in meat production (the policy 'success' legacy) and developing action plans for meat reduction (Machovina et al., 2015; WWF, 2015). As a result, over recent decades, the gap between evidence, policy, and practice has grown ever wider and more fraught. It would be possible, if not wholly true, to argue that the meat industry is now intellectually beleaguered, forced to rely on strong political lobbying and financial influence to retain its favoured policy status.

Such a conspiracy interpretation would be wrong. A sound policy analysis – whatever our personal preferences – has to consider the policy arguments *for* meat, too. Even in a book largely and rightly critical of the 20th-century legacy of meat industrialization, we must note that meat might have a place in ecosystems and culinary culture. It is better for critics of meat (and dairy) to know their opposition truly than to paint a false picture. Indeed, one of the reasons the animal welfare movement has made such remarkable policy inroads into animal management in recent years is because it did its homework properly and came to understand the motivations of farmers and industry. To change policies and policy actors (i.e. people), it helps if you really know them and their differences, and can engage across all the nuances of positions and possibilities. Pragmatically, it is important for meat critics to recognize the fairly consistent message that meat can have a positive nutritional role. The good news is that even mainstream, usually cautious national advice is beginning to recognize the problem of overconsumption. In my own country, the UK, the official nutrition advice since 2016 now includes "[e]at less red and processed meat" at the edge of the advice plate (Public Health England, 2016). This would have been unthinkable a decade ago.

Health is not the only policy concern. Meat is a test case for how and whether policy makers will align the food system with sustainability goals (Garnett, 2009; Tilman et al., 2001). There is strong evidence for behaviour change, for a reorientation of production and for a refinement of supply chain management, land use, and food culture. Meat and dairy consumption is already far too high in high-income countries; is growing too fast in middle-income countries; and is economically aspirational in low-income countries. The evidence, however, suggests that countries at *all* income levels ought to reset their meat and dairy consumption goals.

In my view, this means a new policy goal: to realign animal husbandry with animals' appropriate ecological niche. Cattle didn't evolve in human agriculture to be corralled in feedlots, receiving what the US Department of Agriculture reports as 70–90% of their nutrient intake in the form of grain and protein concentrates

(USDA, 2017). Cattle evolved and were bred mostly to live outdoors but everywhere are increasingly indoors. The rise of concentrated animal feeding operations (CAFO), first in the US and now spreading, is remarkable. CAFOs mean prime land is used to grow crops for animals when they are poor energy converters. It makes more ecologic sense to use land to grow plants direct for human consumption. But CAFOs are an extreme illustration of the 20th-century trend to develop cheaper meat, even though this accelerates the nutrition transition, a term used to describe the shift from simple to highly processed diets that happens when standards of living rise. This nutrition transition is manifest worldwide, bringing a costly health toll in its wake (Monteiro et al., 2013; Popkin, 2003; Popkin and Gordon-Larsen, 2004). Rising meat consumption, particularly red and processed meats, is associated with some cancers (WCRF, 2013; WCRF/AICR, 2009).

As battles over evidence on diet and meat's impact on health or environment rage, official policy makers come under pressure. Meat producers vie with the defenders of health and environment as to which of them best represents the consumer in public policy. The former invoke choice, preference, and individual rights. The challenge, according to this position, is how to unleash ever more production and how to service demand *ad infinitum*. Health and environmental interests, on the other hand, cite public responsibilities, planetary, and health limits. They now ask: what would it take to shift population behaviour to a level where meat-free or low-meat diet is the new normal?

Meat thus unleashes huge philosophical issues. If policy makers favour meat reduction, they are siding with constraint on choice and the whole 20th-century neoliberal consumerist vision. But if they do favour unfettered production and consumption, the critics counter, they consign public and planetary health to ever greater strain. What starts as a scientific matter, supposedly shaped by evidence, rapidly becomes a matter of values and perspective. This is a battle over what we mean by progress. Why is the ubiquity and plentifulness of meat deemed to be a food advance? Why is little attention being paid to epidemiological evidence of the advantages of plant-based diets at the population level, and of the case for rich countries to lower their meat intake, particularly red and processed meat (McMichael et al., 2007)? These are huge and complex questions. No wonder policy makers are somewhat shy of addressing them. But address them, they must. If not now, soon.

This chapter began with a short summary of the evidence against meat or certainly its radical curtailment and policy reorientation. Supporters of meat production and consumption view the situation very differently. Their view is that production and consumption must be encouraged to rise. And 20th-century history suggests that population behaviour has been on their side. Partly, this has been facilitated by the astonishing 'efficiencies' of industrial output. This has not just been due to animal breeding improvements or the industrialization of farms by CAFOs and other methods, but also of the inputs – grain, energy, land, water, minerals, buildings, pharmaceuticals. An army of scientific, technical, and engineering advice has underpinned this. The result has been meat price reduction, which has made everyday meat affordable in those economies where consumers' disposable incomes have risen. The moment their incomes rise, they consume more. Here lies the policy lock-in to the *status quo*. There may be a mismatch of evidence, policy, and practice, and a terrain crisscrossed by competing demands – consumer choice, culinary history, industry economic might, moral dilemmas, public health, and environmental protection – but the hard reality is that few if any politicians dare to enter this policy terrain.

The case for animals goes wider. Animals can convert food waste; this has been an historic use of domestic pigs and poultry (Stuart, 2009). Modern nutritionists also confirm the importance of red meat as a rich source of iron, along with minerals and vitamins such as zinc and vitamin B12 (Fairweather-Tait, 2007). Animals can make use of land otherwise inappropriate for primary production – uplands, marsh, wild terrain (Fairlie, 2010). They are vital income earners for huge populations, particularly in the developing world where a cow or some goats can be a passport to better incomes, family health, and well-being.

The ace in meat proponents' policy pack is that a large majority of consumers like meat (and dairy) (Fairlie, 2010). The drop in meat prices has thus been a boon. Meat has moved from 'feast day' food to 'everyday' food. Social status plays a part in this. Meat (more than dairy) has been historically high status, something reserved for festivals, something which symbolized the exceptional access and choice available to rich people everywhere (Rogers, 2004). Modern marketing and advertising fuels the status appeal of meat. Supermarketization sells itself as offering cheaper meat but always 'fine' or 'choice' cuts. They have to be careful not to say the meat is suspiciously cheap because most consumer cultures have experience of food industries' capacity to adulterate food and sell frauds (Wilson, 2008).

How has this messy policy situation come about? Where now?

Unless one believes that consumers are deluded and don't know what they are doing or have become the pawns of the marketing and advertising industries, one has to accept that consumers buying meat all the time are doing so out of some element of volition. This is why meat reduction becomes so tricky for policy makers. Politicians don't like to attack their voters. And their voters are consumers, the very same meat eaters.

People, organizations, and scientists who want to reduce meat's central role in food culture thus have a hard task. Raising meat and dairy consumption has been an indicator of progress. In the mid-20th century, a consensus had emerged between agricultural policy makers, who saw the economic advantages for farmers of cattle rearing, and the increasingly influential science of nutrition, whose advice was to use milk in particular as a social fix for poor nutrition. John Boyd Orr, who became first Director General of the new UN Food and Agriculture Organisation post–World War II, was no exception. He was one of the most influential food scientists of the day, later recipient of the Nobel Peace Prize for his food work, and the researcher who had shamed the British government with his data on the shocking state of UK food poverty in the 1930s (Boyd Orr, 1936). He was a key government policy advisor in World War II but in 1943 was a wonderfully clear if trenchant 'angry professor' when he wrote *Food and the People*. This was a visionary and powerful policy appeal to tackle child ill-health by instituting school meals (including meat) and providing daily cow's milk for growing children (Boyd Orr, 1943). These were to be the new food welfare, and to reduce malnutrition and stunting. It is possible, he and others argued, to raise food production and get good, quick-fix foods available to all the people.

This kind of intellectual support for animal and dairy production helped frame the 'productionist' policy architecture of the post–World War II food system (Lang and Heasman, 2015). Largely vegetarian India was the exception, of course (Stuart, 2006), but even there massive policy support shifted it from low production to becoming the biggest dairy herd in the world by the end of the 20th century (Punjabi, 2009). Meat or dairy were to take an important place in meals. This ushered in changes to the older traditional pattern of the meal. Sidney Mintz, the great US food anthropologist, has noted that traditional meals almost everywhere used to have three basic elements: a core food item such as rice (C), a fringe item such as a sauce (F), and a legume (L) (Mintz, 1996). This CFL pattern was even recently common in developing economies but has changed to a different recipe: meat (M) plus a staple (S) such as potatoes and two vegetables (V): M + S + 2V. Meat has triumphed, central to the meal, rather than providing flavouring or being the exceptional. It has moved from feast day to every day.

But today, meat is a powerful drag on progress. It is undermining food system success. So what would the goal of a food system framed for sustainable development look like? The scientific consensus is to reduce meat from the Western high, and to cap the aspirations of the low-income-country consumers – what is called a 'contract and converge' policy (Royal Society, 2012). This would be a seismic policy shift.

Consider the figures. In 2014 US consumers ate on average 90 kilos (kg) of meat per year, nearly three times the world average of 34 kg. But average figures disguise remarkable variation in what kind of meat and how much different countries eat. Israel, for example, leads the world in chicken consumption at 57.7 kg per capita per annum (kg/pc/pa) compared to India's 1.7 kg/pc/pa (OECD Data, 2017). The European Union's consumers eat 33 kg/pc/pa of pork meat a year, marginally more than China's 31.6 kg, compared to Mozambique's 3.9 kg or Mexico's 11.5 kg. The broad policy support for meat, therefore, is taking different forms across the world. In 1992, Jeremy Rifkin could argue in *Beef Culture* that the food system is now geared to serve cattle (Rifkin, 1992). Today, a mere quarter of a century later, meat production is hydra-headed: pushing pig production in some, chicken in others, and beef in yet others.

There is a particularly important cultural element here. By 'culture' I mean the mix of aspirations, norms, meanings, and values which people bring to the table, i.e. the set of assumptions and everyday 'rules for living' which we all apply to our food choices. These rules are learned, and shaped overwhelmingly by family, religion, location, and income. So if we want to recalibrate meat culture – and ask policy makers to help that – we enter the moral, not just scientific, world. And on meat, possibly like no other in the world of food, moral philosophers have been particularly effective and noisy over the last half century. Partly in horror at the intensification of meat production, and partly reconnecting with older analysis of the case for respecting animals (most famously Aristotle) (Spencer, 1993), moral philosophers have articulated the modern case for meat reduction or eradication (Singer, 1975; Singer and Mason, 2006; Ricard, 2016). Historically, most religions have set rules of everyday life for meat consumption and the killing of animals. In a consumerist world, those cultural rules have been shown to be malleable. Inherited moral codes come up against neoliberal choice culture. New cultural segmentation occurs, with conflicts between thought leaders on all sides. This moral dimension to modern life is highly political, of course, in contemporary geo-politics. That conflict between hardline or liberal interpretations of the great religions is beyond the scope of this book, but it happens that what matters for meat policy is that the new moral case against meat is secular. It is replacing (or revising) existing moral rules. Food ethics and welfare standards may transform how animals are reared, handled, and killed before consumers see the meat, but the new secular rules are also beginning to shape meat consumption. One of the most famous, barely a decade old, is Prof. Michael Pollan's simple dictum: "Eat food. Not too much. Mostly plants" (Pollan, 2008, p. 35).

This brief summary of the arguments pushing at policy makers' doors suggests a complex picture of arguments about meat, mostly for a new constraint or contract-and-converge, but also reminding us of the case for meat. Table 19.1 provides a brief summary. No wonder politicians are wary of taking a lead on meat policy. Leave well alone! Stay in the post-war comfort zone, championing market forces or consumer rights and the 'freedom to choose'! Can we blame policy makers for seeing meat as something to leave in the 'too hard to deal with' box or for ministers to 'leave for my successor to deal with'? This, however, is to bury heads in the sand.

Multi-level, multi-actor, multi-sector policy responses

How could policy makers engage with this complexity? Since the 1970s, a policy framework has emerged for almost all issues – not just food, let alone meat – which policy academics describe as multi-level, multi-actor, and multi-sector. Gone are the days when 'policy' was only what governments did or thought. In this section, I sketch how this complex modern policy world emerges and shapes what can or might be done about meat policy.

In 2006 the FAO published *Livestock's Long Shadow*, an ambitious audit of the role and impact of livestock (Steinfeld et al., 2006). This sent an official UN signal into the meat policy terrain that there is a significant problem. Meat critics saw this as validating the unsustainability of meat, but the report also recommended a policy push to reduce the CO_2 emissions from meat production without necessarily

TABLE 19.1 Summary of significant policy arguments for and against meat

Issue	*Salient factor*	*Argument for meat*	*Argument against meat*
Ecosystems	Land use	Can use grasses and other food not directly available to humans	Gross waste of land producing grain for animals
	Water	n/a	Heavy direct and indirect use of water in animal rearing
	Biodiversity	Some value in protecting marginal lands	Big driver of biodiversity destruction
Health	Nutrition	Direct source of iron, folates, zinc; indirect source of income which improves health	Competes with plant production for direct human use; significant role in non-communicable diseases
	Safety	Value depends on good levels of hygiene	Can be source of communicable disease unless optimum hygienic production, slaughter, and cooking
Economic	Employment	Huge employer	Some jobs working on animals are degrading (e.g. abattoir work)
	Supply chain	Major source of value-adding	Mass industrialized meat is too cheap
	Costs	Profitable product to some sectors	Huge externalized health and environmental costs
	Waste	Animals can use food waste if hygienic	Waste should be reduced anyway and the rest can be composted
Socio-cultural	Pleasure	Long-term cultural appeal	21st century food culture needs to de-emphasize meat
	Consumer choice	Strong consumer support	Consumer tastes can be reshaped
	Inequalities	Animal production can be source of significant income for low-income small producers	Meat consumption reflects grossly unequal distribution of wealth within and between societies
Morality	Values	Neoliberal belief in primacy of individual choice	Inhumane and unethical
	Religion	Most religions condone meat; Hinduism is one exception	Some meats are proscribed by some religions, as are some slaughter methods

confronting high or rising meat consumption. The report also sidestepped the role of ruminants in sequestering carbon through grass (see other chapters in this volume). The meat industry, equally, demanded a 'recount' and seven years later, the sequel report appeared. This showed that the most efficient farm systems could reduce greenhouse gas emissions by up to 30% (Gerber et al., 2013). But it also noted that if world consumption continued to rise, those efficiency gains would be cancelled out.

Food products vary widely in where their main greenhouse gas emissions are concentrated (Munasinghe et al., 2009). For cooked vegetables, it is the consumer cooking them at home that contributes most. For meat and dairy, the largest source of emissions is before the farm gate. This is why the big retailers with such a grip on milk supply chains are exploring the impact of changed feeding regimes, more efficient use of grazing (also to keep carbon in the soil), and improving agricultural practices. There is parallel thinking about how to reduce greenhouse gases in meat production. The motive is partly self-interest – fear of being blamed later – and partly because the corporate sector recognizes that while governments and policy makers come and go, and are shaped by electoral cycles, they and their shareholders have an eye on long-term market growth and share. Their technical managers see the logic and want to do the right thing. As a result, they have increasingly adopted a 'choice-editing' approach (Gunn and Mont, 2014; National Consumer Council and Sustainable Development Commission, 2006). In choice-editing, the retailer or manufacturer shapes change before the consumer sees the food product. The product is reformulated; or its size altered; or its supply chain is re-engineered; or all of these. The net effect is to change the product *before* consumers can exert their 'right to choose'.

Strategies such as choice-editing expose the role of governmental policy makers. Here are the big companies taking meat's negative role seriously, so what are you governments doing? Choice-editing can actually let governments off the hook, leaving matters to their beloved market forces. Some theoreticians argue this hands-off role for government is right; government has no place in shaping consumer policy. Others, not least companies, know this is not wholly true. Markets work well only if there are some common terms of reference, standards, legal duties, and fairness.

There is governmental policy at five levels: global, inter-governmental or continental, national, sub-national (local), and domestic. In each, different actors vie for influence. This patchwork policy world is complex and is why NGOs may lobby at the EU or national or global level for law changes or governmental commitments, while companies lobby for something different, and all eye how mass consumer behaviour works. To make things even more complex, there can be little congruence between policy actors even within nominally the same family of agencies. Within the UN, for instance, UNEP has been more openly critical of the environmental consequences of meat, and the WHO has come ever clearer in its recommendations to keep consumption of red and processed meats low, while the FAO has tended to support meat production, even while producing evidence which undermines that. At the UN level, i.e. at the New York–based UN itself, rather than at FAO in Rome or UNEP in Nairobi or WHO in Geneva, there has emerged an important set of overarching goals which ought to shape new meat policies.

The 2015 Paris Climate Change Accord committed governments to strong reduction actions (UNFCCC, 2015), and the 2015 Sustainable Development Goals agreed upon the same year also had a thread of food throughout their 17 goals and following 163 targets (United Nations, 2015). Without specifying meat, these policies point to meat reduction, or certainly a dramatic alteration in meat production. These positive policy pointers came after disappointment with the long-arranged 2014 International Conference on Nutrition (ICN2), the first UN reconvening on nutrition since the first ICN in 1992 (FAO and WHO, 1992). In the run-up to 2014, there had been much pressure from scientists and NGOs for ICN2 to set clearer linkages between environment, health, and production, but it did so only in broad terms (Brinsden and Lang, 2015). It did however promise a Decade of Nutrition Action (FAO and WHO, 2014) through which more might follow.

Why ICN2 mattered so much is that for decades nation states have been encouraged by the UN to set dietary guidelines as frameworks for public and commercial policy. In Sweden, Australia, the Netherlands, the UK, Germany, and elsewhere, scientific advisors began to try to create a new generation of sustainable dietary guidelines, expanding the nutrition advice (Lang, 2014). Most attempts were rebuffed, unless left at fairly soft advice, without hard targets or KPIs. As the ICN2 process met, the US was becoming the policy frontline in this long tussle. Since the 1980s, by law the US has to revise its official Dietary Guidelines for Americans (DGA) every five years. The 2012–15 US revision received clear advice from its scientific advisors – in a huge, comprehensive literature review (since updated) (Nelson et al., 2016; US Dietary Guidelines Advisory Committee, 2015) – that the DGA should inject environmental considerations into dietary advice. This was furiously lobbied against by the US meat industry which persuaded the Secretary of State for Agriculture to its side, despite loud consumer and health lobbying (over 30,000 submissions from the public supporting the change). Productionism triumphed over commitments to tackle meat-related non-communicable diseases.

The health policy case for controlling meat is not simply a battle over nutrition, but also over meat's role as a vector in communicable disease. In 2015, the WHO produced its first ever estimate of the cost of foodborne disease (WHO, 2015). Almost 1 in 10 people fall ill every year from eating contaminated food and 420,000 die as a result. Children under five years of age are at particularly high risk, with 125,000 children dying from foodborne diseases every year. Africa and Southeast Asia have the highest burden of foodborne diseases. The WHO report went far wider than meat, of course, but meat is a thread running throughout the analysis. (The precise connection warrants amplification.) The policy response here does not automatically point to meat reduction but could be pharmaceuticals and better farm practices, which are indeed the default policy response.

Food safety directly threatens not just consumers but also commercial reputation and trust. It underpins food culture. Food quality scandals can and do destabilize governments (Smith et al., 2005). For over two decades, for example, UK politics was peppered with animal health–related incidents: *salmonella* in eggs exposed hidden food poisoning rates (Agriculture Committee, 1989); BSE (mad cow disease) exposed unsavoury feeding practices (Zwanenberg and Millstone, 2005); foot and mouth disease exposed poor farm practice (and some hints of illicit trade) (National Audit Office, 2002); and deaths induced by *e. coli* showed poor butcher hygiene standards (Pennington, 1996; Pennington, 2009). In the US, the Centers for Disease Control and Prevention estimate is that one in six people got sick from foodborne illness (CDC, 2016).

Within the food industry, there is clear recognition of the dangers posed by meat. Reputations can be damaged, and sales hit. The policy framework within which most work is Hazards Analysis Critical Control Point (HACCP), first developed from the 1950s to prevent food poisoning in food for US astronauts (who can hardly get to a local hospital) (US FDA, 2015). HACCP encourages management and workers to identify where the most likely source of risk lies and to focus on prevention there. It is a tool for cleaning up rather than stopping supply chains. Some food companies have seen the market opportunities in meat reduction, not just its cleanup. Since the 1990s there has been a rise and now explosion of plant-based processed food products, with a rush of technical innovation today. Some giant food companies now recognize the ecological impact of their supply chains.

This mix of motives is why there has been a slow but steady acceptance of the policy approach known as Sustainable Consumption and Production (SCP). SCP emerged from the 1992 Rio UN Conference on Environment and Development (UNCED), where the EU offered to take the global lead in fleshing this policy thinking out, with Sweden offering to be lead. It culminated in the EU's 2008 Communiqué (European Commission, 2008). Many food companies saw the value of this as creating a new level playing field and a rationale for choice-editing. For a while it looked as though this could create a new level playing field in Europe, with the food industry doing important assessments of the carbon footprint of their products. Inevitably, meat and dairy emerged as key, if not *the* key, foods in not just climate change but water and nutrition in these audits (IGD, 2013; IGD ShopperVista et al., 2013).

The picture I am painting is of slow development – useful preconditions, perhaps for wider change. But the elephant in the room has been consumers. Few want to confront them, certainly not on the mass scale the scientists have long been suggesting (McMichael et al., 2007). Arguably it is civil society which has taken the clearest lead in confronting meat habits. As often happens in food policy, NGOs are the policy scouts, mapping future directions and encouraging mass consumption to follow. Animal welfare organizations have been in the front of this process, but are now accompanied by large conservation and public health bodies. WWF's Livewell project charting a sustainable diet and modelling it across Europe warrants particular credit (World Wildlife Fund, 2015). The largest conservation organization in the world has recognized that it will not protect biodiversity unless it encourages consumers to cut back on meat (Gladek et al., 2016). This spawned many internal arguments but continues to be rolled out. Across the world, many NGOs have made this policy leap. Some new campaigns and collaborations have emerged, such as the Square Meal Coalition (RSPB, 2014) and WWF's annual report with the Zoological Society of London (WWF and Zoological Society of London, 2015), or the Eating Better coalition in the UK (Eating Better, 2016). Meatless Monday, now a global campaign, has encouraged school cooks to reduce meat offerings since it began in the US in 2003 (Meatless Monday Global, 2016). Such coalitions can open up policy space, encouraging evidence-gatherers to speak out, creating room for progressive policy makers to act. Without such outside pressure, it is unlikely official bodies could take the step such as Public Health England's revised Eatwell advice in 2016 to "[e]at less red and processed meat", cited earlier (Public Health England, 2016).

In summary, a complex range of strategic options now exists and is being populated by diverse actors. Gone is the policy era where governments governed from on high. In its place is this messier policy world where companies may be more powerful than governments, and where policy is overtly not just covertly ideological, and where there are multiple actors, ranging across a spectrum of possibilities. This range of options for meat futures is summarized in Table 19.2. These go from

TABLE 19.2 The range of strategic options for meat futures

Option	*Intention*	*Comment*
Increase production	Build meat industry and encourage consumption	This is happening but storing up future trouble
Technical development	Meet increased demand through new technology, taking a variety of forms from laboratory-grown meat or intensive fish tanks to novel plant proteins	This approach requires consumer acceptance and carries risks to trust and market stability.
'Freeze' at current levels	Maintain status quo	This exposes policy makers to accusations of policy drift and complacency; offers little public interest gain but is the default position for meat trades
Reduce production	Ration consumption by various means including pricing and taxation	This would raise prices but heighten unequal access, possibly increasing desirability
Reduce consumption	Stimulate change to more sustainable diets, sending signals from consumers to supply	This implies that supply chain would not respond to increase uptake
Ban or rationing	Reduce negative impacts drastically	Enforced veganism is politically unacceptable even in vegetarian cultures

supporting more production and consumption (undesirable today but the default) to their restriction and reorientation (desirable). On a positive note, the health and environmental evidence has begun to affect the discourse. And official guidelines ought to be one means to set targets to meet SCP, and to switch from policy being at the upper end of Table 19.2 to being farther down. Academic modelling has also begun to suggest global targets of around 90g of meat per capita per day (Weis, 2013; Smil, 2013; McMichael et al., 2007), but most analysts recognize such figures need to be nuanced according to the meat type and its mode of production – grass-fed versus grain-fed, etc. – and to be created to suit local and national conditions. There is simply not enough or effective pressure yet to get these goals agreed upon, let alone implemented. This is now the urgent task on meat.

To meet sustainable development and health goals, we need to put pressure on policy makers to start climbing a progressive 'ladder' of achievement, which must include the commitment to: (1) produce a solid evidence base that meat and dairy are problematic; (2) develop global/national/local/domestic 'meat reduction/change' strategies; (3) identify alternative land use and livelihoods for current producers; (4) develop population change strategies; (5) identify industry winners and losers, supporters and opponents; and (6) reposition meat and dairy consumption as seasonal or exceptional, i.e. to become 'feast day' not 'every day'. Table 19.3 outlines policy measures which could be invoked to reshape meat production and consumption. The table outlines which actor tends to use each measure and what its implications or potential for meat might be. 'Soft' measures

TABLE 19.3 The range of public policy measures available to shape meat supply and consumption

Measure	*Main sources*	*Implications for meat policy*
Advice	Tends to be state or companies	Tends to be weak and with low impact
Labelling	State or company	Puts onus on consumers, who can feel information overload; labels are used by producers to convey mode of production
Education	Used to be a state role, but is increasingly used by corporations and e-media	Takes a long time to be effective; works best when coupled with other measures
Public information	Increasing corporate involvement; legacy of 'old' top-down governance	Currently dominated by commercial advertising and marketing, and increasing virtual and web-based media presence
Endorsement and sponsorship	Corporate	Increasing role of celebrity culture; some blurring of lines between media content and advertising
Welfare	State welfare e.g. school food	Opportunities for state sector to take a lead in shaping attitudes

Measure	*Main sources*	*Implications for meat policy*
Product/ compositional standards	This used to be the preserve of the state but increasingly set through supply chain contracts and specifications	Rise of animal welfare and organic farm movements has had a significant effect on championing process orientations in standards-setting
Licensing	Traditionally state, but now used by companies, and by NGOs negotiating their own standards	Consumers may not be aware of such measures
Subsidies	State	Deeply opposed by neoliberal theoreticians as market distorting
Competition rules	State	Competition bodies could conduct inquiries into the level of market concentration in the meat sector
Research and development	State and private sectors	Programmes to explore alternatives to meat and meat reduction are needed
Taxes and fiscal measures	State can incentivize 'good' and penalize 'bad' actions	Can become highly politicized, but are the most feared measures by vested interest, as they mean real change and can add direct costs; critics see this as market distortion
Bans	Used to be preserve of state, but companies do increasingly exert bans although almost always only on 'own-label' products	These exemplify overt 'choice-editing' and usually require clear PR handling by companies
Rationing	Preserve of state, usually in times of crisis	Meat can be rationed in times of war or market shortage; conventional peace-time markets also ration by creating equilibrium between supply and demand

are at the top of the table, and 'hard' ones towards the bottom. In practice, meat policy and actions tend to be accompanied by soft measures because the default position has been won by the productionist agenda – more and cheaper meat for all. This is the challenge.

Conclusion

This chapter has outlined the new complex policy world in which meat policy is a sub-section. This is a multi-level, multi-actor, multi-sector world. The evidence for tackling runaway meat production and consumption is strong. There is a gap between evidence, policy, and practice, a gap which sadly is not unusual in policy. It took half a century for the evidence (and much campaigning by doctors and NGOs) on tobacco, for instance, to create intergovernmental support for the WHO's global 2003 Framework Convention for Tobacco Control (WHO, 2003). Still today, however, tobacco is legal, and public behaviour remains in thrall to the ideology of consumer choice, albeit now happily constrained in part. The good news is that sudden policy changes can and do happen. Smoking was banned on the London Underground after a fire in 1987 (Fennell, 1988), and people obeyed the ban. In the 2000s, a ban on smoking in public or work buildings indoors spread worldwide. Suddenly governments were prepared to act, and people prepared to obey. Commerce and the giant tobacco corporations were put on the back foot; enough businesses supported controls for there not to be a commercial backlash. Culture changed.

In the case of meat, too few policy makers so far are prepared to act so strongly. But then in 2016 the Chinese government showed some leadership, taking the remarkable step by announcing a commitment to constrain meat (Milman and Leavenworth, 2016). Time will tell how this will work. Meanwhile, few governments talk even privately of 'hard' measures, although they are beginning to recognize the urgent need to act on climate change. I see this policy situation as one of precondition for big change, rather than that big change actually happening. But the preconditions have taken much work and much evidence. Slowly, the pressures are building up and some policy frameworks which cover meat have begun to emerge. The movement to create Sustainable Dietary Guidelines continues to grow. Policy commitments to sustainable consumption and production (SCP) are nominally accepted by companies and governments. The big challenge remains how to get the significant shift among consumers and how to change behaviour sufficiently for animals to be back into their ecological niche, and for meat production and consumption to be downgraded after decades, if not centuries, of policy support. There is much to do before we can say that meat policy is evidence-based.

Note

1 This extensively rewritten chapter replaces that by Lang, Wu and Caraher in the first edition of this book, and draws on thinking in Mason and Lang (2017).

References

Agriculture Committee (House of Commons). (1989) *Salmonella in Eggs: A Progress Report*, London: Her Majesty's Stationery Office.

Aune D, Chan DS, Vieira AR, et al. (2013) Red and processed meat intake and risk of colorectal adenomas: A systematic review and meta-analysis of epidemiological studies. *Cancer Causes Control* 24: 611–627.

Bailey R, Froggatt A and Wellesley L. (2014) *Livestock: Climate Change's Forgotten Sector: Global Public Opinion on Meat and Dairy Consumption*, London: Royal Institution of International Affairs.

Bouvard V, Loomis D, Guyton KZ, et al. (2015) Carcinogenicity of consumption of red and processed meat. *The Lancet Oncology*. http://dx.doi.org/10.1016/S1470-2045(1015) 00444-00441.

Boyd Orr J. (1936) *Food, Health and Income: Report on Adequacy of Diet in Relation to Income*, London: Macmillan and Co.

Boyd Orr SJ. (1943) *Food and the People*, London: Pilot Press.

Brandt K. (1945) *The Reconstruction of World Agriculture*, London: George Allen & Unwin.

Brinsden H and Lang T. (2015) Reflecting on ICN2: Was it a game changer? *Archives of Public Health* 73, doi: 10.1186/s13690-015-0091-y.

CDC. (2016) Attribution of Foodborne Illness: Findings Atlanta: Centers for Disease Control and Prevention, www.cdc.gov/foodborneburden/index.html [accessed 22 April 2017].

Chan DS, Lau R, Aune D, et al. (2011) Red and processed meat and colorectal cancer incidence: Meta-analysis of prospective studies. *PLoS ONE* 6: e20456.

Eating Better. (2016) Statement Welcoming the New Public Health England Eatwell Plate, March 17 2016, Brighton: Eating Better Coalition.

Elferink EV and Nonhebel S. (2007) Variations in land requirements for meat production. *Journal of Cleaner Production* 15: 1778–1786.

European Commission. (2008) Communication from the Commission to the European Parliament, the Council, the European Economic and Social Committee and the Committee of the Regions on the Sustainable Consumption and Production and Sustainable Industrial Policy Action Plan COM/2008/0397 Final, Brussels: Commission of the European Communities.

Fairlie S. (2010) *Meat: A Benign Extravagance*, East Meon, NH: Permanent Publications.

Fairweather-Tait SJ. (2007) Iron nutrition in the UK: Getting the balance right. *Proceedings of the Nutrition Society* 63: 519–528.

FAO and WHO. (1992) *International Conference on Nutrition: Final Report of the Conference*, Rome: Food and Agriculture Organisation, and World Health Organisation.

FAO and WHO. (2014) ICN2 International Conference on Nutrition: Better Nutrition, Better Lives. 19–21 November 2014, Rome. Rome: Food and Agriculture Organisation.

Fennell D. (1988) *Investigation Into the King's Cross Underground Fire: Report to the Department of Transport*, London: Her Majesty's Stationery Office.

Garnett T. (2009) Livestock-related greenhouse gas emissions: Impacts and options for policy makers. *Environmental Science & Policy* 12: 491–503.

Gerber P, Steinfeld H, Henderson B, et al. (2013) *Tackling Climate Change through Livestock: A Global Assessment of Emissions and Mitigation Opportunities*, Rome: Food and Agricultural Organisation. www.fao.org/3/i3437e.pdf [accessed March 3 2014].

Gladek E, Fraser M, Roemers G, et al. (2016) *The Global Food System: An Analysis: Report to WWF*, Amsterdam: WWF Netherlands, 188.

Gunn M and Mont O. (2014) Choice editing as a retailers' tool for sustainable consumption. *International Journal of Retail & Distribution Management* 42: 464–481.

Hoekstra AY. (2010) The water footprint of animal products. In: D'Silva, J. and Webster, J. (eds). *The Meat Crisis: Developing More Sustainable Production and Consumption*, London, UK: Earthscan, pp 22–33.

Holm L and Møhl M. (2004) The role of meat in everyday food culture: An analysis of an interview study in Copenhagen. *Appetite* 34: 277–283.

IARC. (2015) *The Carcinogenicity of the Consumption of Red Meat and Processed Meat*. IARC Monographs Volume 114 *IARC Monographs*, Lyons: The International Agency for Research on Cancer of the World Health Organization.

IGD. (2013) *Sustainable Diets Working Group* (chair: Cathryn Higgs), Letchmore Health (Herts): IGD.

IGD ShopperVista, Arnold H and Pickard T. (2013) *Sustainable Diets: Helping Shoppers*, Letchmore Heath: IGD.

Lang T. (2014) Sustainable diets: Hairshirts or a better food future? *Development* 57: 40–256.

Lang T and Heasman M. (2015) *Food Wars: The Global Battle for Mouths, Minds and Markets.* 2nd edition, Abingdon: Routledge.
Larsen J. (2012) *Plan B: Meat Consumption in China Now Double That in the United States.* Earth Policy Institute. www.earth-policy.org/plan_b_updates/2012/update102 [accessed January 21 2017].
Machovina B, Feeley KJ and Ripple WJ. (2015) Biodiversity conservation: The key is reducing meat consumption. *Science of the Total Environment* 536: 419–431.
Mason, P and Lang T. (2017) *Sustainable Diets: How Ecological Nutrition Can Transform Consumption and the Food System,* London and New York: Routledge.
McMichael AJ, Powles JW, Butler CD, et al. (2007) Food, livestock production, energy, climate change, and health. *The Lancet* 370: 1253–1263.
Meatless Monday Global. (2016) Meatless Monday Global. www.meatlessmonday.com/the-global-movement/ [accessed January 21 2017].
Milman O and Leavenworth S. (2016) China's plan to cut meat consumption by 50% cheered by climate campaigners. *The Guardian.* Beijing and London, 20 June. www.theguardian.com/world/2016/jun/20/chinas-meat-consumption-climate-change [accessed January 22 2017].
Mintz S. (1996) *Tasting Food, Tasting Freedom: Excursions Into Eating, Culture and the Past,* Boston: Beacon Press.
Monteiro CA, Moubarac J, Cannon G, et al. (2013) Ultra-processed products are becoming dominant in the global food system. *Obesity Reviews* 14: 21–28.
Munasinghe M, Dasgupta P, Southerton D, et al. (2009) *Consumers, Business and Climate Change: Report by SCI With the CEO Forum of Companies,* Manchester: Sustainable Consumption Institute, University of Manchester, 59.
National Audit Office. (2002) The 2001 Outbreak of Foot and Mouth Disease: Report by the Comptroller and Auditor General. HC 939 Session 2001–2002, June 21 2002. London: The Stationery Office.
National Consumer Council and Sustainable Development Commission. (2006) Looking Back Looking Forward: Lessons in Choice Editing for Sustainability: 19 Case Studies into Drivers and Barriers to Mainstreaming More Sustainable Products, London: Sustainable Development Commission.
Nelson ME, Hamm MW, Hu FB, et al. (2016) Alignment of healthy dietary patterns and environmental sustainability: A systematic review. *Advances in Nutrition* 7: 1005–1025.
Nierenberg D. (2005) *Happier Meals: Rethinking the Global Meat Industry.* Worldwatch paper 171, Washington, DC: Worldwatch Institute.
OECD Data. (2017) Meat Consumption (indicator). doi: 10.1787/fa290fd0-en, Paris: Organisation for Economic Co-Operation and Development. https://data.oecd.org/agroutput/meat-consumption.htm[accessed January 15 2017].
Pennington HC. (1996) Report on the Circumstances Leading to the 1996 Outbreak of Infection with E.coli O157 in Central Scotland, the Implications for Food Safety and the Lessons to be Learned, Edinburgh: The Scottish Office.
Pennington HC. (2009) The Public Inquiry Into the September 2005 Outbreak of E.coli 0157 in South Wales, Cardiff: Wales Assembly Government, 355.
Pollan M. (2008) In Defence of Food: The Myth of Nutrition and the Pleasures of Eating, London: Allen Lane.
Popkin BM. (2003) The nutrition transition in the developing world. *Development Policy Review* 21: 581–597.
Popkin BM and Gordon-Larsen P. (2004) The nutrition transition: Worldwide obesity dynamics and their determinants. *International Journal of Obesity and Related Metabolic Disorders* 28: S2–S9.

Public Health England. (2016) *The Eatwell Guide: Helping You Eat a Healthy, Balanced Diet*, London: Public Health England.

Punjabi M. (2009) *India: Increasing Demand Challenges the Dairy Sector*, New Delhi: Food and Agriculture Organisation. www.fao.org/docrep/011/i0588e/I0588E0505.htm [accessed January 20 2017].

Ricard M. (2016) *A Plea for the Animals*, Boulder, CO: Shambala Publications.

Rifkin J. (1992) *Beyond Beef: The Rise and Fall of the Cattle Culture*, New York: Dutton.

Rogers B. (2004) *Beef and Liberty: Roast Beef, John Bull and the English Nation*, London: Vintage books.

Royal Society. (2012) *People and the Planet*, London: Royal Society.

RSPB, Wildlife Trusts, Friends of the Earth, Sustain, et al. (2014) *Square Meal: Why We Need a Better Recipe for the Future*, London: Food Research Collaboration.

Singer P. (1975) *Animal Liberation: A New Ethics for Our Treatment of Animals*, New York: Random House.

Singer P and Mason J. (2006) *Eating*, London: Arrow.

Sinha R, Cross AJ, Graubard BI, et al. (2009) Meat intake and mortality. *Archives of Internal Medicine* 169: 562–571.

Smil V. (2013) *Should we Eat Meat? Evolution and Consequences of Modern Carnivory*, Chichester: Wiley-Blackwell.

Smith DF, Diack HL, Pennington TH, et al. (2005) *Food Poisoning, Policy and Politics: Typhoid and Corned Beef in the 1960s*, London: Boydell Press.

Spencer C. (1993) *The Heretic's Feast: A History of Vegetarianism*, London: Fourth Estate.

Steinfeld H, Gerber P, Wassenaar T, et al. (2006) *Livestock's Long Shadow: Environmental Issues and Options*, Rome: Food and Agricultural Organisation.

Stuart T. (2006) *The Bloodless Revolution: Radical Vegetarians and the Discovery of India*, London: Harper Collins.

Stuart T. (2009) *Waste: Uncovering the Global Food Scandal*, London: Penguin.

Tilman D, Fargione J, Wolff B, et al. (2001) Forecasting agriculturally driven global environmental change. *Science* 292: 281–284.

UNFCCC. (2015) UN Framework Convention on Climate Change (COP21). Paris. November 30–December 11 2015. Bonn, Germany: United Nations Framework Convention on Climate Change. http://unfccc.int/secretariat/contact/items/2782.php.

United Nations. (2015) Sustainable Development Goals, Agreed at the UN Summit, September 27–29 2015, New York: United Nations Department of Economic and Social Affairs, Division for Sustainable Development. https://sustainabledevelopment.un.org/post2015/summit.

USDA. (2017) *Cattle and Beef: Background*, Washington DC: United States Department of Agriculture. www.ers.usda.gov/topics/animal-products/cattle-beef/background.aspx [accessed January 15, 2017].

US Dietary Guidelines Advisory Committee. (2015) Scientific Report of the 2015 Dietary Guidelines Advisory Committee to the Secretaries of the U.S. Department of Health and Human Services and the U.S. Department of Agriculture, Washington, DC: U.S. Department of Health & Human Services.

US FDA. (2015) *Hazards Analysis Critical Control Point (HACCP)*, Silver Spring, MD: United States Food and Drug Administration. www.fda.gov/Food/GuidanceRegulation/HACCP/ [accessed August 2 2016].

WCRF. (2013) *Red and Processed Meat and Cancers*, London: World Cancer Research Fund.

WCRF/AICR. (2009) *Policy and Action for Cancer Prevention: Food, Nutrition, and Physical Activity: A Global Perspective*, London and Washington, DC: World Cancer Research Fund/American Institute for Cancer Research.

Weis T. (2013) The meat of the global food crisis. *The Journal of Peasant Studies* 40: 65–85.
WHO. (2003) *WHO Framework Convention on Tobacco Control*, Geneva: World Health Organisation.
WHO. (2015) *WHO Estimates of the Global Burden of Foodborne Diseases: Foodborne Diseases Burden Epidemiology Reference Group 2007–2015*, Geneva: World Health Organisation, 225.
Wilson B. (2008) *Swindled: From Poison Sweets to Counterfeit Coffee: The Dark History of the Food Cheats*, London: John Murray.
World Wildlife Fund. (2015) Livewell: A Balance of Sustainable and Healthy Food Choices. http://assets.wwf.org.uk/downloads/livewell_report_jan11.pdf [accessed May 20 2015].
WWF. (2015) *On Our Plate Today: Healthy, Sustainable Food Choices: LiveWell Final Recommendations*, Gland: WWF-UK.
WWF and Zoological Society of London. (2015) *Living Blue Planet Report 2015: Species, Habitats and Human Well-Being*, Gland, Switzerland: WWF and ZSL.
Zwanenberg P van and Millstone E. (2005) *BSE: Risk, Science, and Governance*, Oxford and New York: Oxford University Press.

20

THE IMPACT OF LEGISLATION AND INDUSTRY STANDARDS ON FARM ANIMAL WELFARE

Carol McKenna

In 1965 a Government committee investigating the welfare of factory-farmed animals in the wake of the publication of Ruth Harrison's *Animal Machines* recommended that animals should have the freedom to "stand up, lie down, turn around, groom themselves and stretch their limbs" (Brambell, 1965). These freedoms provided the inspiration for the now internationally recognised 'Five Freedoms' that provide a framework for animal welfare that has been adopted in legislation and industry standards around the world (freedom from hunger and thirst; freedom from discomfort; freedom from pain, injury and disease; freedom to express normal behaviour; and freedom from fear and distress).

Half a century on, industrialised production systems that often deprive animals of the five freedoms have come to dominate global commercial meat and dairy production. This has occurred despite growing public concern for farm animal welfare and scientific revelations about the complex behaviours, emotions, needs and drives of farm animals, each one of which is an individual sentient being. Historian Dr Yuval Noah Harari has described domesticated cows and chickens as being among "the most miserable creatures that ever lived", citing the discrepancy between their evolutionary success and their individual suffering, as "one of the most important lessons of history" (Harari, 2015).

Whilst public opinion in support of farm animal welfare has become overwhelming in some parts of the world with a poll of European Union (EU) residents finding that 82% believe animal welfare standards need to improve (Eurobarometer, 2016), so-called agricultural progress has seen farm animals not only being treated as machines but transformed into machines by selective breeding. For example, chickens have been selectively bred for high breast yield and fast growth with adverse welfare and health impacts. Today new technologies – cloning, genetic engineering, gene editing – are posing new threats that risk animals being born to endure not only a life not worth living but suffering inflicted by their own genetics.

The worst systems for animal welfare in widespread use around the world include caged systems for rearing egg-laying hens (barren battery, so-called enriched and colony cages), intensive indoor systems for pigs (sow/gestation stalls,[1] farrowing crates), caged and standard indoor production of broilers (meat chickens), indoor and feedlot production of beef cattle, indoor tethered and free stall systems for dairy cows, caged systems for rabbits and veal crates[2] for calves.

Higher welfare alternatives for all these animals include well-designed, well-managed free-range systems, or indoor housing in well-ventilated buildings, with ample space, appropriate and adequate environmental enrichments, comfortable bedding, such as straw, as well as natural light. Higher welfare systems also avoid routine mutilations of animals and genetic selection of animals for fast growth and high yields where this results in compromised welfare such as ill-health, pain or limits on behavioural expression.

This chapter will explore what has been achieved so far through both legislative and voluntary industry approaches to move away from some of the worst farming systems for animal welfare towards higher welfare alternatives. It will also suggest where efforts might most effectively be targeted to realise a world where animals kept for food experience a good life with steadily reducing numbers being reared in systems that are better for animals, people and the planet.

Urgent action is needed because whilst a combination of legislation and international codes of practice covers billions of individual animals, many, many billions of farm animals continue to suffer appalling cruelty in intensive systems around the world, and sadly, legislators are increasingly leaving the issue for business to resolve.

Food industry momentum for change

Over the last few decades, consumers and campaigning groups have made effective use of emerging media technologies to raise the profile of farm animal welfare issues, piling pressure on governments, retailers and other businesses to move from farming systems that are bad for animal welfare towards those that are better, as outlined in Table 20.1. Public demand for improved farm animal welfare has led to the introduction of legislation and a number of voluntary farm welfare assurance schemes in many countries. It has also brought about initiatives between NGOs and global companies, working together to bring about sustainable animal welfare policy changes. While this approach has the potential to improve the lives of billions of farm animals, a lack of guaranteed enforcement in the absence of buttressing legislation and reliance on voluntary change alone risks empty promises.

Announcements by major international food companies of significant policy changes have fuelled an unprecedented ripple effect throughout the food industry in recent years. Since the landmark decision made by McDonald's in 2015 to reject eggs from caged hens, scores of other US companies – including retail giant Walmart with its 25% market share of the US grocery market – have declared their intention to go cage-free too, either on their shell eggs or their entire egg supply. In June 2016, the United Egg Producers, a cooperative representing egg producers

TABLE 20.1 Welfare potential of various farming systems for chickens, pigs, cattle and rabbits

Species	*Bad*	*Better*	*Best*
Egg-laying hens	Caged systems: barren battery, so-called enriched and colony cages.	Indoor barn with nest boxes, litter on floor, perches scratching areas, with or without natural light.	Free range with nest boxes, litter on floor, perches, scratching areas, natural daylight. Includes outdoor access for whole of laying period. Shade/shelter may or may not be provided. Organic* Nest boxes, litter on floor, perches, scratching areas, natural light outdoors, shade and shelter*. Outdoor access for whole of laying period*, smaller flock size (usually 2,000 birds in a house). *depending on the certification scheme.
Sows	Intensive indoor standard production with sow/ gestation stalls and farrowing crates.	Higher welfare indoor production. Group housing used throughout gestation and free farrowing. Nesting material (from 24 hours prior to farrowing) and bedding and manipulable material (edible fibrous material) provided.	Free-range outdoor grouping throughout gestation. Provision of: outdoor arks, bale tents, farrowing arks. Nesting material (from 24 hours prior to farrowing). Loose bedding material and manipulable material (edible fibrous material) provided throughout life, as well as wallows, rooting, vegetation, shade.
Meat pigs	Intensive standard indoor production. There is no enrichment. All and any of the following mutilations may occur: castration, spaying, tail docking, teeth clipping/grinding.	a) Higher welfare indoor b) Outdoor bred (born outside and fattened indoors) c) Outdoor reared (reared outside for about half their lives). For each of these systems loose bedding and manipulable materials are provided throughout life.	Free range. No routine mutilations. A minimum space allowance of at least $12m^2$/pig where accommodation is moved to new paddocks after each batch; a minimum of $40m^2$/pig where accommodation is not moved to the new paddocks after each batch.

(Continued)

TABLE 20.1 (Continued)

Species	*Bad*	*Better*	*Best*
		In b and c shelter and shade are provided outdoors and wallowing in hot climates. No routine use of mutilations permitted.	Outdoor access, loose bedding material and manipulable materials provided throughout life, wallowing in hot climates, shade and shelter outdoors.
Broiler chickens	Cage production and standard indoor production on floor.	Higher welfare indoor with stocking density of 30kg/m^2 or less in house and enrichment provided permitting perching, pecking of substrates, straw bales. Natural light provided.	Free range (27.5kg/m^2 in housing and 1m^2/bird outdoor. Outdoor access for half of life, natural cover/woodland and indoors: perching, straw bales Organic – 30kg/m^2 inside house plus access to 4m^2/bird outdoor area. One third of lifetime with outdoor access and limits on flock size, natural cover/woodland and indoors: perching and straw bales.
Beef cattle	Fully slatted indoors. Concentrated animal feeding operation (feedlot). Indoor part slatted floor. Straw barn/yards. Grain or other concentrate forms significant proportion of diet.	Semi-extensive system. Pasture reared in grazing season. Shade and shelter depending on climatic conditions. Grass is a significant part of the diet and may be supplemented.	Pasture reared/extensive. Grass grazing (silage, concentrate or suitable other supplement).
Dairy cattle	Tie stall. Free stall.	Free stall with pasture access for varying times of day according to scheme (e.g. RSPCA Freedom Food scheme requires at least four hours a day, and Beter Leven one-star scheme in the Netherlands requires eight hours a day for 150 days a year).	Free stall or deep-bedded barn with cows having free choice of access between housing and pasture. Extensive with year-round access to pasture that is well drained with shade and shelter provided.

Species	*Bad*	*Better*	*Best*
Meat rabbits	Caged systems.	Outdoor mobile runs (mobile cage on grass with a covered area, moved daily to provide fresh grass for grazing). Park system/barn system – cage-free indoor pen with no height restriction. Provision of platforms, gnawing blocks, hiding tubes, hay rack/compressed straw tube, non-wire flooring, natural light.	Free range: large outdoor enclosure with covered shelters and good fencing against predators. Provision of gnawing items, tubes (preferably), shelter with solid flooring, hay rack, bedding material (preferably).

owning more than 95% of all egg-laying hens in the US also announced its intention to phase out the culling of all male chicks in its entire egg-laying operation.

Some of Europe's biggest retailers have also announced that they are going cage-free. Summer 2016 saw unprecedented retail moves in the UK with Aldi, ASDA, Lidl, Morrison's, Iceland and Tesco's announcing that they would go cage-free on all their shell eggs by 2025. They followed in the footsteps of other companies that had already moved to a cage-free egg supply chain: Marks and Spencer in 1997, Waitrose in 2007, the Co-operative in 2007/8 and Sainsbury in 2009. Giants Unilever, Nestlé and Heinz have also made animal welfare commitments, including on cage-free eggs. July 2016 saw Sodexo, a leading food service company announcing that by 2025 it would be sourcing cage-free whole eggs and liquid eggs from local producers in all of its 80 countries of operation by 2025 (Food Ingredients First, 2016). September 2016 saw international contract caterer Compass Group announcing a global commitment to go cage-free on all its shell and liquid eggs by 2025.

The vast majority of the world's farmed animals are broilers. They represent, for example, 95% of farm animals slaughtered each year in the US. Two very important commitments to improve broiler welfare occurred in 2016 by the Global Animal Partnership (GAP) and Perdue Farms. GAP, the country's most comprehensive farm animal welfare standards body, announced its intention to replace 100% of its fast-growing chicken breeds with slower-growing breeds in order to address the root of the chicken welfare problem (Global Animal Partnership, 2016). Perdue, the third-largest chicken producing company in the US, introduced a detailed animal welfare policy aiming to create "an environment where chickens can express normal behaviours" (Perdue Farms, 2016). The company cited its reasons for change as including farmer support for improved husbandry methods and consumer interest in how animals raised for food are treated. The move followed a 2015 announcement by the company's chairman, Jim Perdue, that what the company needed was "happier chickens" (*New York Times*, 2015).

In stark contrast to this corporate momentum, the appetite for progress through legislation appears to have waned in the EU in recent years and has never really existed in the US, where, for example, poultry are exempt from most animal protection legislation. The European Commission has made it clear that it does not intend to introduce any new legislation. Indeed, I was present at a June 2016 speech in Brussels by the Commissioner responsible for animal welfare, where he made it clear that animal protection organisations shouldn't come knocking on his door but should seek to work with relevant stakeholders and develop voluntary solutions. To this end the EU has been discussing establishment of an Animal Welfare Platform to bring together stakeholders: an approach that will either prove fruitful or kick animal welfare issues into the long grass.

Table 20.1 contains information adapted from Compassion in World Farming Welfare Potential Matrices for different species.

International and national laws and standards for farm animal welfare

Since the world's first modern, national animal protection law was passed in the UK parliament in 1822 to prevent "the cruel and improper treatment of cattle", campaigning groups, businesses and legislators around the world have each played a part in improving the lives of farm animals. National animal protection legislation now exists in many countries, and the EU has taken a lead in introducing regulations and directives applicable across all its Member States. International standards relating to the health and welfare of farm animals have also been set by the World Organisation for Animal Health (OIE), but there is no mandate requiring implementation of the standards by its 180 member countries.

UK legislation

The UK Government is proud of its status as a world leader in animal welfare and has extensive legislation and guidance on farm animal welfare covering rearing, transportation and slaughter. The country has an 'A' rating from the Animal Protection Index (API), which classifies 50 countries according to their commitments to protect animal welfare in policy and legislation. The UK was one of only four countries to achieve an 'A' rating along with Austria, Switzerland and New Zealand.

The UK led the way internationally by banning the veal crate in 1990, which followed a court case taken by Peter Roberts, founder of Compassion in World Farming (CIWF) and high-profile campaigning by CIWF and other animal protection organisations. Further sustained pressure and campaigning brought about a ban on the keeping of pregnant sows in stalls in 1999, in advance of the 2007 and 2013 Europe-wide bans.

The main legislation relating to farm animals is the Animal Welfare Act 2006 (for England and Wales), the Animal Health and Welfare Act (Scotland) 2006 and the Welfare of Animals Act (Northern Ireland) 2011. In some areas, UK legislation exceeds the minimum standards required by the EU, for example, in relation to pigs and calves.

The Five Freedoms, which now inform international animal welfare legislation and standards, were established by the UK Government's independent advisory committee, the Farm Animal Welfare Council (FAWC), which led the development of farm animal welfare protection for many years. All UK Codes of Practice for the Welfare of Farm Animals include the five freedoms and provide detailed guidance to farmers and industry. Failure to comply with the Codes can also be used as evidence in prosecutions under certain primary legislation. The compulsory sections of these Codes are legal requirements set out in other legislation. The 2009 report "Farm Animal Welfare in Great Britain: Past, Present, Future" produced by the independent Farm Animal Welfare Committee, reports that animal welfare legislation in the UK is strong and that there is good compliance among farmers (FAWC, 2009).

Overall, the UK Government has forged a reputation for excellence in animal welfare legislation, but this is principally the result of the success of high-profile campaigns and enormous public pressure generated by CIWF and other animal protection organisations. Whether the UK government can retain its 'A' classification under the API remains to be seen. Its attempt – reversed in 2016 following high-profile opposition – to remove responsibility for the codes of practice for farm animals in England from Defra, the responsible government department, and replace them with guidance set by industry, contrasted starkly with its status as a forerunner in animal welfare. Another concern is government reluctance to make further progress through legislation, instead placing responsibility for action squarely at the foot of business and industry.

In the light of the Brexit decision the UK has the opportunity to demonstrate leadership to the rest of the world with respect to the future of food and farming. A move away from the Common Agricultural Policy presents possibilities to incentivise moves away from industrial agriculture towards a farming system that promotes public good by protecting the environment, public health and animal welfare. It will be important for the government to avoid a Brexit bonfire of EU legislation and to maintain and build on its existing legislation promoting a strong emphasis on shaping legislation and standards around the needs of each species of farm animal. The absence of cruelty and suffering does not equate to good animal welfare. A life worth living should be the absolute minimum standard for farm animal welfare moving forward, with the aim being for each animal to experience a good life (FAWC, 2009).

EU legislation

Since 1974, the EU has introduced several important pieces of legislation relevant to farm animal welfare, enforceable throughout the Member States. Most are

Directives, some are Regulations – both are legally binding and enforceable in all Member States. These laws have provided basic protection to billions of farm animals throughout the region and have a number of benefits as they establish welfare standards for farm animals during rearing, transport and slaughter, as well as banning some of the most inhumane aspects of industrial livestock production.

All EU legislation is underpinned by the Treaty on the Functioning of the European Union, which recognises animals as 'sentient beings'. This legal recognition of animals as sentient beings was first agreed in a landmark decision in 1997 and followed a ten-year-long campaign initiated by Compassion in World Farming's founder, Peter Roberts, and later supported by animal welfare organisations all over Europe. It means when considering any new legislation, the EU must "pay full regard to the welfare requirements of animals" (EU, 2007).

A core piece of EU legislation is Council Directive 1998/58, which lays down key principles and some minimum standards for the protection of all farmed animals, while other legislation relates to the welfare of animals during transport or at slaughter. Further detailed rules are in place relating to specific species such as pigs, laying hens, calves and broiler chickens.

The Pigs Directive (EU, 2008b), laying down minimum standards for the protection of pigs, bans the use of sow stalls/gestation crates for most of the sow's pregnancy, thanks to long-running consumer and NGO lobbying and campaigning, as well as strong scientific evidence (European Commission, 1997). This ban has created a ripple effect and similar bans and phase-outs are now being introduced in other parts of the world including in Australia, New Zealand and in some US states.

Unfortunately, the Directive still allows sows to be confined in stalls for the first four weeks of pregnancy, and it does not address the issue of barren environments and all-slatted floors for rearing pigs, which has had lasting knock-on effects for the provision of straw for bedding, although manipulable material must be provided. Tail docking also continues to occur routinely, despite the included ban on routine tail docking. Also relevant is the 2011 European Declaration on Alternatives to Surgical Castration of Pigs, which states that from 1 January 2012, surgical castration of pigs, if carried out, shall be performed with prolonged analgesia and/or anaesthesia; and surgical castration should be abandoned by 1 January 2018. Around 250 million pigs a year are affected by the EU Pigs Directive (FAO, 2012).

The Calves Directive (EU, 2008a), laying down minimum standards for the protection of calves, abolished veal crates in the EU following long-running campaigns by NGOs and considerable consumer pressure. Disappointingly, veal calves are still allowed to be reared in intensive conditions, without straw, and on an inadequate diet that enables 'white veal' to be produced. Just over 6 million calves every year are affected by this legislation (FAO, 2012).

The Laying Hens Directive (European Union, 1997) outlawed the keeping of the EU's 500 million laying hens in barren battery cages with the introduction of mandatory egg labelling acting as a key driver for change. EU hens' eggs must be labelled as either 'eggs from caged hens', 'barn eggs', 'free range' or 'organic', promoting consumer choice. In the UK this has led to an increase in production of cage-free eggs from 31% in 2003 to over 50% at present. Encouragingly, since the EU ban was introduced, there have been moves in other countries around the world to go cage-free.

Unfortunately, the Directive still allows laying hens to be kept in so-called 'enriched' cages that offer few significant welfare benefits for hens. This is because the space and height required are too small and the facilities for perching, pecking and scratching are too meagre to enable hens to properly engage in natural movements and behaviours. Furthermore, although the Directive prohibits all mutilations, it goes on to permit the cruel practice of beak trimming in certain circumstances. The EU legislation affects the lives of some 500 million hens – around 7% of the world's laying hens (FAO, 2012).

The Broiler Directive (European Union, 2007) contains a number of provisions designed to prevent some of the worst welfare problems arising from industrial broiler production. For example, it requires training for persons in charge of chickens, all chickens to have permanent access to dry and loose litter and all chickens to be inspected twice a day. Unfortunately, despite years of campaigning, the Directive has done little to significantly improve the welfare of broiler chickens; for example, the stocking density is little different from what many producers would have been using before the legislation was introduced and chicken growth rate is not addressed. The Directive has not resolved the welfare problems of broiler breeding chickens. The Poultry Meat Marketing Regulations specify the conditions for using higher welfare labels for various poultry meats; however there is no mandatory labelling of standard, low-welfare chicken meat. Around 7 billion broiler chickens are reared in the EU every year (FAO, 2012).

The Slaughter Regulation (European Union, 2009) provides that: "Animals shall be spared any avoidable pain, distress or suffering during their killing and related operations". It also requires slaughterhouse operators to draw up standard operating procedures, have monitoring procedures in place and to designate an animal welfare officer to assist them in ensuring compliance with the welfare rules. The Regulation requires that all animals, including poultry, are stunned before slaughter but regrettably exempts religious slaughter, which permits the killing of animals while they are fully conscious, causing suffering that competent stunning would avoid. Around 7 billion chickens, 160 million ducks, 300 million rabbits, 200 million turkeys, 27.5 million cattle, 250 million pigs and 6 million sheep are slaughtered annually in EU (FAO, 2012).

The Transport Regulation (European Union, 2004) lays down an overarching requirement that transporters must not transport any animal, or cause any animal to be transported, in a way which is likely to cause injury or undue suffering to that animal. It affords some worthwhile protection to animals in that it prohibits the transport of ill or injured animals, transporters are required to have an authorisation and drivers must have a certificate of competence. However, despite massive campaigning and lobbying, it still permits prolonged journeys and the scale of live transport remains worryingly high, presumably because of economic advantages for producers and traders. Thousands of live animals are exported from the EU on long journeys to the Middle East and other non-EU regions where even OIE minimum standards on animal handling, transport and slaughter are ignored.

Enforcement of the Regulation remains a major challenge, partly because of differences in interpretation of the requirements and because of lack of controls by the Member States. The quality of monitoring data, submitted to the Commission by Member States, is often insufficient to provide a clear analysis of the situation and to allow planning of specific corrective measures at EU level (European Commission, 2011).

US legislation

The API classifies the US as 'D' rated along with countries including Argentina, Indonesia, Peru, Tanzania, Uruguay and South Africa. The US has no federal (national) laws on the conditions in which farm animals should be kept, and farmed animals are often excluded from existing state anti-cruelty laws. Farmed animals are excluded from the federal Animal Welfare Act. On transport, the federal 28 Hour Law requires vehicles transporting animals for slaughter to stop every 28 hours to allow animals exercise, food and water. This law is rarely enforced, and the USDA advises it does not apply to birds. The Humane Methods of Livestock Slaughter Act requires animals to be stunned into unconsciousness and rendered insensible to pain prior to slaughter but has been interpreted as not applying to birds. However, some states have commenced introduction of legislation covering farm animal welfare (Humane Society of the United States, 2016).

Laws to end the use of gestation crates (sow stalls) have been passed in nine states – Arizona, California, Colorado, Florida, Maine, Michigan, Ohio, Oregon and Rhode Island. However, it must be said that these are not major pig producers. Iowa, North Carolina and Minnesota are the main pig producing states, holding 55% of the 66 million US pigs alive at any one time (USDA, 2012). Nevertheless these limited state bans have saved 16,000 breeding pigs from stalls in Arizona and almost 150,000 breeding pigs from stalls in Colorado (Humane Society of the United States, 2016). Eight states now have legislation to ban or end veal crates and five states have legislation banning battery cages. Dairy cow tail docking is banned in California, Ohio and Rhode Island. California is the top dairy state, with 1.8 million dairy cows, around 15% of whom were docked before the ban. It is estimated that as many as 80% of dairy cows nationally may be docked. It should be noted that this practice is not permitted under the OIE's standards.

International legislation

Animal welfare was first identified as a priority in the OIE Strategic Plan 2001–2005, aiming for 'recommendations and guidelines' covering animal welfare practices. All 180 member countries have to date adopted the OIE's guiding principles, its ten animal welfare standards in the OIE's Terrestrial Code and four animal welfare standards in the OIE's Aquatic Animal Health Code. Importantly the OIE's guiding principles for animal welfare outlined in the introduction to the Terrestrial Code include the statement that "the use of animals carries with it an ethical responsibility to ensure the welfare of such animals to the greatest extent practicable".

The OIE standards largely reflect what is considered normal good industry practice. They consist mostly of general principles and educational guidance about handling and husbandry, rather than specific requirements. OIE appears to treat all conventional rearing systems as equally acceptable if the general principles are followed and outcomes are acceptable within conventional good farming practice. However, this approach implicitly accepts factory farming and normalises the reduced quality of life that is inevitable in intensive conditions. Disappointingly the OIE Codes are merely voluntary and there is no requirement for them to be implemented by member countries.

Nevertheless, the OIE standards are important in setting global baselines and demonstrating consensus in principle that welfare is an important aspect of animal production. The existence of these standards and codes also illustrate that it is possible to set global criteria and agree on unacceptable practices. However, the OIE's response to calls for it to act following gross breaches of the Codes, such as the recent US plan to kill poultry by turning off ventilation in the case of disease outbreak, has been extremely disappointing. Another area of considerable and recurring concern is the transportation of animals. For example, in June 2016, Australia suspended cattle exports to Vietnam after NGO investigators revealed that cattle were being bludgeoned to death with sledgehammers in one Vietnamese slaughterhouse. The investigators found that only two out of 13 slaughterhouses visited met requirements (*Daily Mail*, 2016).

The influence of the OIE is limited because implementation and enforcement and quantitative standards are left to member countries, and many countries, including wealthy countries like the US, fail to take action (Animal Protection Index, 2014). For example, the US Government has failed to enact legislation on a number of OIE standards, including on humane slaughter of poultry, humane transport of poultry and welfare in beef cattle production systems. If they were to be implemented globally, the OIE's guiding animal welfare principles and standards have the potential to greatly improve the health and well-being of billions of animals. For example, according to FAO figures (FAO, 2012), more than 69 billion land animals are slaughtered worldwide each year: 62 billion chickens, 2.9 billion ducks, 1.5 billion pigs, 1.2 billion rabbits, 630 million turkeys, 530 million sheep, 440 million goats and 300 million cattle. In addition, 10–100 billion farmed fish are slaughtered every year (Fishcount, 2010).

Voluntary producer and food business schemes

Background

There is evidence of increasing interest and concern among consumers to know more about where their food has come from and to have the option to purchase products that ensure higher welfare for farm animals (Eurobarometer, 2016). Unfortunately, the lack of mandatory method of production labelling means that labelling on meat and dairy products can often be bewildering and often fails to provide consumers with the information they need to make an informed choice (*The Times*, 2016). Generic, meaningless phrases – such as 'farm fresh' or 'natural' – and images of rolling landscapes and happy animals are often displayed on factory-farmed products when the reality of how they were reared couldn't be more different.

Consumer desire for higher welfare products and the lack of proper, accurate labelling has driven the emergence of several voluntary assurance schemes – such as RSPCA Assured in the UK and Global Animal Partnership in the US – with the aim of raising farm animal welfare while helping consumers buy higher welfare products. Alongside these voluntary producer schemes, NGOs and big business have come together. Collaboration between major food businesses and NGOs such as CIWF and the HSUS has instigated the announcement of a number of major corporate policy changes.

There are significant differences between and also within voluntary producer schemes with respect to the animal welfare benefits experienced by difference species of farm animals. The best schemes go beyond minimum legal requirements and attempt to ensure that animals experience either a life worth living or a good life.

Voluntary producer schemes

UK

RSPCA Assured (formerly Freedom Food) is a UK food labelling scheme aiming to improve the welfare of animals farmed for food. RSPCA Assured assesses farms, hauliers and abattoirs to the RSPCA's welfare standards, and if they meet the standards the RSPCA Assured label can be used on their products. The RSPCA Assured website states the scheme covers 9 million meat chickens (around 1% of meat chickens slaughtered in the UK), 18 million laying hens, 2.5 million pigs, 3 million turkeys, 198 million salmon and 35.5 million trout.

The Red Tractor (Assured Food) labelling scheme offers few welfare benefits beyond compliance with minimum legal requirements, although it doesn't permit the castration of pigs. Red Tractor covers over 800,000 broilers, 1.7 million dairy cows, 8.5 million pigs and 1.6 million of the beef cattle and calves slaughtered during the year (Defra, 2014).

US

The Global Animal Partnership (GAP) is a US based 5-Step® animal welfare labelling system. It starts with Step 1 – no cages, crates or crowding – and goes up to Step 5 and 5+ – equivalent of European organic standards or higher. Products are available through retailers and foodservice in the US and Canada. The 5-Step®

ratings were launched in every Whole Foods Market store in the United States and Canada in 2011.

By the end of 2015 more than 3,000 farms were reported to be operating under GAP, supplying more than 400 Whole Foods stores. At that time Whole Foods was the largest purchaser of GAP-certified products with more than 300 million animals being covered under the scheme (Pacelle, 2016).

In 2016 GAP made a ground-breaking commitment to tackle the welfare of broiler chickens by announcing that by 2024 it would work "to replace 100 per-cent of fast-growing chicken breeds with slower-growing breeds for all levels of its 5-Step® Rating Program" (GAP, 2016).

Retailer own-brand standards

UK

Compassion in World Farming's Good Farm Animal Welfare Awards celebrate the commitment of leading food businesses to improve animal welfare standards. As of June 2016, a total of 342,717, 311 farm animals are set to benefit each year from the Awards, including: 53 million hens, 284 million broilers, 276,000 dairy cows and calves, 2.6 million pigs and 3 million rabbits.

Sainsbury is one of the UK's biggest supermarkets, and in February 2009 it became the first of the UK's larger retailers to stop selling eggs from caged hens. Sainsbury has also eliminated the use of caged eggs in ingredients.

Waitrose, one of the UK's leading supermarkets, advises on its website that it believes "animal welfare and good business go hand in hand". Waitrose 'Essential British chicken', its cheapest own-brand chicken, has 25% more space than the industry standard and meets RSPCA stocking standards. All Waitrose breeding sows are outdoor all their lives and all pigs are outdoor bred. No farrowing crates are used. Waitrose high welfare veal comes from one supplier who rears veal calves on straw in barns.

US

According to a March 2016 article in *World Poultry*, the shift to cage-free among US food business companies has reached 'tipping point'(World Poultry, 2016). The HSUS lists on its website around 60 major food companies that have announced phase-outs of gestation crates and/or battery cages, including major companies McDonald's, Compass Group, Sodexo, Burger King, Subway, Wendy's, Starbucks, Unilever and Taco Bell (Yum! Brands). According to HSUS, around ten grocery supermarkets have made similar commitments or expressed aspirations to end the use of confinement systems for hens or pigs or veal calves.

Around a dozen food manufacturers, including Kraft Foods, Heinz, Unilever, Nestlé, General Mills and ConAgra Foods, plus ten animal producers, including Cargill, Hormel Foods, Tyson Foods, Smithfield Foods, Strauss Veal, Wolfgang Puck and Maple Leaf Foods, have also made similar commitments. Not all have switched or made concrete commitments to end the use of confinement systems. Their statements may, for example, acknowledge that current confinement systems are undesirable or becoming unacceptable and that change should be beginning. Tyson, for example, is urging, rather than requiring, its pig suppliers to move to systems where sows can turn around and improve 'quality and quantity of space' (Tyson, 2014).

Walmart has committed to a 100% cage-free egg supply chain by 2025. Cargill has agreed to move to 100% group sow housing by 2017 in the US. Sodexo's switch to cage-free hens for its shell eggs has already benefited 150,000 hens, and by 2020 it will switch to cage-free for its liquid eggs, benefiting a further 750,000 hens per year. Sodexo has also committed to end supplies from veal crates within two years from 2015. HSUS also lists five hotel/hospitality groups that have made similar commitments, including Hyatt, Marriott International and Hilton Worldwide.

The grocery arm of the Retail Council of Canada has announced a switch to cage-free eggs by 2025 (a ten-year phase out) (Canadian Grocer, 2016).

Animal welfare rating and scoring systems

The Welfare Quality project

The Welfare Quality assessment protocols have been devised and tested by an EU-funded group of European scientists, led by Wageningen University. The project aimed to find a way of integrating animal welfare into the food quality chain. The scoring systems measures 30–50 detailed aspects regarding the animals, for example, evidence of disease or injury and expression of normal behaviour, their environment and their management, and then rates these against 12 welfare criteria and finally four principles of good welfare (feeding, housing, health and behaviour) to give an overall score for the farm. The 12 welfare criteria appear to be an expanded version of the Five Freedoms and include the provisions that animals should have comfort for resting and enough space to move around freely. The overall farm scores (for the species) are then banded into 'unclassified', 'acceptable', 'enhanced' and 'excellent'. Protocols were published in 2009 for poultry, cattle and pigs, and require a very detailed examination of both animals and farm and would give a clear picture of the state of the animals on any farm. It is difficult to ascertain what impact they have had on the food chain or how many food companies use them.

Future progress in farm animal welfare

Over the last 20 years, much has changed in the pursuit of a better life for farm animals. The principal aim of campaigners used to be to see new or improved legislation ban inhumane farming practices such as the use of veal crates or the long distance live transport of animals. Sustained and hard-hitting campaigns, often over years or even decades, which grabbed the attention of both politicians and the public, were essential to persuade policy makers to act.

There is no doubt that a great deal has been achieved through such traditional campaigning. The UK now has some of the best animal protection laws in the world and is matched by only Austria, Switzerland and New Zealand in the API's 'A' classification. EU legislation has prohibited some of the worst aspects of industrial livestock production such as veal crates, barren battery cages and sow stalls. However, very considerable strengthening of the law is required before the EU can take the view that it has put in place a body of law that fully protects the welfare of farm animals and indeed legislates for a positive state of well-being for them.

Legislation and improved enforcement of current legislation is desperately needed to end all, not just some, of the abuses of industrial animal production. Some of the key issues that need to be tackled are the keeping of fattening pigs and chickens reared for meat in barren, overcrowded sheds and the genetic selection of animals for very fast growth and high yields. Furthermore, the transport regulation is inadequate in that it still permits prolonged journeys over huge distances across Europe and beyond. A staggering 2 million cattle and sheep are exported from the EU every year to the Middle East, North Africa and Turkey. They experience terrible suffering during the journeys and those that survive the ordeal are often subjected to appalling, archaic slaughter practices. In 2015, the European Court of Justice (ECJ) ruled that EU law on the protection of animals continues to apply even after the animals leave the EU, but despite this the suffering continues with little enforcement or action by the responsible authorities (Animals' Angels, 2016). Clearly, profits come before animal welfare in the eyes of the EU despite its recognition of animals as sentient beings.

Nonetheless, campaigners will continue to urge the EU to act, as a matter of urgency, to enforce existing laws and to protect animals that are not covered by species-specific EU legislation such as cattle, turkeys, ducks, rabbits and farmed fish. For example, a staggering 330 million EU rabbits spend their entire lives in barren wire cages, yet there is currently no specific EU legislation for farmed rabbits. In the EU alone, as many as 700 million animals spend all, or a significant part, of their lives imprisoned in cages – from sows in farrowing crates to egg-laying hens in so-called 'enriched' cages. The use of cages should be ended in all EU farming, and policy makers need to help bring about that change by initiating and supporting new legislation to bring farming into the 21st century.

Yet the prospect of further new or improved legislation is doubtful. The current European Commission has made it clear that it will not consider introducing any new legislation and has even failed to update its own animal welfare strategy. Instead, it points to voluntary initiatives to bring interested parties together in stakeholder initiatives. Sadly it appears that even if we were to succeed in getting prospective legislation to a vote, the likelihood of getting it adopted has diminished since the EU expanded to 28 countries. Worryingly, I estimate that countries with higher animal welfare records now represent only 34% of the EU Council votes with some 60% of votes being largely opposed to animal welfare progress. Even getting the

EU to enforce existing legislation is slow and laborious. Take, for example, the issue of the inherent need for pigs to have access to proper materials for enrichment for rooting and exploring. This requirement has existed in EU legislation since 2003, yet since that time most of the EU's 250 million pigs have had either no enrichment or been given inappropriate objects such as chains. It took an astonishing 13 further years of sustained pressure, until March 2016, before the EU produced a Recommendation aimed at securing improved compliance with its Directive (European Union, 2016).

On the international landscape, the hope is that jurisdictions will now look carefully at the EU's legislation in this field and embark upon their own legislative provisions to protect farm animals. There are signs that the international situation is slowly improving. Animal protection legislation now exists in most countries around the world and there are international animal welfare codes in place through the OIE, albeit ones which the OIE itself is powerless to enforce. Sadly, at the moment they are generally the bare minimum of what is needed and the OIE's lack of remit to tackle blatant breaches of its Code simply compounds the problem.

What is needed is proper investment and mechanisms to ensure that member countries a) incorporate the guidelines into their policies, including in legislation and standards, and b) ensure that they are observed in practice. As a first step, I would suggest that the OIE expand its remit to require member countries to report on an annual basis their progress on transposing the OIE's principles and standards in national policies and legislation.

Decades of campaigning and awareness-raising of the plight of farm animals have certainly succeeded in engaging the public, especially in the EU where opinion on farm animal welfare is overwhelmingly clear. Most people want to see improvements to the welfare of farm animals and a majority are prepared to pay more for higher welfare food products. The 2016 Eurobarometer survey, which gauges the opinions of European citizens, shows that 94% of people believe it is important to protect the welfare of farm animals and that 82% believe the welfare of farmed animals should be better protected than it is now. Support for change also appears to be increasing. Since the 2006 Eurobarometer survey, there are nine countries where there has been a greater than five percentage points increase in the proportion of people who believe the welfare of farmed animals should be better protected. In the US, there seems to be a move towards eating less meat – its consumption has dropped by 12% in recent years (Earth Policy Institute, 2012).

There is now compelling support for action and it is affecting shopping habits. More than half of those who responded to Eurobarometer surveys say they look for animal welfare labels when shopping and nearly six in ten are willing to pay more for higher welfare products. Since the EU introduced mandatory labelling of eggs in 2004, the UK's production of cage-free eggs has increased dramatically, showing that given clear information about the production method, people are rejecting caged eggs. Such strong demand for higher welfare products has inspired the launch of several different farm animal welfare assurance schemes – such as RSPCA Assured in the UK, Beter Leven in the Netherlands, the RSPCA Approved Farming Scheme in Australia and GAP in the US. They have clearly had a positive impact on animal welfare and there is great potential for them to achieve much more, as long as standards are constantly improved.

Interestingly, there is a new form of collaboration with the corporate sector that is creating an exciting ripple effect around the world – working with global retailers and producers to commit to policy changes, with the potential to improve the welfare of billions of animals. This is especially important in jurisdictions such as the US that lag behind other developed countries with respect to legislative protection for animals.

It is incredible to see the effect that the announcement of just one food service organisation can have. When McDonald's announced in 2015 that it was rejecting eggs from cages, an astonishing 130 other companies followed suit within just a few months.

Global businesses have the ability to change things fast. Within a couple of years, policy changes can be fully implemented without any cost to the taxpayer. For any corporate commitments to be truly meaningful, processes must be in place to properly fulfil them, ideally backed up with legislation designed to provide for an animal's needs.

CIWF's Good Business Awards, which celebrate the commitment of leading food businesses around the world to improve animal welfare standards, have produced some exciting results through collaboration as far afield as South America, as mentioned above. In 2014, the Good Pig Production Awards were launched, which recognise Chinese producers for improving pig welfare, food safety and environmental standards. Working with a Chinese Government-backed organisation – the International Cooperation Committee of Animal Welfare (ICCAW) – CIWF is encouraging Chinese farmers and producers to improve animal welfare standards. As China is the world's largest producer of pigs (at more than 726 million a year), efforts to encourage and improve animal welfare can make a difference to the lives of an enormous number of individual animals. In June 2016, the Chinese Government announced plans to cut meat consumption by a massive 50%, and as 28% of the world's meat is currently consumed in China, it is a move that, if realised, has the potential to bring about huge animal welfare, environmental and health benefits, for example, if China were to move to sustainable systems with high animal welfare as an integral component (*The Guardian*, 2016). The idea of eating less meat, but better meat from higher welfare pasture-based production systems is one that, if replicated worldwide, would have far reaching benefits for animals, people and our planet.

Another great example of what can be achieved when NGOs and industry stakeholders work side by side is the Calf Forum, which operated between 2006 and 2013 in the UK. The forum was established to tackle the treatment of male dairy calves, which was a cause of public concern. The calves – a by-product of the dairy industry – were either being killed at birth or exported to veal crate systems in mainland Europe. The aim of the Forum was to cut the number of calves being killed at birth, increase uptake of male calves into the UK beef food chain and to reduce the number of live calves being exported. Through the Calf Forum – a collaboration between CIWF, the RSPCA, the UK beef and dairy industry, UK supermarkets, producers and farmers – the number of male calves kept in the UK rose from 59% to 86%, those killed on farm dropped from 21% to 12% and exports fell from 20% to 2% (CIWF/RSPCA, 2013).

The relationships that evolved during the Forum's life, particularly between retailers and farmers, means there is now a continued market solution to the problem. As project manager and then co-chair of the Forum I witnessed how a true collaborative spirit in aid of commonly agreed upon goals inspired every stakeholder to take action that has benefitted animal welfare; for example, McDonalds set itself – and then met – a target of provisioning 10% of its supply in the UK from male dairy calves (CIWF/RSPCA, 2013). There is absolutely no reason why this partnership between industry and campaigners cannot be extended to other farm animal issues.

In more general terms, I believe it's time for a fresh approach in which animal welfare is measured in terms of how well we provide for an animal's needs. While the Five Freedoms have provided a sound framework since they were developed in the 1990s, scientific understanding of animal welfare has increased significantly in recent years, and as we understand more about the sentience of farm animals, our laws and policies should also reflect those findings and be updated accordingly. There are signs that it's starting to happen – during the last ten or 20 years, national and international welfare regulations have begun to include provisions that go beyond the basic survival needs of farm animals – but we are a long way off properly providing for their needs.

All the while we live in a world where people choose to eat meat, we have a moral duty to do everything possible to ensure farm animals lead a good life, do not suffer on farm or during transport and experience a stress- and pain-free death. Whether that's achieved through innovative uses of technology, simple natural objects or pioneering new husbandry practices, NGOS, farmers, business and legislators alike must work together to find sustainable solutions that make farm animals' lives more satisfying and rewarding as an integral part of a farming system that restores and then protects soils, water and wildlife whilst providing healthy, nutritious food for all, as well as decent livelihoods for farmers. This may appear to be a very tall order, but huge strides towards these aims might be made by addressing overproduction and overconsumption of meat and dairy and by urging consumers to eat less and better meat produced from animals that have been put back into their ecological niche – living on pasture and converting food that humans cannot eat into human edible animal products.

In the UK a coalition has been formed – Eating Better for a Fair, Green Healthy Future, or "Eating Better" – for short, which promotes this very aim – that people are encouraged to eat less meat, but when buying meat, to opt for the higher welfare product. The coalition now has 50 NGO members, drawn from the animal welfare, environment and health sectors.

The inevitable consequence of an eating less and better approach towards meat, eggs and dairy would be a vast reduction in the number of farmed animals, enabling those fewer farm animals to be given a higher quality of life and sparing animals, people and our planet from the devastation being caused by today's industrial agriculture that has been so well documented elsewhere.

Notes

1 A pregnant sow is confined in much of the world to a sow stall (also called a gestation crate) for the whole of her 16-week gestation period. A sow stall is a metal crate or cage, usually with a bare slatted floor, which is so narrow that the sow cannot turn around and can only stand up and lie down with difficulty.
2 The veal crate, banned in the EU but still used elsewhere, confines calves individually inside farm buildings either tethered by the neck in partial stalls (open at the rear) or enclosed in boxes, sometimes called pens. The crates are traditionally made of wood with a slatted floor. The sides may be solid so that the calves cannot normally see or touch their fellows or they may be barred, permitting visual and some tactile contact. The calves are fed a diet of milk from buckets attached to the front.

References

Animals' Angels, 2016. The myth of enforcement.
Animal Protection Index, 2014. api.worldanimalprotection.org
Canadian Grocer, 18 March 2016. Big grocers make cage-free egg pledge.
CIWF/RSPCA, 2013. The modern solution to the exports of calves: Working in black and white: The beyond calf exports stakeholders Forum: A final report on progress.
Daily Mail, 16 June 2016. News article: Horrific abattoir footage shows cattle bludgeoned to death with sledgehammers – and one bull collapsing in fear before it has even been struck after watching the fate of its pen mates.
DEFRA, 2014. Agriculture in the UK 2014.
Earth Policy Institute, 2015. Peak meat: US meat consumption falling.
European Commission, 30 September 1997. Scientific veterinary committee, animal welfare section: Report on the welfare of intensively kept pigs, official journal L 47, 18 February 2009, p. 5–13.
European Commission, 2011. Report on the impact of Council Regulation (EC) No 1/2005 on the protection of animals during transport.
European Commission, 2016. Eurobarometer 442, attitudes of Europeans towards animal welfare.
European Union (EU), 2004. Council Regulation (EC) No 1/2005 of 22 December 2004 on the protection of animals during transport and related operations and amending Directives 64/432/EEC and 93/1.
European Union (EU), 2007a. Consolidated versions of the Treaty on European Union and the Treaty on the Functioning of the European Union, official journal C 326, 26 October 2012, p. 0001–0390 19/EC and Regulation (EC) No 1255/97 L3, 5 January 1991, pp. 0001–0042.
European Union (EU), June 2007b Council Directive 2007/43/CE laying down minimum rules for the protection of chickens kept for meat production.
European Union (EU), 2008a. Council Directive 2008/119/EEC of 18 December 2008 laying down minimum standards for the protection of calves.
European Union (EU), 2008b. Council Directive 2008/120/EC of 18 December 2008 laying down minimum standards for the protection of pigs.
European Union (EU), 2009. Council Regulation (EC) No 1099/2009 on the protection of animals at the time of killing.

FAO, 2012. FAOSTAT.
FAWC, 2009. Farm animal welfare council: Report on farm animal welfare in Great Britain: Past, present and future, defra.
Fishcount, 2010. Summary Report, *Worse things happen at sea.* http://fishcount.org.uk/
Food Ingredients First, 2016. NFU warns of cage-free egg conversion challenges.
Global Animal Partnership (GAP), 2016. www.globalanimalpartnership.org/about/news/post/our-commitment-to-improving-bird-welfare-with-100-slower-growing-chicken-breeds
Guardian, 2016. Milman, O & Leavenworth, S., 20 June 2016. News article. China's plan to cut meat consumption by 50% cheered by climate campaigners.
Harari, Y. N., 2015. *Sapiens: A brief history of humankind*, Vintage, April 2015.
H.M.S.O., 1965. Report of the technical committee to enquire into the welfare of animals kept under intensive livestock husbandry systems.
Humane League, 2016. United egg producers announces elimination of chick culling, humane league press release, 9 June 2016.
Humane Society of the United States, 2016. (HSUS) major advancements in farm animal protection.
New York Times, 31 July 2015, Stepanie strom "perdue sharply cuts antibiotic use in chickens and jabs at its rivals".
NFU, 2016. Egg producers need clarity on retailer cage-free promises.
Pacelle, W., 2016. The humane economy: How innovators and enlightened consumers are transforming the lives of animals.
Perdue Farms, 2016. Perdue announces industry-first animal care commitments. Press Release.
Stevenson, P., 2012. European Union legislation on the welfare of animals, compassion in world farming.
Tyson, 2014. Tyson foods letter to Hog Farmers.
USDA, 2012. Census of agriculture.
Webster, B., 6 February 2016. The Times. News article. Shoppers misled by meat labels with images of idyllic farm life.
World Organisation for Animal Health, 2016. OIE, Terrestrial Animal Health Code (2016) Section 7 animal welfare.
World Poultry, 2016. Continued shift to "cage-free" in US egg market.

21

CONFRONTING POLICY DILEMMAS

Jonathon Porritt

Apart from much of today's idiotic "conspicuous consumption", there are only two facets of current human behaviour which simply cannot be squared with any reasonable scenario of a genuinely sustainable future for humankind as a whole. The first is the continuing growth in demand for air travel, and the second is the continuing growth in demand for meat consumption. However contested the transition from a carbon-intensive way of life to an ultra-low carbon way of life may prove to be (and the longer we delay, the more contested it *will* be), there are no other *insuperable* barriers from either a technological or a socio-economic point of view.

Aviation's contribution to total greenhouse gas emissions is still relatively small (anywhere between 2.5% and 5%, depending on how the calculations are done). Livestock production, by contrast, contributes around 15% of total greenhouse gas emissions – though here again the figures are complex.

Interestingly, that 15% is almost exactly the equivalent of total greenhouse gas emissions from continuing deforestation. After years of neglect, what is known as REDD (Reducing Emissions from Deforestation and Degradation) is now very high up the list of priorities for world leaders, powerfully reinforced in the historic Paris Agreement at the end of 2015. Ever-larger sums of money are being talked about in order to get a series of global deals in place, particularly to help developing and emerging countries address still chronic levels of rural poverty whilst avoiding unacceptably high levels of deforestation.

By contrast, policy makers' attention to the 15% of greenhouse gas emissions from meat eating remains as close to zero as it is possible to get. But for how much longer can that deplorable state of affairs continue? As the data gets more robust (as mapped out in Tara Garnett's chapter in this collection), academics and NGOs are now beginning to flex their muscles in terms of forcing the issue into the public domain. Twelve years ago, through its Eat Less Meat campaign, Compassion in

World Farming was pretty much a lone voice advocating decisive interventions by government to restrict projected increases in per capita meat consumption. Today, it's far from being a lone voice. Major food retailers and manufacturers are starting to face up to their own responsibilities in this area, and more and more people inside governments in the EU now acknowledge that the meat consumption challenge just cannot be ducked for very much longer.

In a previous publication for CIWF, I felt it important to state my own personal rationale as a consumer of meat:

> I write these words as a meat-eater. I've never been a vegetarian, and as a prominent exponent of all things sustainable, have often been attacked by vegetarians for what they see as inconsistency at best and outright hypocrisy at worst. I don't see it that way, though I'm aware that my own personal response to this dilemma (which is to try and eat a lot less meat and buy almost all the meat we consume as a family from organic suppliers) won't work for most people for reasons of price, availability and so on.
>
> Whilst I will always continue to campaign actively to improve the welfare of farm animals, and to eliminate all forms of cruelty from the food chain, I'm reconciled – with those caveats – to the moral acceptability of the human species using other animal species for their own benefit. By contrast, I'm far from reconciled to the grotesque misuse of the earth's resources that our current pattern of meat-eating demands.
>
> *(CIWF Trust 2004)*

Building on that rationale, I *still* believe it's perfectly possible to produce meat on a strictly sustainable basis and according to the strictest ethical criteria. But the implication of taking both of those two concepts seriously (sustainability and ethics) is that the total amount of meat consumed in the world will be massively reduced.

Exactly the opposite is happening today. According to the Food and Agriculture Organisation, total global meat consumption is projected to grow from around 300 million tonnes today to 465 million tonnes in 2050. Producing another 165 million tonnes by 2050 will require the growing of at least 1 billion tonnes of additional feed. Even if such growth were "a good thing" (and this book has demonstrated just how dreadful a thing it would in fact be), it simply won't be physically possible – in terms of availability of land, water and low-carbon energy. So why do we permit chronic "impossiblism" of this kind to dominate our worldviews and our policy deliberations?

The power of industry

Many of the reasons for this deeply unsatisfactory state of affairs have been surfaced in preceding chapters. Politicians are hugely reluctant to incur substantial political risk where the upside in addressing the challenge is not as yet (for most of them) as clear as it needs to be, let alone for most of their voters.

That risk resides in a number of different areas. First, the industry itself has become increasingly concentrated. With fewer companies commanding an ever-greater share of the marketplace, the food industry has simultaneously become increasingly powerful, particularly in the US. A loose coalition of industry trade groups deploys armies of lawyers and lobbyists to protect their own interests – and tried to make the supremely influential Oprah Winfrey back down when she started championing some of the industry's critics. They did not succeed (Independent 27/2/98). US democracy is a strange beast, and the role of the pork barrel (and indeed the beef barrel and the chicken barrel) remains disturbingly present.

Second, there will undoubtedly be substantial consumer resistance to any concerted measures to reduce average meat consumption. This may be an uncomfortable truth to surface in a book of this kind, but the majority of people rather like their meat, and a substantial minority like it a lot. It has taken years to raise concerns about the health effects of excessive meat consumption, and education campaigns to date have had little effect. The average US citizen, for instance, *still* consumes four times as much meat per annum as is recommended for dietary purposes.

Third, there is a whole set of legitimate concerns about the potentially regressive impacts of policies designed to reduce meat consumption. "Cheap meat" has been built up as one of the great achievements of the last two or three decades – and so it is, just so long as you avoid doing a more detailed cost-benefit analysis. Meat is now so cheap that in both the US and (to a lesser extent) in the EU, it has somehow become "culturally embedded", the default dietary option as much if not more for the poor than for the rich. China and other emerging economies are following rapidly in those ill-advised footsteps.

Lastly, there's now an important equity issue in terms of food as a globally traded commodity. The huge expansion in meat consumption in the rich world has opened up unprecedented opportunities for countries like Brazil and Argentina to provide the feedstuffs on which the livestock industry depends – soy, wheat and so on (as outlined in Joyce D'Silva's chapter in this volume). The future prosperity of these nations has become dangerously dependent on continued growth in meat consumption in emerging economies – and particularly in China.

Against that backdrop, politicians' finely honed survival skills are inevitably going to predispose them to inertia rather than to the kind of leadership that the evidence now demands. My nine years as Chairman of the Sustainable Development Commission (2000 to 2009) taught me that Ministers' enthusiastic advocacy of "evidence-based policy making" pretty quickly evaporated once that evidence turned out to be either inconvenient or totally unpalatable. So even if today's Chief Scientific Advisor in the UK were to take to Ministers the kind of comprehensive dossier of evidence to be found in this collection, he or she would still get very short shrift.

Eventually, however, evidence wins the day. You can't permanently suppress a body of solid evidence – it will out. But even that, of itself, is not necessarily enough to ensure the kind of policy-making process required for such a deeply controversial area. Seduced though I would happily be by Colin Tudge's eloquent account of how increased meat consumption has *not*, historically, been a principal indicator of status and affluence, I fear that history is against him on this one. As societies work their way out of poverty, meat consumption correlates with increased income in almost all circumstances where religious constraints (as with Hinduism) and cultural norms (as in Buddhist cultures) do not obtain. In discussions with Colin, I've always been amused by his anecdote that the Emperors of China infinitely preferred the skin of the duck to the flesh of the duck, but you can guarantee that hundreds of millions of their subjects would have loved to dine on duck each and every day. And right now in China, that's pretty much what they're doing, where the correlation between increased income (and the status that brings) and increased meat consumption could not possibly be clearer.

Criteria for successful policy making

In such circumstances, policy makers will have to focus single-mindedly on one simple objective: to reduce per capita meat consumption. In recent years experts and health bodies have made varying recommendations for the maximum daily amount of meat one should eat, such as the UK Department of Health advocating no more than 70 grams a day of red meat, which is similar to the World Cancer Research Fund's not more than 500 grams a week (WCRF, 2016). This is against a 2010 baseline of around 300g a day, which on current projections would keep on gently rising rather than declining.

Personally, I'm not sure that the 70g threshold is sufficient from a climate change perspective. Achieving such a threshold will do little more than stabilise the emissions associated with meat consumption at today's baseline. The likelihood is that meat consumption, as a generic human activity, will have to take a bigger share than that if we're to get anywhere close to the 80% cut in greenhouse gases required by 2050. And let's not forget that this 80% figure is based on the objective of restricting the average temperature increase by the end of the century to no more than 2°C. For the first time, the Paris Agreement has acknowledged that even 2°C will not deliver a stable climate: we need to be doing everything in our power not to exceed an average temperature increase of 1.5°C.

There's an increasing amount of good public health research showing that even 70g per day may not be a sufficiently low baseline. And we certainly don't want people to shift all their consumption to chicken as today's meat chickens have such a huge variety of health and welfare problems (see Andy Butterworth's chapter in this book). The 2014 study (referred to in the Rayner chapter) shows that a diet of below 50g per day results in a 35% reduction in greenhouse gas emissions as compared with a diet of over 100g per day (Scarborough et al., 2014). So we'll go with 50g as the optimum global figure – I'm going to use the UK here as a policy maker's proxy for all countries with unsustainably meat-intensive diets.

If I was the Permanent Secretary in Defra, listening to the Chief Scientific Advisor and recognising that the challenge of excessive meat consumption could no longer be avoided, I would recommend to the Prime Minister of the day that he/she should promptly set up a high-level Advisory Council to determine "how best to get from 300g to 50g a day within the next ten years". Such a Council should include no representatives of the different vegetarian/vegan advocacy groups and no representatives of the meat industry or farmers' bodies. It should be made up of people with impeccable scientific and non-scientific credentials, to ensure that their resulting conclusions/recommendations would give plenty of "cover" for whichever Ministers happened to be in the firing line when the going gets tough. Let's call it the "50g Advisory Council".

They will have a lot of material to play with. The astonishing truth is that there can be few theoretical "single-policy objectives" (i.e. reduce per capita meat consumption to 50g per person per day) for which there are more supporting evidence bases: health, food hygiene, animal welfare, climate change, wider environmental impacts and equity issues all have a crucial part to play. Any one of these might (and, from an ethical point of view, *should*) suffice on its own – so the combination should surely be overwhelming.

The first thing to do would be to develop some kind of policy matrix. Such a matrix would need to assess the value of different policy interventions against a set of overarching criteria: *effectiveness* (just how substantive is the contribution any policy might make to the 50g objective?); *practicality* (just how easy will it be to implement and enforce any particular policy?); *acceptability* (just how intense are the objections to any particular policy likely to be?); and *desirability* (just how important would any policy intervention be, in the best of all possible worlds, from an ethical or values-based perspective?).

It is clear, as far as Kate Rawles is concerned, that once the science has been "signed off", any such policy-making process should be *primarily* values based, rather than geared to effectiveness and practicality, let alone public acceptability. And she is, of course, right. But world-weary Permanent Secretaries would dutifully point out that this is not the "best of all possible worlds", and that even the best of policies can sometimes be derailed by a combination of vested interests, ignorance and crude political prejudices.

To reduce the risks of any such backlash on the reduced meat consumption front, the 50g Advisory Council would need, quite ruthlessly, to assess the correlation between any proposed policy instruments and people's *raw self-interest*. Though Colin Tudge is right to point out that the vast majority of people do indeed demonstrate significant "natural sympathy" (to retrieve the long-overlooked phrase that Adam Smith used regularly to explain what would actually make the "invisible hand" of the market work) for other people and other creatures, that natural sympathy is never quite as powerful as the sympathy that people have for their own interests and the interests of those nearest to them. Successful policy making is always as much about perceived self-interest as it is about the national interest, let alone global interest.

Working with self-interest

So how would the hierarchy of self-interest look as the 50g Advisory Council settled into its first few months of work? Which potential areas of concern are likely to be more material? They'd probably argue like hell about it, but having no particular vested interests to deal with, I suspect they'd come up with something like the following:

1 Individual Health
2 Climate Change
3 Wider Environmental Impacts
4 Animal Welfare
5 Equity/Fairness Issues

I appreciate, from an ethical point of view, that such a hierarchy is probably deeply offensive to animal welfare campaigners. But how else can we account for the grindingly slow process of change over the last few decades to establish the bare minimum of "decency" standards for animals kept in captivity? Very few people condone suffering or cruelty to animals when confronted by it, but not enough of them feel sufficiently concerned to have encouraged politicians to have raised standards faster and more comprehensively.

But they *do* care about their own health, and with a serious education campaign (think of smoking as the analogy here, or possibly alcohol consumption), there's no reason why more people would not start to think much more seriously about the impact of their personal meat consumption on their own health. The evidence linking excessive levels of meat consumption (particularly of processed meat products) with both heart disease and certain kinds of cancer gets stronger all the time (Pan et al., 2012; Crous-Bou et al., 2014; Van Dooren, 2013). It's just that we haven't had a serious education campaign as yet.

As spelled out in Part III, there's now a particular emphasis on obesity in terms of current public health issues. Both the Cabinet Office's "Food Matters" report (Cabinet Office, 2008) and the "Healthy Lives, Healthy People" report ("A Call to Action on Obesity in England", 2011) have demonstrated just how serious a policy challenge this has now become. An earlier Foresight Report in 2007 predicted that 40% of UK citizens will be obese by 2025, and 60% by 2050 on current projections Foresight (2007).

In the US, it's even worse: the US Centers for Disease Control estimates that there are already 112,000 premature deaths every year arising from complications from obesity and related problems, amounting to around $75 billion in medical costs – that's nearly 5% of total healthcare costs in the US (US CDC, 2006).

Tentatively, a few commentators *are* beginning to make some direct connections between obesity and climate change. The World Health Organisation published some data in 2009 showing that each overweight person causes an additional 1 tonne of CO_2 to be emitted every year. With 1 billion people judged to be overweight around the world – of whom at least 300 million are obese – that's an additional 1 billion tonnes (Edwards and Roberts, 2009).

This is still very controversial territory. But on the whole question of accelerating climate change, opinion has changed dramatically over the last ten years. For more and more people, it's moved out of the "possibly, but not in my lifetime" category of concern to the "we need to be doing more about this *right now*" category. Whereas the rhetoric was once geared almost entirely to appeals on behalf of "our children and our children's children" (eloquently invoking the spirit of intergenerational justice), now it's all about *us*, in our lives, in our own backyards – as reinforced by ever more frequent extreme weather events.

As regards the wider environment, moving down the policy makers' hierarchy, I'm not sure that this collection of essays has done full justice either to the range or the seriousness of the impacts of intensive meat production on the environment. But the chapter by Arjen Hoekstra on the "Water Footprint of Animal Products" makes an extraordinarily convincing case as to this particular environmental issue. With delicious irony, one of the best overall summaries of these cumulative impacts can still be found in the FAO's (2006) Report *Livestock's Long Shadow* (FAO, 2006) although the FAO has come under constant pressure since publication to disavow its own report!

As to animal welfare, I think it's important to subdivide this into "impacts on human health" and "impacts on the animals themselves". Quite frankly, having taken in the full analysis of the chapters by Greger and Nunan in this book, it's perfectly clear that potential impacts on human health could go straight to the top of the 50g Advisory Council's hierarchy at any point in time. As we contemplate the full extent of a potential "catastrophic storm of microbial effects", either directly or indirectly associated with intensive livestock production systems, it wouldn't take much to spill public opinion over from "don't like the sound of that" to "no more intensive systems of that kind *now* – and we don't care how much more our meat will cost".

There's one aspect of this which is particularly potent: the continuing, widespread use of antibiotics in livestock production systems on a sub-therapeutic or even prophylactic basis. More and more senior medical advisors are warning that we're on the brink of a major health crisis, and the nightmare vision of a world where antibiotics no longer work looms larger and larger. It's already been calculated that around 25,000 people in the EU die every year of resistant infections (ECDC and EMEA, 2009), and there are some who believe that this figure could rise to around a million by 2025 (ECDC/EFSA/EMA, 2015).

As concern about different multidrug-resistant bacteria becomes ever more acute, pressure on Ministers to regulate and even ban such practices is growing all the time. Here in the UK, the new "Alliance to Save Our Antibiotics" (set up by Compassion in World Farming, the Soil Association and Sustain) will be seeking to make visible what is still largely invisible to the majority of meat-eaters – and, for once, will be able to call on the influence of the mass media to help get that message across. (See Cóilín Nunan's chapter for the details.)

It is, to be sure, a rather indirect route to our 50g objective (banning the sub-therapeutic use of antibiotics would substantially raise costs of production, which would raise costs through the supply chain, which may contribute eventually to people turning away from meat and meat-based products), but it would be highly influential in terms of subtly transforming the whole cheap meat debate.

On the straight animal welfare issues themselves, I only wish that what Andy Butterworth describes as "the margin for care" for animals held in captivity mattered far more to far more people. I'm persuaded this *will* happen in time, and the indefatigable efforts of animal welfare organisations the world over will in the meantime keep chipping away at raising standards and eliminating some of the cruellest practices. But I would be very surprised if the 50g Advisory Committee suggested to Ministers that they should spearhead their new policy interventions primarily on the basis of improved welfare standards.

And that's also why concerns about the impact of *our* meat consumption on the lives of some of the world's poorest and hungriest people still come at the bottom of my list – despite the fact that in this age of cornucopian plenty there are still around 35 million hunger-related deaths a year. There is of course the most powerful moral argument (spelled out a number of times in this collection) that the grain and other feedstuffs that currently feed animals should instead directly feed people. As Colin Tudge points out, by 2050 (on current projections), the livestock we eat will then be consuming the same amount of food as would be sufficient to feed 4 billion people directly, in effect increasing total human numbers at that time from an estimated 9.5 billion in 2050 to 13.5 billion. I fear that's not the way most people see things.

Policy interventions

Armed with its necessarily Machiavellian matrix, our intrepid 50g Advisory Council would then move to the consideration of specific policy interventions available to governments, working their way along a conventional policy spectrum with voluntarism at one end to outright interdiction at the other. Given that our objective is 50g a day rather than "no meat at all", we need not concern ourselves with a total ban. At the voluntary end of things, this is obviously the relatively easy place to start, with a commitment to a substantial and ongoing public education campaign to enable citizens to understand the full personal and societal implications of today's meat-intensive diets. "Meat-free Mondays" and other "Eat Less" campaigns are early signals of just how big this could be.

If past dietary challenges (on salt, for instance, or fat or artificial colourings) are anything to go by, the government will seek to shift as much of the burden involved in such a campaign onto our food retailers and (of increasing importance today) the catering industry. Portion size is already part of many retailers' "healthy meals initiatives". Alternatives to meat could be marketed much more aggressively, and there's considerable scope for further innovation here. For an industry that brings out around 20,000 new products *every year*, the opportunities for a whole new family of "I can't believe it's not meat!" products must be enormous! As the *New Scientist* reported in October 2015:

> The market for meat substitutes is taking shape, with multiple start-ups, mostly in the US, coming on to the scene. Los Angeles-based Beyond Meat uses pea protein to mimic meat structure, for example, and Impossible Foods in Redwood City in California is developing a mixture of plant-derived proteins to make meat-like patties. Dutch company Beeter and British firm Quorn both have sizeable market shares in imitation meat.
>
> *(Hodson, 2015)*

And let's not overlook the possibility that more and more of the demand for meat will be met by artificially grown substitutes, produced in industrial bioreactors, with just a fraction of the impact of real meat on the environment, and a fraction of greenhouse gas emissions. In "The World We Made", published back in 2013, I provided one possible scenario here, looking *back* from the vantage point of 2050:

> A rather different kind of breakthrough came in the early 2020s with the widespread take-up of artificial meat, made by culturing stem cells from cows, pigs, sheep and chickens. This was promoted at the time as a major health innovation; most cultured meats are nutritionally enhanced with Omega-3 fatty acids and other good things. However, environmentalists remain pretty sceptical – on the grounds that people should go the whole hog (excuse the pun!) and become proper vegetarians. But artificial meat is here to stay: nearly a third of all meat consumed today is already cultured, and with pressure on good farming land getting even more intense, my bet is that this will soon be up to 50%.
>
> *(Porritt, 2013)*

(By the way, sticking with that 2050 vision, artificial meat proves to be only one of the factors which slows growth in overall demand for meat: "Back in 2015, the experts were confidently predicting that meat consumption would grow to around 465 million tonnes in 2050. Well, that didn't happen: instead, public opinion began to change for both health and environmental reasons. Per capita meat consumption actually plateaued in 2030 at around 355 million tonnes in total – the 'peak meat' moment, if you like!")

But let's get back to today's reality for our hard-pressed policy makers. The next area for decisive intervention is for any government to take responsibility for its own actions and for its use of public money. Throughout the world, billions of dollars of agricultural subsidies directly and indirectly promote increased meat consumption. In 2013, specific livestock subsidies across all 34 OECD countries amounted to around £35 billion, including an unbelievable average of around £150 for each and every cow!

An end to all such perverse subsidies (let alone to specific government-funded meat-promotion campaigns) would have a huge impact on the economics of meat production. What is the logic of using taxpayers' money to promote patterns of behaviour that translate directly into an increased burden for the taxpayer in terms of health, environmental pollution, disease, climate change and so on? The case against production-related subsidies within the CAP is of course one that has been diligently pursued by the UK for many years. With the combined fire-power of the health lobby and the climate change lobby weighing in behind that campaign, things could just move a little faster from now on.

Closer to home, the government would need to get its own food procurement policies sorted out. In its own climate change strategy, the National Health Service (NHS) has started to think through the implications of all this in terms of hospital food:

> The actions needed to develop a more sustainable food system in the NHS, as well as maintaining nutritional value, include the use of seasonally adjusted menus, increased use of sustainably sourced fish, and a reduction in the reliance on meat, dairy and eggs.
>
> *(NHS, 2009)*

And that would be just the start. Predominantly meat-free school dinners; reduced meat consumption in prisons; 100% meat-free government canteens: there is absolutely no reason why this should not be taken completely for granted in ten years' time.

Next up would be unambiguous regulatory interventions – on pollution controls, higher welfare standards, a ban on the use of sub-therapeutic antibiotics and so on. As already discussed, the effect of all this would be to raise the cost of meat for consumers – in effect to start consigning the concept of "cheap meat" to the dustbin of history.

But it's at this point that a couple of "wicked issues" raise their ugly heads. First, how could we do this in the UK without further disadvantaging our own farmers, at the hands of intensive livestock operations elsewhere in the world, free to carry on in the same old cruel, polluting and environmentally unsustainable way that we had just put behind us?

Our farmers should in every respect be compensated as pioneers in the transition to genuinely sustainable and ethical meat production systems. Unfortunately, under WTO rules, that's not possible – just as we can't do a lot of other sustainable and ethical things under the wretched WTO rules. So how far might we here in the UK be prepared to go to reassert our right to pursue our own health, environmental and welfare interests?

The second wicked issue is, of course, social justice. Rationing meat consumption by price is a deeply regressive approach. For instance, David Pimentel of Cornell University has for a long time advocated some kind of "sustainability tax" that would be applied to all foods on the basis of the external costs involved in bringing them to the market (Pimentel and Pimentel, 2008). Meat and dairy products would be taxed most heavily, whilst legumes, fresh fruit and vegetables wouldn't be taxed at all. But the problem here is a simple one: this would still hit the poorest hardest.

Personal meat quotas

For the Advisory Council, this is where the going gets tough, and where that overarching objective (50g a day per person) begins to look somewhat elusive. After all the regulation and the education and the incentivisation, there are only two ways of further reducing demand. First, by raising prices until the inherent inelasticity in this particular market disappears. But meat is now so cheap that prices would have to rise very substantially indeed for that to happen, and the regressive impacts would be very severe.

Alternatively, governments could move to set "personal meat quotas" along the lines of the kind of personal carbon quotas proposed as a way of reducing individual carbon footprints. Were that to be the recommendation of the 50g Advisory Committee, the response would undoubtedly be something along the lines of "are you all out of your tiny minds?!" But science and logic are great bulwarks against accusations of insanity. And let's just remind ourselves of the science that lies behind all this, from the perspective of what is and what isn't physically possible. In his admirable book *The End of Food*, Paul Roberts puts it like this:

> Under any model for a future food system that is both sustainable and equitable, the meat-rich diets of the West and especially the United States, simply don't work on a global scale. If the American level of meat consumption – about 217lbs per person per year – were suddenly replicated world wide, our total global grain harvest would support just 2.6 billion people – or less than 40% of the existing population.
>
> Even if we use a more modest level of Western meat consumption such as that of Italy, where per capita meat consumption is about 80% of the United States, world grain supplies would still be adequate for just 5 billion people. In fact, according to the Earth Policy Institute, it's only when the world adopts an Indian level of meat consumption – that is, around 12lbs of meat per person per year – that current global grain supplies would be adequate to feed 9.5 billion people.
>
> *(Roberts, 2008)*

Which sets that kind of incontrovertible *physical reality* at odds with today's *political reality*. But if the science is robust, and the imperative to do something about it without further delay is as strong as more and more people believe it to be, then personal meat quotas (PMQs) would provide an elegant and effective policy intervention. Every citizen would receive the same quota, eliminating any regressive effects; it would be set on a sliding scale, starting with current consumption levels for Year 1, reducing down to 50g in Year 10, allowing people plenty of time to adapt;

quotas could be made tradeable, although any such resale market would obviously favour rich carnivores over poor carnivores; and the whole thing would be done electronically, via a smartcard from which deductions are made automatically at the butcher, supermarket or restaurant.

Scary prospect for our politicians? Of course. For people who see cheap meat as part of their latter-day birthright, such a proposal is a total anathema. For people like Colin Tudge (whose simple maxim is "plenty of plants, not much meat and maximum variety") it's just common sense, based on a sound understanding of the role that meat has played in our lives over the entire evolution of the human species. For those somewhere in the middle, their first response is quite likely to be one of resistance. However logical such an approach might be, it would still be seen to be non-viable. Psychologically, there doesn't seem to be that much difference between PMQs and the kind of meat rationing we had back in the Second World War.

And that's true! But that's exactly the point. Very few people have yet grasped the fact that combating the threat of accelerating climate change will, in many respects, entail going onto some kind of "war footing". As I said before, most of the changes that need to happen could be driven through by technological innovation, radical fiscal shift and integrated policy interventions that will make low-carbon living relatively pain-free and positively benign from all sorts of environmental, health and well-being perspectives. But aviation and meat consumption are not amenable, I fear, to that kind of relatively conventional policy portfolio. Hence the need for sterner measures!

References

Cabinet Office UK Government, "Food matters: Towards a strategy for the 21st Century", July 2008.

Crous-Bou, M., Fung, T., Prescott, J., Julin, B., Du, M., Sun, Q., Rexrode, K., Hu, F., De Vivo, I., 2014. "Mediterranean diet and telomere length in Nurses' Health Study: Population based cohort study". *BMJ* 2014: 349:g6674.

Edwards, P. and Roberts, I. (London School of Hygiene and Tropical Medicine), March 2009. *International Journal of Epidemiology*.

ECDC and EMEA, 2009. "The bacterial challenge: Time to react. A call to narrow the gap between multidrug-resistant bacteria in the EU and the development of new antibacterial agents", www.ecdc.europa.eu/en/publications/Publications/0909_TER_The_Bacterial_Challenge_Time_to_ React.pdf

Executive Summary only. http://webarchive.nationalarchives.gov.uk/+/http:/www.cabinetoffice.gov.uk/media/cabinetoffice/strategy/assets/food/food_matters_es.pdf

FAO, 2006. "Livestock's Long Shadow: Environmental Issues and Options".

Foresight, "Tackling Obesities: Future Choices", Cabinet Office, Chief Scientific Advisor's Foresight Programme, 2007.

Full Report. www.ifr.ac.uk/waste/Reports/food%20matters,%20Towards%20a%20Strategy%20for%20the%2021st%20Century.pdf

Hodson, H., "Massive Vats of Fake Meat Browed in Goo Could Change How We Eat", *New Scientist* pp10–11, 31 October 2015.

Independent, The, "Oprah Triumphs Over the Texas Cattle Ranchers", 27 February 1998.

Porritt, J., 2013. *The World We Made*, Phaidon.

NHS Sustainable Development Unit, "Saving Carbon, Improving Health", January 2009.

Pan, A., Sun, Q., Bernstein, A., Schulze, M., Manson, J., Stampfer, M., Willett, W. and Hu, F., 2012. "Red meat consumption and mortality: Results from two prospective cohort studies". *Archives of Internal Medicine* 172(7):555–563. doi:10.1001/archinternmed.2011.2287. Red Meat Consumption and Mortality Results from 2 Prospective Cohort Studies, p1.

Pimentel, D. and Pimentel, M., *Food, energy and society*, CRC Press, 2008.

Press release: "ESCMID warns that Europe may surpass one-million deaths due to ineffective antibiotics by 2025", www.efsa.europa.eu/en/efsajournal/pub/4006.htm

Roberts, P., 2008. *The End of Food*, Bloomsbury.

Scarborough, P., et al., 2014. "Dietary greenhouse gas emissions of meat-eaters, fish-eaters, vegetarians and vegans in the UK". *Climatic Change* 125:179–192. doi: 10.1007/s10584-014-1169-1.

UK Government, "Healthy Lives, Healthy People", October 2011 www.gov.uk/government/publications/healthy-lives-healthy-people-a-call-to-action-on-obesity-in-england

US Centers for Disease Control, "Overweight and Obesity: Economic Consequences", March 2006.

Van Dooren, C., Marinussen, M., Blonk, H., Aiking, H., and Vellinga, P., 2013. "Exploring dietary guidelines based on ecological and nutritional values: A comparison of six dietary patterns". *Food Policy* 44(2014): 36–46.

World Cancer Research Fund International, 2016. "Animal foods", http://wcrf.org/int/research-we-fund/cancer-prevention-recommendations/animal-foods

INDEX

Page numbers in italic indicate a figure, table or box on the corresponding page.